D0946181

Natural Healing

from Head to Toe

TRADITIONAL MACROBIOTIC REMEDIES

Cornellia Aihara
Herman Aihara
with Carl Ferré

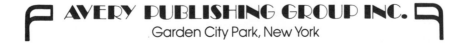
AVERY PUBLISHING GROUP INC.
Garden City Park, New York

The procedures in this book are based upon the research, personal and professional experiences of the authors. Should the reader have any questions regarding the appropriateness of any procedure or material mentioned, the publisher and author strongly suggest consulting a professional health-care advisor.

Because any material or procedure can be misused, the author and publisher are not responsible for any adverse effects or consequences resulting from the use of any of the preparations, materials, or procedures suggested in this book. However, the publisher believes that this information should be available to the public.

Cover design: Rudy Shur and Bill Gonzalez
Illustrator: Cynthia Beers Briscoe
In-house editor: Linda Comac
Typesetter: Kay Rangos
Printer: Paragon Press, Honesdale, PA

Library of Congress Cataloging-in-Publication Data

Aihara, Cornellia.
    Natural healing from head to toe : traditional macrobiotic
remedies / Cornellia Aihara and Herman Aihara, with Carl Ferre.
        p. c.m.
    Includes bibliographical references and index.
    ISBN 0-89529-496-6
    1. Macrobiotic diet. I. Aihara, Herman, 1920– . II. Ferré,
Carl. III. Title.
RM235.A344 1994
615.8'54—dc20   93-4659
                                                 CIP

Copyright © 1994 by Cornellia Aihara

All rights reserved. No part of this publication may be reproduced, stored in a retrieval system, or transmitted, in any form or by any means, electronic, mechanical, photocopying, recording or otherwise, without the prior written permission of the copyright owner.

Printed in the United States of America

10 9 8 7 6 5 4 3 2

CONTENTS

ACKNOWLEDGMENTS

We owe our knowledge of macrobiotic remedies to the following persons: George Ohsawa, Lima Ohsawa, Shuzo Okada, Toshi Kawaguchi, Michi Ogawa, Hideo Ohmori, and Noboru Muramoto. Their teachings and inspiration brought this book to realization. Therefore, we give to them our most deep appreciation. We sincerely thank as well Nippon Center Ignoramus and the Osaka Seishoku Kyokai (Macrobiotic Association) for publishing the many books and magazines that have helped to further our understanding of traditional macrobiotic remedies. It is our utmost wish that this book will bring health and happiness to you and your families.

PREFACE

George Ohsawa introduced the modern-day version of the macrobiotic approach to healing in 1928 for the benefit of everyone, everywhere. My story is only one of thousands upon thousands of stories of people who have changed their lives through macrobiotic principles.

I was born in 1926 with a heart condition—patent ductus arteriosus. This condition causes arterial blood to recirculate through the lungs because of an open channel that normally closes after birth. It causes a shortage of oxygen, fast breathing, and a fast pulse. I was a very weak child because of this condition; as a teenager, I was so weak I could not even wash clothes by hand, as was then the custom in my country. Medical practitioners told me that I would probably not live past the age of eighteen. But I did.

In 1955, at age 29, I came to the United States to meet and marry Herman Aihara, a student of George Ohsawa. After the birth of my first baby, I caught a cold and had difficulty breathing. Herman took me to St. Luke's Hospital in New York City, where the doctor was surprised to find that my pulse rate was 240 per minute. All of the doctors, interns, and nurses at the hospital and all of the medical students from New York University came to visit me to check my unusual pulse. To them, it was a miracle—not only was I alive, but I was also pregnant with my second child.

The doctor insisted that I undergo surgery to cure my condition. I agreed and in 1958 I had the operation, which was not successful. The artery that had been tied during the operation reopened. My doctor believed that I would not live unless I had a second operation. I refused. I had already lived more than thirty years with my heart condition, and I did not understand why I would not be able to live another thirty without another operation. I have, in fact, now lived beyond that time. I believe the operation I underwent damaged my kidneys and brain, and I really regret having agreed to it. The experience has taught me a very important lesson about life.

My heart had adapted to an inferior condition by strengthening itself. Not only did it adapt to beating faster than normal but it also grew to twice the normal size. This adaptability is the result of homeostasis—the body's ability to maintain constant internal conditions, such as body temperature, oxygen supply, water and salt content of the blood, etc.

In my opinion, each of us is born with this adaptability or homeostasis. It is our healing power. However, we can lose this healing power through incorrect eating and drinking habits, too much stress, and/or environmental hazards. The purpose of this book is to provide remedies and dietary suggestions that will show you how you can do away with uncomfortable symptoms and suffering so that you can feel better and your body can manifest its own natural healing ability

Many illnesses can be overcome without the use of chemical drugs, which cause a multitude of side effects and ultimately weaken the body's healing power. One of the reasons I wrote this book is to tell you that a diet of simple natural foods and the use of non-invasive remedies made from natural food products will eliminate many of your symptoms of sickness in a short time and will strengthen your healing power (a more complete cure) in the long run. Once you experience such healing and begin practicing a macrobiotic dietary approach, you will be much healthier and happier than ever before. You will no longer need to fear sickness. Giving you the ability to attain such power and control is the ultimate goal of this book.

The book is organized in four parts. Part One contains a brief and concise explanation of macrobiotic principles and the macrobiotic dietary approach as applied to healing. Part Two contains an alphabetical listing and a head-to-toe listing of disorders of the body.

The head-to-toe list appears at the beginning of the disorders section because it is often helpful to read about illnesses that affect the same organ or area of the body. If you have symptoms and don't know the name of the illness they indicate, read about the area of the body where your symptoms or pains are most prominent and look for a description that fits them. Then you can determine your best course of action. By studying whole groups of disorders, you can begin to understand macrobiotic thinking.

If you know the name of your illness, you can look it up in the alphabetical list and follow the suggestions. If you have an ailment that is not listed in the text, refer to the index for possible references. In Part Two, each disorder is described together with its common symptoms and causes, an explanation based on our macrobiotic understanding, helpful suggestions, and dietary recommendations.

External remedies are described in Part Three and recipes for foods and beverages that are used as remedies are in Part Four. The glossary includes a brief description of foods, products, and procedures that may be new to you.

While we have tried to make this book as complete as possible, there is a limitation that will become clear to you if you read the whole book thoroughly. The book is written so that you can correct illnesses; it does not provide a complete daily macrobiotic approach to diet and living. In other words, this book is not adequate if you want to study the macrobiotic approach more seriously in order to achieve even better health. To learn more about the macrobiotic approach, please refer to the suggested readings and resources for further study. Two very good books for those new to macrobiotic thinking are *Acid and Alkaline* and *Basic Macrobiotics*, both by my husband, Herman Aihara. For in-depth study, I recommend most highly George Ohsawa's books, all of which have inspired and helped so many people.

The danger in writing this type of book is that someone may think the suggestions listed here are the only ones to try. This is not the case. One thing is clear from my many years of experience; each person's illness is unique and requires that remedies be tailored to that person's current condition. At first, you may need to consult a number of books or health-care advisors. As your experience increases, your intuition will become sharper and, with further study, you can become the master of your own health. I know this to be true from my own life experience.

Because I was a very fragile child, my mother treated me with many traditional home remedies long before I heard of macrobiotics. Since learning about the macrobiotic approach, I have combined these traditional home remedies with macrobiotic remedies for the many people who have asked for my help. Thus, I have continued to learn about natural healing at home. With this experience, I hope to help many people eliminate their symptoms and re-establish their own body's natural healing power.

INTRODUCTION

In 1953 bills for doctors and medicine cost 1,500,000 United States families one half or more of their entire income.

Of these families 500,000 spent all or more than all of their income on medicinal bills. . . .

Drugs worth $14,000,000,000 (14 billion dollars) are purchased annually by the American public in its quest for health.

Millions of dollars are solicited and spent every year by research foundations with the avowed purpose of finding cures for the diseases which plague the nation.

. . . It is estimated that there are in our country today 45,000,000 chronic sick (over one quarter of the population), few of whom will ever be completely cured! The number is growing steadily and such major diseases as heart diseases and cancer, on which so much is spent, far from decreasing, are taking an ever greater toll of life.

Who Is Your Doctor and Why?
Alonzo J. Shadman, M.D.

Such were the United States expenditures for medicine in 1953. Table I below shows recent medical expenditures in the United States and a prediction for the year 2000. Health expenditures as a percentage of GNP (gross national product) in the United States are the highest in the world.

Isn't this situation horrible? And to make matters worse, health expenses are increasing at even greater rates each year. Do we get even an adequate return on such tremendous expenditures? Are we going toward better health and happiness?

The answer is "no." In 1900, infectious diseases took many lives, and pneumonia, influenza, and tuberculosis were the leading causes of death in the United States.

Infectious diseases, especially tuberculosis and polio, are better controlled by today's medicine, and diseases of the heart and blood vessels are the number one cause of death, according to recent statistics. Even so, the death rates from heart disease have declined in recent years, partly because many people have reduced the amounts of meat and other sources of cholesterol and saturated fat in their diets.

The incidence of and death rates from cancer have increased steadily to the point where cancer and AIDS are now two of the most feared diseases. Modern medicine has been unable to find a solution to either, and the future doesn't look any more promising.

Aren't we justified in asking questions about the effectiveness of our research and the drugs that are so universally used? I wonder if the whole medical system is wasting immeasurable effort and money because of possible and widely-held misconceptions on the nature of disease and the means of cure.

Since I came to the United States, I have been hospitalized only once, and that was for stomach pain. Even this was not something I chose; I was taken to the hospital by mistake. During the forty years I have lived in this country, I have spent only $800 for doctor's bills, hospitalization, and all medications. I think both my overall good health and low medical expenditures are the result of my following a macrobiotic approach to life.

The basic ideas of macrobiotics come from ancient times and are thousands of years old. The present-day macrobiotic movement is commonly thought to have originated with George Ohsawa, who introduced the modern version of the macrobiotic approach in 1928. Several thinkers influenced Ohsawa and provided the

TABLE I NATIONAL EXPENDITURES FOR HEALTH CARE 1970–2000						
	1970	1975	1980	1985	1987	2000
Total expenditures *(in billions of dollars)*	$ 75.0	$132.7	$ 248.1	$ 419.0	$ 500.3	$1,529.3
Per capita amount	$349	$591	$1,055	$1,596	$1,987	$5,551

From *The Universal Almanac*, 1990

1

building blocks upon which he constructed his approach.

One of these was certainly Ekken Kaibara (1630–1716), a pioneer in botany, herbal medicine, and geography. His belief that physical health, happiness, and longevity are the natural order for humans became one of the cornerstones of macrobiotic theory. Kaibara also felt that sickness occurs only when one breaks the natural order. Literally, we create our own sicknesses. He taught moderation and self-control in his principles of health: Eat small, sleep small (enough but not too long), and desire small, which means satisfying ego desires only to 80 percent. Many of his ideas about food were also picked up by Ohsawa, such as making brown rice the main daily food, using fresh seasonal vegetables as side dishes, refraining from overeating, showing appreciation before eating, and avoiding heavy, fatty meats since they decrease one's life span.

In the late 1700s, another important figure appeared named Nanboku Mizuno, the most famous fortune teller in Japanese history. Nanboku was a homeless wanderer when he was told by a fortune teller that he had only one year to live. He was also told that the only way to change his fate was by eating a diet of mostly brown rice and miso soup. Nanboku did this and thereby completely changed his future. He became a masseur at a public bathhouse where he learned the relationship between one's body and one's profession. Then he became a cremator and learned the relationship between diet and sickness. After studying diet more, he could predict someone's fortune with almost 90 percent accuracy just by analyzing that person's diet. Nanboku, like Ekken, emphasized the eating of less luxurious foods. He taught that by eating simple foods and by eating less, one could become rich in health.

About 100 years ago, Sagen Ishizuka (1851–1910) founded what is now known as macrobiotics. From childhood on, he had suffered from a skin disease similar to eczema that was caused by weak kidneys. Since his doctor couldn't help cure his condition, Sagan decided to study Western medicine. In order to study Western medicine, he learned to read and write in four Western languages, and later became an army doctor. Even though he helped many people, he still couldn't cure his own eczema. When he retired, he began to study Oriental medicine. It was not, however, until he found the traditional Japanese brown rice diet that his skin recovered. He became a very famous doctor in Tokyo and wrote a couple of popular books on nourishing the body and mind through proper eating.

Ishizuka maintained that the way to live a happy and long life is through the proper balance of sodium salts and potassium salts in the body. He believed that eating the proper foods is the most important and critical factor in maintaining this balance. Thus, a proper diet is most important for maximum health.

From his observation of people's teeth and digestive systems, Ishizuka came to the conclusion that the proper food for humankind is vegetable-quality foods. He theorized that our body and the soil are really one because the soil produces the foods that become our body after we eat them. Cereal grains, because of their abundance and sodium potassium ratio, became the principal food in his dietary scheme. Ishizuka also insisted that the proper preparation of foods is as important as proper selection. He came to understand that not only one's physical condition but also one's mental, emotional, and spiritual condition are influenced by food. After Ishizuka died in 1910 from a stomach catarrh, believed to have been caused by overwork, his disciples (many of them military officers) founded Shoku-Yō Kai, a society based on using food to cure sicknesses.

When George Ohsawa was eighteen and suffering from tuberculosis, he read Ishizuka's books. Although he never met him, Ohsawa followed Ishizuka's diet and was completely cured in one year. From that time on, Ohsawa devoted his life to spreading Ishizuka's diet and philosophy.

George Ohsawa (1893–1966) was a very good businessman and leader. He began using the name "macrobiotics" and reintroduced Oriental concepts such as yin and yang to enlarge the concept of "complementary antagonism" as evidenced by potassium salts and sodium salts. Since yin and yang can be applied to all of life, Ohsawa expanded macrobiotic principles into the fields of science, ethics, philosophy, and religion. He then spread these ideas to India, Africa, France, Vietnam, and the United States. He wrote hundreds of books and articles in Japanese, French, and English. Since his passing in 1966, his disciples have continued to make the macrobiotic approach available to people throughout the world.

Simply stated then, the macrobiotic approach to healing is based on the fact that health and happiness are natural as long as you eat and live simply and naturally. This includes reducing stress in your life and living in as natural an environment as possible (free from chemicals, air pollutants, and such). Natural eating and living work because the body's adaptability or healing power is strong as long as the foods proper for humankind are selected and prepared correctly. These foods are whole grains and fresh vegetables. In theory, if you become sick, all you have to do to become well is to return to eating simple natural foods. Thus, by following a daily macrobiotic dietary approach, you can increase your healing power so that your recovery from sickness will be faster and more complete.

PART ONE

MACROBIOTIC APPROACH TO HEALING

THE PRINCIPLES OF MACROBIOTICS

INTRODUCTION

Macrobiotics is the study of life and the natural laws of change. Since macrobiotics deals with all of life, there are too many principles to explain even briefly in this book. Suggested Reading on pages 249–250 lists many excellent books for your further study. However, the seven basic underlying principles related to the healing process are given in this section.

1. *Individual physical life is a manifestation of Infinity or Oneness*

Macrobiotic theory considers all phenomena from a wholistic large-scale perspective rather than from a fragmented analytical view. Thus, we begin by looking at Life itself. According to George Ohsawa, founder of the modern-day macrobiotic movement, Life is another name for Infinity, Oneness, Universal Consciousness, Nature, or God. Since Life is the originator and ultimate power that creates the visible and invisible worlds, it follows that individual beings are created by the power of Life. Furthermore, creation occurs in an orderly way from the Infinite World to the inorganic (yin and yang, energy, particles, and earth) world and finally to the organic (plant and animal) world.

The primary characteristic of the Infinite World is Oneness. This Oneness cannot be touched and is invisible, formless, colorless, soundless, and odorless. In order to manifest itself into the finite or visible inorganic world, Oneness polarizes into positive and negative energy (yin and yang in macrobiotic terminology). These two opposite poles attract and repel each other, producing vibrations that are manifest as light, heat, magnetism, electricity, chemical and atomic energy, and gravitation. These energies condense and materialize into electrons, protons, and neutrons. These particles combine in an orderly way to form atoms or elements. These elements make up water, air, soil, stones, and rocks.

Organic material is created from air, soil, and water (inorganic materials) with the energy of light. This is the beginning or origin of biological life—the plant world.

From the plant world, the animal world is created. By eating sea vegetables and land plants, animals have evolved. Over billions of years of evolution, the plant world has developed grains as its highest stage of evolution, and the animal world has evolved to humans as its highest stage. Thus, the proper food for humans as the main daily food is whole grains with other vegetable foods as side dishes.

2. *Individual consciousness is a manifestation of Universal Consciousness or Infinity.*

There are two types of genesis. Just as there is an orderly genesis of our physical life, there is an orderly genesis of our spiritual life. Spiritual life (or consciousness) begins with conception, the uniting of egg and sperm. Fetal development in terms of consciousness is mechanical or instinctive. After birth, sensorial development—seeing, hearing, smelling, tasting, and touching—occurs. Later, the ability to discriminate between liking and disliking develops. Next, intelligence—the ability to count and reason—develops. Then, the ability to distinguish self from others and to become aware of family, community, and friends (social consciousness) develops. And finally, religious consciousness—the ability to judge good or bad, right or wrong—develops. These stages of consciousness begin at different times with different children, depending on the parents, especially the mother.

These six stages of consciousness are all relative types of consciousness or judgment and are connected to or are part of Life or Universal Consciousness. Our development of consciousness or our spiritual life is a growth process through these stages. Universal Consciousness can be described as unconditional love. Unconditional love is shown by being grateful for difficulties and sicknesses because they teach us about Life. It is also shown by giving up things that we like; that is, by not satisfying all our ego desires so that others may have more of their desires fulfilled. When people express such unconditional love, they show their connection to Universal Consciousness.

3. Physical, mental, emotional, and spiritual health and happiness depend largely on the quality of our food.

Foods are also manifestations of Infinity or Oneness and include air, water, light, heat, radiation, etc., in addition to all the things we put in our mouths to eat. Once the definition of food has been widened to include all that we take in for nourishment, we realize that our environment, what we read or watch on television, and our thinking or attitudes greatly affect our health. When appropriate foods are consumed or taken in, our physical condition is healthy and our mental, emotional, and spiritual condition is peaceful and sound.

Use of appropriate foods involves proper selection, preparation, and consumption, all of which are discussed in The Macrobiotic Dietary Approach (see page 11). Here is a brief summary:

- Choose naturally produced foods of good quality.
- Choose locally grown and seasonal foods as much as possible.
- Eat mostly whole grains and fresh vegetables.
- Avoid chemicalized foods and those with artificial additives or preservatives.
- Select and prepare foods based on your condition and purpose.
- Learn how to change the effects of foods with cooking.
- Chew well and control liquid intake.
- Do not overeat. Moderation and simplicity are the keys to a happy and healthy life.

4. Everything changes in this relative world.

If there were no change in our lives, life would be very boring. Fortunately everything is constantly changing. Climatic changes are perhaps easiest to see. Just as the seasons change, our activities change, our emotions change, and the amounts we eat and drink change. This is common sense. However, this principle presents us with a problem.

Macrobiotics is not and cannot be a prescriptive approach as is nutritional/medical theory. What works one day for an individual may not work the next because we change every day. In other words, a macrobiotic approach requires a change in thinking from a static, prescriptive view of life to a dynamic and flexible one. This leads to real freedom. Changing your diet as conditions and desires change may sound complicated at first, but the end result is worth the effort. And the first step, the most important one, is to change to a diet based on whole grains and fresh vegetables.

5. Everything is different in this relative, finite world.

This principle is very important because many mistakes are made by not fully understanding it. For example, we may think we need a certain amount of proteins, fats, carbohydrates, vitamins, and minerals each day based on nutritional charts that reflect an average of people's needs. While charts make the recommended daily allowances easy to comprehend, averages do not allow for the uniqueness of each individual. On the other hand, the macrobiotic approach maintains that what works for one person will not necessarily be beneficial for another. Therefore, according to our macrobiotic understanding, individuals must determine the most appropriate foods for their own unique needs at any given moment.

6. Yin and yang are the two poles of Infinity or Oneness that allow the invisible infinite world to manifest as the visible finite world.

This principle teaches us the most important lesson in our life: opposites or antagonisms are complementary because they are the two sides (poles) of Oneness. There can be no day without night, no hot without cold, no male without female, and vice versa. In macrobiotic thinking, these opposites can be represented by yin and yang. Thus, yin and yang are a means of referring to any pair of opposites. In comparing opposites, one of the pair is considered more yin and the other is considered more yang.

It is important to note that yin and yang are only used for comparison; they are not absolute labels. Think for a moment about hot and cold. Something that is hot would generally be termed yang. But, what is "hot"? Say "hot" means 95°F, as in a hot day. In this case, "hot" would be termed yang compared with a cold day of 20°F. But, if "hot" means 212°F, as in boiling water, then the "hot" of 95°F would be cooler and thus yin by comparison. The fact that something may be termed yang in one case and yin in another, or yang one day and yin another, is a big stumbling block for people new to this kind of thinking.

The yin-yang principle is like a guiding compass. It shows direction in life in much the same way as a compass shows geographical direction. The principle that all opposites are complementary teaches us that there is no health without sickness and that there is no sickness without health. The yin-yang unifying principle is a very useful tool in sickness. If you are too yin, choose more yang foods and more yangizing preparation. If you are too yang, choose more yin foods and more yinizing preparations. Table 1.1, which shows the yin or yang state of various characteristics, will help you to make your choices.

The classification of foods into yin and yang is somewhat subjective since many factors are involved. Tables 1.2 and 1.3 show the factors used to determine yin and yang classifications while Table 1.4 gives you an overview of ying and yang characteristics in sickness. Table 1.5 gives a sample listing of fruits, beans, and vegetables classified from yin to yang as written by George Ohsawa over 45 years ago. These tables are included to deepen your understanding of macrobiotic principles. There are charts in most macrobiotic theory and cooking books and since each author varies the list by his or her experience, there are slight variations. By paying attention to how you react to different foods, you can produce your own charts, which will be the most accurate for you. But always remember, the most important characteristic of yin and yang is that they are terms of comparison and not terms of definite units.

7. The final macrobiotic principle is continuation.

The principle of continuation seems to contradict the principle that everything changes. In this finite world, everything *does* change. What you start has to end. That is the reason why it is so difficult to continue the things you start. People break promises; marriages break up; most businesses last about ten years; people don't stay long in one place, etc.

Why is it difficult to continue for *even* one month—much less for our lifetimes or forever—something we've decided to do? I believe it is due to our brain function. Our brain has two functions—consciousness and subconsciousness. Consciousness receives stimulation from the ever-changing outside world and analyzes, evaluates, and remembers the material for future reference.

Consciousness is happy and excited by this stimulation from the changing world. Therefore consciousness is always looking for new and different things. Consciousness gets bored if everything stays the same.

Subconsciousness is the opposite. Subconsciousness maintains our body's internal, stable conditions. Subconsciousness doesn't like change or different situations. It is our instinct and reflects more of our Supreme Consciousness. When we have clear instinct, we can continue with our resolutions and promises. Continuation depends on our highest consciousness (judging ability) or what George Ohsawa called Supreme Judgment. This highest consciousness reflects Infinity, Oneness, or the Eternal Spirit that doesn't change. If one can continue something promised or planned, one's highest consciousness is working. The macrobiotic way of life helps us to reach the Eternal Spirit or Supreme Consciousness and guides and supports us in staying healthy and happy our whole life.

THE BODY'S WISDOM—HOMEOSTASIS

The macrobiotic dietary approach does not cure any sickness, but neither does any medication or doctor. The body heals itself by its own healing power. This is very important. It is natural to be healthy. Deviation from the natural state results in sickness. Curing is the process of returning unnatural conditions to natural ones. Since the macrobiotic dietary approach is to eat natural foods and to live simply in as natural an environment as possible, followers find their physiological condition returns to its natural healthy condition. This seems too simple to be true. However, in the view of nature, that which is true is always simple.

TABLE 1.1   YIN AND YANG CLASSIFICATIONS

Characteristics	Yin		to				Yang
autonomic nerves	sympathetic						parasympathetic
behavior	passive						active
blood	cold						warm
color	violet →	blue →	green →	yellow →	orange →		red
emotions	fear →	grief →	sympathy →	joy →			anger
heat	cold →		warm →				hot
hormones	epinephrine →		adrenocortical →				acetylecholine
length	long						short
living things	plants						animals
minerals	phosphorous →	potassium →	magnesium →				sodium
size	large						small
taste	pungent →	sour →	sweet →	salty →			bitter
tropism	upward						downward
voice	groan →	weep →	sing →	laugh →			shout
weight	light						heavy

TABLE 1.2   YIN AND YANG CLASSIFICATION OF VEGETABLE-QUALITY FOODS

Characteristics	More yang	More yin
Color	Yellow, orange, red, brown, black	Green, blue, purple, white
Cooking method	Cold water	Boiling water
Cooking time	Long time	Short time
Geographic area	Northern	Southern
Growing direction	Downward and inward	Upward and outward
Above-ground direction	Horizontal (parallel to earth)	Vertical
Underground direction	Straight downward	Horizontal (parallel to earth)
Growing speed	Slow	Fast
Height	Low	High
Reaction to cooking	Slowly becomes soft	Quickly becomes soft
Season	Harvested from October to March	Harvested from April to September
Water content	Less water	More water

TABLE 1.3   YIN AND YANG CLASSIFICATION OF ANIMAL QUALITIES

Characteristics	More yang	More yin
Action	Swift	Slow
Blood quality	Thick	Thin
Breath and pulse	Quick	Slow
Build or physique	Chubby	Slender
Character	Active	Passive, gentle
Environment most conducive to growth	North	South
Growth rate	Slow	Fast
Height	Short	Tall
Hibernation	No hibernation	Complete hibernation
Musculature	Hard	Soft
Oxygen required	More oxygen	Less oxygen
Preferred climate	North; cold	South; warm
Preferred food	Flesh	Plants
Temperature	High	Low

TABLE 1.4   YIN AND YANG CLASSIFICATION OF CHARACTERISTICS DURING SICKNESS

Characteristics	More yang	More yin
Attitude	Aggressive	Passive
Body tendency	Contracted or hardened	Expanded or softened
Color of face	More red	More pale
Energy level	Excessive	Tired
Headache position	Back of head	Forehead or temple
Tendency of fists	Clenched	Open palms
Time of fever	Higher from midnight to morning (noon)	Higher from afternoon to midnight

TABLE 1.5   VEGETABLES, BEANS, AND FRUITS LISTED FROM YIN TO YANG

Vegetables		Beans	Fruit
Potato	Mustard greens	Soybean	Any tropical fruit
Eggplant	Kohlrabi	Green split pea	Lemon
Tomato	Cabbage	Lima bean	Orange
Shiitake mushroom	Cauliflower	Black-eyed pea	Fig
Mushroom	Turnip greens	Black soybean	Peach
Green pepper	Brussels sprouts	Kidney bean	Pear
Albi potato	Turnip	Pinto bean	Grape
Cucumber	Rutabaga	Great Northern white bean	Prune
Sweet potato	Parsnip	White bean	Plum
Summer squash	Parsley	Navy bean	Watermelon
Spinach	Winter squash	Mung bean	Cantaloupe
Asparagus	Daikon	Lentil	Apricot
Celery	Scallion	Chickpea	Cherry
Yam	Onion	Azuki bean	Blackberry
Beet	Garlic		Persimmon
Lettuce	Lotus root		Pomegranate
Swiss chard	Burdock		Apple
Kale	Carrot		Strawberry
Collard Greens	Watercress		
Chinese cabbage	Jinenjo (wild mountain		
Bok choy	potato)		

This natural healing power of our body has been called homeostasis by Walter B. Cannon, physiology professor at Harvard University, in his book *The Wisdom of the Body*. What is homeostasis? According to Dr. Cannon, homeostasis is the ability of the body to control its internal conditions and keep them constant. We don't always know very much about how we do this, but the inner conditions are always controlled and kept constant. This is most important. It may be hot and humid or cold and dry outside. But inside the body, in any weather, conditions are amazingly constant.

We perceive and react to the outside world with information provided by our senses. All our senses are very, very sensitive. Our noses are very sensitive; if there are only a couple of drops of vanilla extract in a room, we can smell vanilla. Our eyes are very sensitive; we can detect candlelight from far away. The tongue is very sensitive; we can distinguish even minute and subtle changes in taste. The whole body is very sensitive, but its internal conditions are maintained incredibly constant.

In a healthy person, the amount of oxygen in the body is constant. The amount of glucose is constant. Body temperature is relatively constant. Acidity and alkalinity are maintained at constant levels. All this is homeostasis, the body's wisdom. During the evolutionary process that moved from amoebas to human beings, this homeostatic ability was developed and improved. Without homeostasis, man as a species would have become extinct long ago. Homeostasis, then, is the first

and most vital stage of our healing power.

Our internal temperature is normally around 98.6°F. The body's skin condition is very important because internal temperature is controlled by sweating. Sweating helps us stay at this temperature even if it is 110°F outside. It's as if we have an automatic thermostat in our body set for 98.6°F. If you have a fever, your temperature goes up. Most modern people go to the drugstore right away and take some pills or use ice to lower their temperature. That's a big mistake. Why? Because the purpose of a fever is to kill certain microbes causing an infection. It's part of the body's wisdom or healing power. Once the microbes are gone, the fever goes down naturally. Lowering the fever artificially protects the microbes. They don't die. We lose the natural healing process.

Homeostasis also works to control the pH of the blood. Science measures acidity and alkalinity by pH. A neutral pH is 7.0. A substance with a lower pH is more acid; a substance with a higher pH is more alkaline. Our blood is always maintained around 7.4 or 7.5. The brain and nervous system stop functioning in an acidic condition. A blood pH of 6.9 results in a coma—we're finished. At a blood pH of 7.8, we may have a seizure because this condition is too alkaline. So our body must maintain its blood pH around 7.4—slightly alkaline. This pH is controlled by the kidneys.

Another organ that is important to homeostasis is the lungs. The amount of oxygen in the body is constant. This is controlled by the lungs. The amount of fluid and the amount of carbon dioxide must also be constant and controlled. This control is achieved by the circulatory system.

Blood circulation is very interesting. According to Chinese medicine, curing power comes from good blood circulation. Why is this so important? The body contains about 60 trillion cells. These cells need oxygen to be supplied every three minutes if they are to survive; this oxygen is carried by the blood. So blood circulation maintains a constant level of oxygen and nutrients inside the cells. If the blood doesn't circulate well, inadequate nutrients are supplied and sickness results. In a similar way, blood circulation helps the body maintain a constant level of carbon dioxide. Blood circulation depends on the condition of the heart and circulatory system.

The level of sugar in the blood is also a constant in a healthy individual. When the blood sugar level is too high, the pancreas produces insulin that changes to glycogen to reduce the amount of blood sugar to the proper level. When the blood sugar level is too low, the adrenal gland produces cortical hormone that changes glycogen in the liver to glucose so that the amount of blood sugar is raised to the proper level. Thus, two hormones, insulin and cortical hormone, maintain the constancy of the blood sugar level in the body.

These are all examples of homeostasis, the body's healing power. By homeostasis, our body maintains constancy in body temperature, acidity and alkalinity levels, oxygen and carbon dioxide levels, blood circulation, blood sugar level, etc. This constancy is our body's natural condition. When we maintain this constancy or natural condition, we are healthy. When we cannot maintain this internal stable condition, we are sick.

Modern civilized society weakens homeostasis because air conditioning replaces our body's temperature control system. Medications, including antibiotics, have replaced our natural immunity or healing power. When one cannot produce enough insulin or cortical hormone, medicine substitutes for these hormones with those from animals. With these substitutions and many others, our homeostasis need never have existed. The distinguishing characteristic of modern civilized society is that medicine is necessary to maintain homeostasis.

The macrobiotic healing approach is to strengthen our ability to maintain homeostasis by limiting the use of external means of control such as air conditioners, antibiotics, pain killers, sleeping pills, laxatives, etc. Even so-called macrobiotic external remedies such as ginger compresses and albi plasters are only used when necessary. In other words, we should live in environments that are constantly changing like nature does so that our automatic nervous system and hormonal system constantly have to work hard. Thus they will be strong enough to maintain constant internal conditions in most

weather, during times of infection, or while we are eating strange foods and drinking unhealthy water. This strength includes the ability to maintain constancy in emotions and behavior so that one is not easily upset under any circumstances. Maintaining this constancy depends on the functioning of all of the body's organs.

How can we maintain these organs in topnotch condition? It seems to me that modern medicine has no idea about how to do this. Not only that, medicine has never really tried to find out how to achieve a healthy condition of the organs. Modern medicine is too busy trying to eliminate the symptoms of sicknesses and exchanging healthy organs for sick ones. Therefore, once sick people receive such treatment, they have to continue that medication or treatment almost their entire lives because those medications and treatments are not intended to bring the organs to a natural healthy condition. One sickness follows another.

Homeostasis developed over millions of years of evolution, as Walter Cannon mentioned in his book. However, he does not explain how it developed. According to our macrobiotic understanding, this was accomplished by the development of internal organs, including the nervous and hormonal systems. And the development of internal organs was the result of eating foods most adapted to the environment, and foods most highly developed in the plant world. Whole grains are a recent development and the most abundant food plants at this stage of evolution of the plant world. Seasonal, locally grown vegetables are the foods most adapted to one's environment. If people eat such natural foods, they achieve the highest adaptability or homeostasis.

Of course, there is much more to the macrobiotic approach, and there are many more reasons why it works. But, increasing the body's healing power by eating natural whole grains and fresh vegetables is the most important. It is encouraging to see that many doctors and nutritionists now understand the importance of a low-fat-high-complex-carbohydrate approach such as the macrobiotic dietary approach. (For further study, see the suggested readings, especially *Doctors Look at Macrobiotics*, edited by Edward Esko, and *Tired or Toxic?* by Sherry A. Rogers, M.D.)

In conclusion, the human body is truly a miracle. It can adjust to many years of abuse, including the eating of inappropriate foods such as large amounts of fatty meats and refined sugar. However, these adjustments are what are commonly called sicknesses. How you respond to sickness is your choice. The macrobiotic approach is to use the most simple and natural techniques possible. This allows the body's healing power to remedy the current condition and to become stronger so that future adjustments are minor and easily achieved.

THE MACROBIOTIC DIETARY APPROACH

The macrobiotic approach is based on the primary idea that one's physical life depends on the nourishment of food and that foods consumed determine the condition of the vital organs, including the brain. Therefore, our psychological or mental health and happiness are also largely dependent upon the quality and quantity of the food and liquid we consume. Thus, the macrobiotic dietary approach is the study of how to select, prepare, and consume appropriate foods in order to establish health and happiness on Earth.

Selection

1. Choose naturally produced foods and beverages of good quality. Generally, the less processed or refined, the better. Avoid hybrid foods, overly processed foods, and chemicalized foods. The number of natural food stores and mail order companies is increasing, and it is becoming much easier to follow this guideline.
2. Select locally grown and seasonal foods as much as possible. These foods will create the healthiest body condition because locally grown and seasonal foods are the foods best adapted to a given environment. Consequently, these foods will aid your body in adapting successfully to that same environment.
3. Choose whole grains as your main food. It is important that these grains be whole and unrefined. Brown rice, because of its nutritive value and ratio of sodium to potassium, is most often used as a daily staple. In colder climates and seasons, use more buckwheat, millet, rye, and wheat. In warmer climates and seasons, more barley, corn, and beans may be used as main foods.
4. Choose fresh land and sea vegetables, including soups, as side dishes. As a general guideline, the amount of land and sea vegetables in the diet should be one-third to one-half of grains by weight. Those who have consumed many animal foods in the past may wish to increase the proportion of fresh vegetables, especially leafy greens. Refined grains may also be used as side dishes and in soups.
5. Occasional foods may be chosen from fish, fruit, natural dairy foods, organic poultry, and non-chemicalized lean meats. These foods generally comprise from 5 to 10 percent of total intake. They are used more or less often, depending on your condition and purpose. For example, some people who participate in competitive sports find it beneficial to eat more animal foods. Others participating in competitive sports find animal foods totally unnecessary or even harmful because of the high concentration of fat and protein. You must decide on the proper amount for

you by listening to your body's needs.

6. Beer or other alcoholic drinks, processed or enriched dairy foods, high-fat foods, sugary cakes, candies, soft drinks, and chemical sweeteners are luxury foods only. In our macrobiotic dietary approach, we do not restrict these foods for healthy individuals. How often and how much of these foods are eaten is left to the individual. One may wish to eat these foods to relieve stress or in social circumstances. In such cases, select those that don't have chemical or artificial additives or preservatives, if possible. In other words, always seek the best quality and the least artificially processed. In any event, when these foods are eaten, try not to worry or feel guilty because these emotions can be more harmful than the food, especially if your daily dietary practice is sound.
7. In all cases, select foods according to your condition and purpose. If you are sick, avoid luxury and occasional foods until your health returns. Once you decide your purpose in life and realize that what you eat greatly affects your ability to attain that purpose, you are well on your way to realizing all your dreams.

Preparation

1. Proper preparation of food is as important as proper selection. When you cook food, you not only change its quality but also its effect on you. In fact, the art of cooking is the easiest and most practical way to learn the principles of change or yin-yang theory. With study and experience, you learn how to change the effects of foods to balance environmental conditions as well as your own physical and mental condition.
2. Use sea salt and natural miso, soy sauce, and vegetable oils as seasonings in your daily dietary practice. Sea vegetables such as kombu and wakame and small dried fish make very good seasonings and contain many vitamins and minerals, including vitamin B12. Do not use monosodium glutamate, chemically produced seasonings, refined sugar, or vinegar except as occasional luxury foods.

Consumption

1. Chew well. When beginning a macrobiotic diet, try chewing each mouthful at least 100 times. The more you chew your food, the better; saliva is an aid to digestion. Some of the benefits of chewing well are: less tendency to overeat, less craving for sweets and liquids after a meal, better comprehension of how much salt the body needs, and better thinking if you chew quickly (the opposite of how a cow chews).
2. Control liquid intake. This helps to strengthen the

heart and kidneys. On a grain-and-vegetable-based diet, drinking large quantities of liquid is not necessary because grains and vegetables are composed mostly of water. Thus, drinking is more of a luxury. Drinking only when thirsty is a good way to control liquid intake. Men should urinate about four times per day and women should urinate about three times per day. Otherwise, too much liquid is being taken. However, older people usually urinate more often—five to six times per day is not too often. You have to pay attention to what is normal for you.

3. Quantity affects quality. We are conditioned to think that more is better. However, most of the degenerative diseases in civilized society are caused by excesses rather than by deficiencies. The overconsumption of animal foods and overly refined and chemicalized foods has led us to where we are today by overburdening the body's natural healing power. It is possible to overburden it with good-quality food as well, especially when these foods are not chewed properly. For example, minerals are very important, but too many minerals can cause hardness or tightness in the body.

In conclusion and in all cases, moderation and simplicity are the keys to a happy and healthy life. So, our daily practice is the moderate use of simple foods—whole grains and beans and fresh land and sea vegetables with good-quality seasonings. However, it is even important to be moderate about being moderate and thus, when not sick, occasionally consuming luxury foods or eating out is necessary for a healthy and socially active life.

THE WILL TO CURE

No matter what method is used in attempting to overcome sickness, a strong will to cure is necessary. Where does this will come from? How can we produce this will? Understanding or acquiring such will is the most difficult thing for the sick person. However, when the will to cure is found or cultivated, any sickness can be cured.

First, you must understand that natural food is the manifestation or realization of Infinity. Our foods are produced by Infinity only and not in any human factory. Because our foods are the product of sun (heat and radiation), air, water, minerals, microbes, vitamins, and much more, these are our environment and the producers of our life. Thus, food is the source of the will to cure and possesses miraculous power. We are living miracles surrounded by miracles. Consider the following facts:

The Earth rotates on its axis at such a precise rate that our vegetation does not burn up during the day or freeze at night. Our Earth is just far enough away from

the sun so that its heat warms us just enough—not too much and not too little. The slant of the Earth gives us seasons and makes the Earth habitable. And the air is just the right composition to make chemical reactions such as oxidation happen. Life is balanced with oxygen-needing animals and oxygen-producing plants. Without this complementariness, there would be no life on this planet. Plant life would never have existed without insects that could pollinate. By the same token, human life could not have existed without trillions of microbes living in us. These same microbes may create hazards for us if they grow too much or if we produce ones unfavorable to our health. However, this happens because of our mistakes or because we eat improper foods and not because we are cursed by nature or unlucky. In a sense, eating improper foods weakens our will to cure.

The human body is a miracle and a marvel. The first cell that is fertilized in a mother's oviduct divides and becomes two, then four, eight, a thousand, a million, etc. These develop into a brain, a nervous system, stomach, intestines, lungs, heart, spleen, nose, hair, etc. It seems to me that the first cell knows how to build each organ, all tissue, blood, and the whole body. Everything is exactly planned from the very beginning.

We are able to maintain the right temperature all the time, wherever we go or whatever the condition may be on the outside. We can also maintain our body fluids at the proper levels of acidity and alkalinity and our levels of oxygen, carbon dioxide, minerals, microbes, enzymes, vitamins, red blood cells, and white blood cells. These things cannot all happen by accident. We are a living miracle.

An even more miraculous thing is the function of our brain, which can calculate, imagine, interpret the senses, create thought, etc. When I was a university student in Japan, I was a member of the mountain-climbing team. Once, while rock climbing, my holding rock broke and I fell about 20 feet. I was lucky to have landed on a ledge. The fall took only a second or two. Within this short time, my memory flashed back through all my past, from my childhood to that moment. Our memory is wonderful. Its mechanism is miraculous.

But how do these miraculous mechanisms relate to the will to cure? It is my belief that the human body is a minute part of the whole universe or Infinity. The spirit, mind, or consciousness is the other side of this universe or Infinity. It is my view that our thoughts are originated by Infinity. Our brain is comparable to a television set; it can pick up any of thousands of signals radiated from Infinity all the time. Which signals we pick up depend on the condition or constitution of the brain. This condition or constitution is determined by the foods we eat. If we eat synthetic foods, we cannot catch the signals of Universal Mind or Consciousness and Highest

Judgment and then our will to cure is diminished and we cannot cure any sickness.

Physical life is nothing but vanity. One hundred years of it are as nothing. It is the spiritual life that is real. Let us make our bodies healthy with natural, macrobiotic food. We can thus enter into the miracles of the universe and enjoy a wonderful life.

I hope this book will be a guide to help you fix your body when you have made mistakes in the course of your journey to reach the wonderful world of Life. But please remember, to cure the body or to heal sickness is not our real aim. Our real aim in healing the body is to correct and sharpen the brain's function so that we can catch messages from the wonderful, miraculous Universal Mind that is manifested in our life as happiness and health. When we reach such understanding, we will have the Will to Cure.

PART TWO

DISORDERS FROM A TO Z

INTRODUCTION

This section includes explanations of and helpful suggestions for common disorders. If you know the name of the illness you have, you will find it listed here in alphabetical order. If you have an illness that is not listed, see the index for possible references to pertinent material in the text.

It is also helpful to read about illnesses that are related to yours. Thus, we have included Table 2.1 (see page 18), which is a listing of disorders in more or less head-to-toe order according to the body organ or systems involved. For example, if you have a stomachache, you would also benefit from reading the sections on Gastritis, Heartburn, and Stomach Cramps. In addition, this listing is very helpful in cases where you are uncertain as to the specific illness that you have.

Once you have chosen the appropriate sections and read them, you will note that some words appear in small caps. These words refer you to Part Three for more specific directions for preparation and use of remedies. For

example, if you want to find "an APPLICATION of GREEN LEAVES" you would look in Part Three (External Remedies, pages 167 through 191) for the word "APPLICATION" (these words are listed in alphabetical order) and beneath that for "Green Leaves" (also in alphabetical order). Words that appear in small italic caps refer you to the recipes listed in alphabetical order in Part Four.

Specific dietary suggestions are included for certain disorders. This special limited diet should be followed only for a short time, until your condition improves or up to about one month. Then, widen your food choices based on a macrobiotic dietary approach (see Part One, pages 11–12, for an explanation of this approach).

Miso soup is recommended daily for anyone with any disorder. You will find several foods listed as miso soup ingredients. From this list, choose two or three ingredients with which to make your daily soup. This process is described in the recipe section (see pages 193–242).

TABLE 2.1   HEAD-TO-TOE REFERENCE LISTING OF DISORDERS

LOCAL AREA AFFECTED	DISORDER
Scalp and Hair	Hair Loss; Dandruff; Hair, Grey.
Head and Brain	Headache; Headache, Migraine; Sunstroke; Fainting; Convulsions, Children's; Epilepsy; Stroke; Meningitis; Hysteria; Hyperactivity; Depression; Nervous System Malfunction; Beriberi; Malaria; Tetanus; Fatigue, Excessive; Pain, Facial and Nerve.
Eye	Corneal Inflammation; Trachoma; Retinitis; Glaucoma; Cataracts; Night Blindness; Tears, Excessive; Astigmatism; Sty.
Nose	Nosebleeds; Nose, Obstructed; Nasal Polyps; Sinus Infection.
Ear	Eardrum, Ruptured; Ear Infections; Motion Sickness.
Mouth and Teeth	Bad Breath; Chapped Lips; Canker Sores; Cold Sores, Fever Blisters; Thrush; Tongue Trouble; Dental Caries; Periodontal Disease.
Throat	Laryngitis; Stuttering; Tonsilitis; Sore Throat; Mumps; Diphtheria.
Upper Respiratory	Goiter; Thyroiditis; Hypothyroidism; Hyperthyroidism; Bronchitis; Allergies; Asthma; Colds; Whooping Cough; Fever; Flu; Hiccups; Esophageal Stricture; Measles.
Lung and Breast	Pneumonia; Tuberculosis; Pleurisy; Lung Cancer; Fibrocystic Diseases of the Breast; Breast Cancer; Breast Infection; Breast Milk Flow, Inhibited.
Body and Spine	Body Odor; Rheumatism; Arthritis; Osteoporosis; Osteomyelitis; Periostitis; Shoulder Ache; Spinal Curvature; Backaches; Hunchback; Spinal Cord Inflammation; Tuberculosis of the Spine; Sciatica; Muscle Cramps; Finger Infection.
Heart and Circulation	Heart Block; Heart-Rhythm Irregularity; Heart-Valve Problems; Heartbeat, Rapid; Pericarditis; Heart Failure, Congestive; Blood Pressure, High; Heart Attack; Blood Poisoning (Septicemia); Aneurysm; Arteriosclerosis; Thrombosis; Leukemia; Malaria; Anemia; Heavy Metal Poisoning.
Stomach	Gastritis; Stomachache; Heartburn; Stomach Cramps; Gastric Juice, Lack of; Food Poisoning; Stomach Ulcer; Stomach Cancer; Stomach, Downward Displacement of.
Intestines	Parasites; Peritonitis; Enteritis; Diarrhea; Dysentery, Adults'; Dysentery, Children's; Cholera; Typhoid Fever; Typhus, Epidemic; Constipation; Appendicitis; Motion Sickness; Tuberculosis of the Intestines; Small Intestine Cancer; Diverticular Disease; Colon Cancer; Hernia; Rectal Prolapse; Hemorrhoids; Anal Fissure; Anal Itch.
Liver	Diabetes, Insulin Dependent; Diabetes, Non-Insulin Dependent; Hypoglycemia; Hepatitis; Cirrhosis of the Liver; Jaundice; Liver Cancer; Gallstones.
Kidney	Fatigue; Kidney Failure; Uremia; Bed-Wetting; Insomnia; Bladder Infections.
Skin	Skin Infection; Prickly Heat; Skin Cancer; Acne; Skin Abscesses; Skin, Itchy; Skin, Moisture Problems; Ringworm; Rashes (Poison Oak and Poison Ivy); Chickenpox; Scarlet Fever; Leprosy; Measles; Bites and Stings; Warts; Birthmarks; Burns; Bruises.
Sex Organs	Uterine Bleeding; Uterine Tumors; Ovarian Inflammation; Ovarian Cyst; Endometriosis; Menstrual Irregularities; Morning Sickness; Miscarriage and Premature Birth; Vaginitis; Candidiasis; Infertility; Syphilis; Gonorrhea; Nocturnal Emission; Impotence; Prostate Problems; Pain, Penis; Testicular Inflammation; Scrotum Swelling.
Legs	Leg Trouble, Children's; Edema; Varicose Veins; Leg Cramps; Sprains.
Feet	Frostbite; Corns and Callouses; Athlete's Foot.

ACNE

Common acne is an inflammatory condition with skin lesions and eruptions most frequently occurring on the face, chest, and upper back. Acne occurs when oil glands in the skin become clogged, and then infected by bacteria normally found in the glands. The resulting symptoms are blackheads, small black spots about the size of a pinhead; whiteheads, small white spots; small pus-filled lesions; and/or redness and inflammation around the eruptions.

Acne is most common among adolescents, especially among boys. Sex-hormone changes during adolescence play a role but are not considered to be the cause, and sexual activity appears to have no effect on acne. Contributing factors are believed to be allergies, stress, oily skin, drug use (cortisone and oral contraceptives, for instance), exposure to extremely hot or cold weather, endocrine disorders, male hormones, family history of acne, and junk food.

According to our macrobiotic understanding, the major contributing factor is a diet overly rich in protein such as animal foods, which also contain large quantities of fat, along with the overconsumption of refined sugar. This kind of diet adds to the clogging of oil glands in the skin on the face and upper part of the trunk, and contributes to a weakened condition of the kidneys. In the macrobiotic view, the health of the skin is directly related to the health of the kidneys. The skin and kidneys work together to help cleanse the body. The skin is responsible for ridding the body of approximately 20 percent of its waste products. The lungs, through the act of breathing, account for 70 percent while urination and bowel movements account for 7 and 3 percent respectively. Because of the drying effects of the sun in the summertime, acne often improves in the summer and worsens in the winter.

Helpful Suggestions

Since antibiotics kill both beneficial and nonbeneficial bacteria, the macrobiotic approach is to try to solve the problem without their use.

OBJECTIVE	REMEDY
To control acne flare-ups	FASTING for several days is best if your overall condition allows it. *and* You might try a TOFU APPLICATION on the pimples. Cover with a bandage to keep the tofu in place. Change the tofu and bandage 3 times per day.
To remove toxins	Drinking 1 to 2 cups of *HABUCHA TEA* per day for several days until the acne diminishes is recommended because habucha tea helps cleanse the body of toxins.
To minimize oil on skin	Cleanse the skin often by rubbing gently with soap for several minutes. Rinse thoroughly. Do not rub hard because this can spread the condition. Rubbing alcohol can be applied after cleansing to help remove excess oil. *and* Use a fresh washcloth each time as bacteria flourish in damp cloths. Dry the affected area with a hair dryer or pat dry with a clean towel each time you wash. *and* Shampoo your hair several times a week and avoid letting the hair touch the face, even at night. *and* Wash as soon as possible after vigorous exercise. *and* It is best not to squeeze the pimples but if you must, make sure to clean your hands and use rubbing alcohol before and after squeezing. *and* Avoid resting your face on your hands.

Dietary Recommendations

In general, the macrobiotic dietary approach (see page 11) is low in oily foods and refined sugar and is a good way to help clear up acne and lessen its effects on a long-term basis. Follow a macrobiotic dietary approach for a period of at least one month and your acne should improve. If you choose not to continue with a macrobiotic dietary approach, then it is wise to determine your sensitivities to certain foods. In this case, reintroduce dairy foods; oily foods such as nuts, peanut butter, and potato chips; and sugary foods and drinks (including chocolate) one at a time. If the acne flares up two to three days after a certain food is eaten, this indicates a sensitivity to that food and it should be avoided. Also, consult your doctor before taking oral medications, especially if you are pregnant.

ALLERGIES

Allergy denotes an altered capacity of the body's immune system to react to a particular substance called an allergen. The immune system identifies foreign substances and marks them for attack by the white blood cells. If normally nonforeign substances are identified for attack, the white cells can do more harm than the so-called foreign substances. Immediate responses range from watery eyes, itching, frequent sneezing, a tingling sensation around the mouth, a stuffy nose with a clear discharge, and swelling around the mouth or throat to difficulty in breathing, a pounding heart, faintness, and even loss of consciousness. Delayed allergic responses can appear hours or days after exposure and include skin responses such as contact dermatitis and bacterial allergies.

There are several types of allergy conditions and these can be divided into food allergies and environmental allergies. Food allergies result from eating foods to which one is allergic, taking medications of all types, injecting chemicals such as those used in x-rays into the body, and from being stung or bitten by insects such as bees or spiders. Environmental allergies result from a sensitivity to airborne allergens such as pollens, mold, and dust, and to tobacco smoke and other air pollutants. Nowadays, synthetic materials trigger allergic reactions in many people. However, these are not the primary cause of allergies.

According to our macrobiotic understanding, in cases of allergies all the organs are weak and homeostasis cannot be maintained. Specifically, most allergies are caused by protein antigens; however, simple carbohydrates or fat can be the underlying cause as well. In the case of reactions caused by protein antigens, allergies are caused by insufficient hydrochloric acid in the stomach and/or weak kidneys. The body needs to break proteins down into amino acids during digestion. If there is not enough hydrochloric acid in the stomach, the body tries to eliminate the protein that it cannot break down. These proteins then block the bronchial tubes and cause congestion in the lungs. If the protein comes from a food, then a food allergy results. If the protein comes from pollens, molds, or synthetic materials, an environmental allergy occurs.

Be aware that a diet low in salt can cause a shortage of hydrochloric acid. Diets high in protein, fat, and simple carbohydrates produce an overly acidic condition that may weaken the kidneys and the intestines. Weak kidneys also result in reduced sodium in the bodily fluids. In this case, infections start because the body's ability to make antibodies is reduced when there is not enough sodium in the bodily fluids. Without antibodies, the body cannot fend off an invasion of microbes. These microbes then cause an infection that shows up as allergy symptoms. Weak intestines lead to elimination troubles and, in the end, a greater possibility of allergic reactions. Emotional factors such as stress and too much anger also cause the immune system to be suppressed.

Recovery from allergies may take years, but your reaction to allergens should decrease each year while you are following a macrobiotic approach. However, be aware that most people become more sensitive before they become stronger and more able to combat the allergies. If you don't improve, you may want to test for allergies to particular foods or environmental pollutants. Be sure to test for the foods you are actually eating; some people, for example, are allergic to white rice but not to whole, brown rice. You might want to try a rotation diet. Also, make every attempt to rid your house of dust, mold, and toxin-producing products.

Helpful Suggestions

It is important to stop smoking. Also, the daily practice of one or more of the following suggestions makes the kidneys stronger because the procedures improve blood circulation and increase the amount of oxygen available to the kidneys.

OBJECTIVE	REMEDY
To improve kidneys	Apply a GINGER COMPRESS over the kidneys (see Figure 3.8 on page 176) every other day for 20 minutes until the symptoms go away.
	and/or
	Walk barefoot on the grass every day in the early morning for about 20 minutes.
	and/or
	Take a SAUNA at 100–115°F every night until sweat appears.
	and/or
	Take a 1 percent SALT BATH for 30 minutes 3 to 4 times a week.

Dietary Recommendations

Follow a macrobiotic dietary approach (see page 11) with plenty of sea vegetables and miso. Eat four to five small dried fish every day. Eat fewer wheat products.

☐ Avoid especially: all animal foods such as red meat, eggs, fish (except the small dried fish), cheese and other dairy foods, sugary foods such as candy—especially chocolate and ice cream—coffee, caffeine, all fruit, potatoes, tomatoes, eggplant.

See also ASTHMA.

ANAL FISSURE

An anal fissure refers to a crack or tear in the mucous membrane of the rectum or in the skin around the anus. This condition is like a pus ulcer or an ulcer infection. It almost always happens with tuberculosis. Symptoms range from itching around the rectum to streaks of blood and sharp pain following large and bulky bowel movements. According to our macrobiotic understanding, anal fissures are caused by overeating meat, fish, and other animal foods since the body stores the excess sodium (old salt) and the cells become inflexible, resulting in cracking or tearing with the passage of a large, hard stool. If you have this condition along with tuberculosis, having an operation for the anal fissure will worsen the effects of the tuberculosis. Therefore, it is wiser to try changing your diet first instead of having an operation to remedy this condition.

Helpful Suggestions

OBJECTIVE	REMEDY
To eliminate streaks of blood	You might try the traditional Japanese remedy of eating a thumb-sized piece of ginger once a day until bleeding stops. Chew well.
To relieve pain	A DAIKON or ARAME HIP BATH followed by an ALBI PLASTER every day helps relieve the pain. Change the plaster every 4 hours and leave it on overnight.
To relieve pain or infection	Applying good-quality sesame oil to the anus on a small bandage before bowel movements is helpful.
To improve circulation	Taking a warm shower once a day, 10 minutes maximum, until the fissure heals is beneficial.

Dietary Recommendations

The following dietary suggestions may be used until the fissure heals or for about one month, then widen your food choices based on a macrobiotic dietary approach (see page 11).

☐ Main foods: Brown Rice, Brown Rice with Barley served with Gomashio at each meal. Chew each mouthful 200 times.
☐ Side dishes (one fourth of main foods): Sesame Miso, Hijiki Nitsuke, burdock carrot dishes, Vegetable Tempura served with Grated Daikon, Okara Nitsuke, Carp Soup, Eggplant Pressed Salad.
☐ Miso soup ingredients: dried daikon, daikon, eggplant, tofu, Chinese cabbage, green leafy vegetables, cucumbers, Brown Rice Mochi.
☐ Beverages: Brown Rice Tea, Brown Rice Bancha Tea, Bancha Tea, Vegetable Broth, Grain Coffee. Drink two and a half cups maximum per day.
☐ Avoid especially: all animal foods, shellfish, fish (except carp), eggs, meat-based soups, dairy foods, alcohol, sweet foods, all fruit.

ANAL ITCH

According to our macrobiotic understanding, anal itch results from an overly acidic condition of the bodily fluids that is caused by eating too much animal food, sugary food, and fatty food. An overly acidic condition is also caused by weak kidneys. The skin excretes excess acid from the bodily fluids through perspiration, and this can cause topical itchiness, particularly in sensitive skin areas like the anus. Anal itch can also result from pinworms.

Helpful Suggestions

OBJECTIVE	REMEDY
To relieve itching	Take a DAIKON or ARAME HIP BATH for 20 minutes every night until itching stops.
To relieve severe itch	Use a GINGER COMPRESS over the kidneys (see Figure 3.8 on page 176) for 20 minutes every night until the severe itching stops.

Dietary Recommendations

In general, try to eat less, eating only until the stomach is two-thirds full. Use the following dietary suggestions until the itching stops or for about one month, then select foods according to a macrobiotic dietary approach (see page 11).

☐ Main foods: Brown Rice with a little Gomashio as a condiment, Baked Mochi with Soy Sauce or Mochi Soup, Buckwheat Noodles or Buckwheat Groats.
☐ Side dishes (one-fourth of main foods maximum): Tekka Miso, Scallion Miso, Vegetable Stew, Vegetable Stew with Fish, Carp Soup, Small Fish Tempura, Vegetable Tempura served with Grated Daikon, Oyster Tempura, Oysters Cooked with Miso, Burdock Carrot Nitsuke, Hijiki Nitsuke, Takuan Pickles.
☐ Miso soup ingredients: wakame, tororo kombu, onions, scallions, Homemade Agé, Brown Rice Mochi.
☐ Beverages: Brown Rice Tea, Brown Rice Bancha Tea,

Bancha Tea, Sho-Ban Tea, Mu Tea.

☐ Avoid especially: all animal foods including red-meat fish (except small fish as above), shellfish, meat-based soups, all dairy foods (including ice cream), fruit, sweet foods and drinks, all alcohol, rice vinegar, white bread, tomatoes, eggplant, potatoes, mushrooms, commercial sushi, melons, peanuts, hot spices, pressed salad.

See also PINWORMS and PARASITES.

ANEMIA

There are many types of anemia; here we discuss only anemia in general. Anemia means a decreased number of circulating blood cells, insufficient hemoglobin in the cells, or an inadequate volume of red cells in the blood that occurs when the balance between blood loss and blood production is disturbed. Like fever, anemia is a symptom of other disorders and it is important to determine these. The most common symptoms of anemia are shortness of breath, paleness, weakness, faintness, sore tongue, nausea, and fatigue. Other symptoms include headaches, appetite loss, abdominal pain, constipation, irritability, irregular heartbeat, frequent infections, and jaundice.

According to our macrobiotic understanding, an infection in a lung, weak intestines, or a shortage of oxygen can cause anemia because the quality of red blood cells is affected by plasma and oxygen in the intestines and lungs. Other causes include the inadequate intake or absorption of folic acid, iron, or B₁₂; a decrease of hydrochloric acid in the stomach (caused by the overconsumption of proteins) that inhibits the proper digestion of proteins; a weak liver, since the liver controls metabolism and thus overall body energy; radiation that destroys red blood cells; the overconsumption of refined sugar, also damaging red blood cells; improper breathing; and the overconsumption of fatty foods, which causes blood circulation to be reduced.

Helpful Suggestions

OBJECTIVE	REMEDY
To improve red blood cell production	Start by trying 10 to 15 minutes of BREATHING EXERCISE every day to learn how to breathe deeply and completely.
To improve blood circulation	Exercising each day until you break into a sweat is very helpful because sweating helps eliminate excess acids from the blood.
	or
	If you are unable to exercise, then take a SAUNA until you sweat. Continue with the saunas every other day until anemia improves.
In serious cases of anemia	Try eating at least 2 to 3 small dried fish every day. These are a good source of vitamin B₁₂.

Dietary Recommendations

It is most important that you eat plenty of high-fiber foods such as whole grains and fresh vegetables. This enables the intestines to produce good plasma. Following a macrobiotic dietary approach (see page 11) that includes fish up to two times per week is effective. This diet contains foods high in iron such as leafy greens and includes as luxury foods only very small amounts of those foods that contain oxalic acid, which hinders iron absorption. Additives are avoided in general, and these also interfere with iron absorption. Chew very well, especially the whole grains. Eat miso soup and Rice Bran Pickles every day. Eating shiso every day is also helpful.

ANEURYSM

An aneurysm refers to an enlargement or bulge of a segment of a blood vessel, often an artery in the heart. An aneurysm in a heart muscle causes heartbeat irregularities and symptoms of congestive heart failure. A thoracic (chest) aneurysm produces pain in the chest, neck, back, and abdomen. The pain may be sharp and sudden. An abdominal aneurysm produces back and abdominal pain, loss of appetite, and weight loss. An aneurysm in a leg artery causes poor circulation in the leg with weakness and the absence of skin coloration or with swelling and a bluish coloration. An aneurysm in a brain artery produces headache, weakness, paralysis or numbness, pain behind the eyes, and a change in vision or partial blindness.

The most common cause of aneurysm is thought to be hardening of the arteries (atherosclerosis). Other causes are congenitally weak arteries, injury, or syphilis. However, the fundamental cause is the reason that the arteries become hardened or weak in the first place. According to our macrobiotic understanding, this condition is primarily caused by a diet of too much yin food, resulting in a weakened condition overall. Artery problems are also caused by eating too much fatty food and/or cholesterol-rich food that causes a clogging (hardening) of the arteries themselves.

Helpful Suggestions

Any illness affecting the heart is potentially life-threatening and should be understood and dealt with appropriately. Surgery is often the outcome and aneurysms can recur especially if dietary changes are not made. However, a change to a macrobiotic dietary approach before aneurysms develop can be most beneficial and should be considered, especially if you are at risk; for example, if your family has a history of atherosclerosis, if you smoke, are overweight, or have had a previous heart attack or high blood pressure.

OBJECTIVE	REMEDY
To relieve pain and remove toxins	Try using a GINGER COMPRESS on the affected area for 20 minutes 2 times per day until the pain stops. Follow the Ginger Compress with an ALBI PLASTER for up to 4 hours to help remove toxins from the area. Apply a new albi plaster before going to bed and leave it on overnight. Continue with a Ginger Compress for 20 minutes followed by an Albi Plaster for up to 4 hours each day until the pain is gone.
To strengthen a weak pulse	Drink RANSHO DRINK prepared from 1 egg, once a day for 3 days before going to sleep. If once a day is not enough, eat a second 1-egg preparation of ransho per day until the heart becomes stronger (shows a stronger pulse). *and/or* Eat 1 teaspoon of TEKKA MISO once a day at any meal for 1 week.
To improve circulation	MASSAGE the area with GINGER SESAME OIL to stimulate circulation. *and* Apply a MUSTARD PLASTER to the heart (see Figure 3.8 on page 176) until the skin turns a red color (about 15 minutes), then apply an ALBI PLASTER for up to 4 hours. Apply these plasters for 1 week.
To help make the heart stronger	Eat 1/2 teaspoon of EGG OIL 3 times per day for 1 week.
To eliminate (melt away) fats and crystalized salts	Take a SAUNA (FAR-INFRARED) several times per week.

Dietary Recommendations

Follow a macrobiotic dietary approach (see page 11) with plenty of whole grains, fresh vegetables, sea vegetables, and miso soup.

☐ Avoid especially: sugar, alcohol, fruit, rice syrup, molasses, honey, and vinegar.

See also ARTERIOSCLEROSIS *and* STROKE.

APPENDICITIS

Appendicitis is an inflammation of the appendix, a small tube that extends from the cecum, the first part of the large intestine (ascending colon). The disease begins with a vague discomfort in the navel area. Then, within a few hours, it shifts to the lower right abdomen and the pain becomes severe. It worsens with moving, breathing, coughing, sneezing, walking, or simply being touched. Other symptoms include a loss of appetite, constipation, fever, and an increase in the white blood cell count from 10,000 to 16,000. Appendicitis is sometimes accompanied by nausea, vomiting, or diarrhea.

The cause is thought to be an infection but the reason for the infection is unknown. Also, the appendix is thought to serve no function and to be nothing more than an appendage left over from an earlier stage of biological evolution. However, according to macrobiotic theory, all parts of the body are necessary. The appendix is not only an important part of the body's immune system, but is also responsible for vitamin B_{12} production. Removal of the appendix would, therefore, be detrimental. It is a good idea then to avoid subsequent flare-ups of appendicitis by finding and eliminating the fundamental cause. According to our macrobiotic understanding, the primary cause is eating too much animal protein such as fish, eggs, beef, chicken, and pork along with too many simple carbohydrates such as candy, cakes, and other sugary foods.

Helpful Suggestions

In all cases, it is best to avoid hot baths.

OBJECTIVE	REMEDY
To prevent toxic infection	Try drinking 1 tablespoon of BURDOCK JUICE 3 times per day for 1 to 2 days. If you are a large person, 5 times per day is okay. *or* If burdock is out of season, chop and grind chickweed leaves or any dark green vegetable, including leafy greens, in a suribachi or blender. Squeeze out the juice and drink 1/3 cup 3 times per day for 1 or 2 days.
To reduce fever	Applying a TOFU PLASTER over the appendix (see Figure 3.8 on page 176) and changing it every hour is helpful until the fever is down.

and

Several days of FASTING are recommended if your condition allows it, especially if the fever comes from eating too much yang food.

To aid in cases of appendicitis without fever	Try a GINGER COMPRESS for 20 minutes followed by a 1-inch-thick ALBI PLASTER. Apply a new Albi Plaster every hour for one day. The ginger will help improve the circulation and the albi will help draw out toxins.
To alleviate pain, with or without fever	Use a BUCKWHEAT PLASTER for 20 minutes at a time as often as needed for pain. Keep the plaster warm by placing a ROASTED SALT PACK on top. *and* Drinking up to 3 cups of *BURDOCK CHICKWEED TEA* per day is helpful for pain, especially if there is constipation. Gas will come and feces should be eliminated. *and* Drinking 1 cup of *HABUCHA TEA* 2 or 3 times per day until pain stops is effective if prepared strong and taken for several days.

Dietary Recommendations

The following dietary suggestions may be followed until the appendicitis has subsided or for about one month. Then widen your food choices using a macrobiotic dietary approach (see page 11).

☐ Main foods: Brown Rice Balls, Mochi Soup with Miso, Brown Rice Gruel with Mochi, Brown Rice Cream, Brown Rice Gruel with Potato. Chew each mouthful 200 times.

☐ Side dishes (one-fourth of main foods): Tekka Miso, Oily Miso, Burdock Nitsuke, Carp Soup, Vegetable Tempura served with Grated Daikon, Baked Yams or Sweet Potatoes, Cucumber with Kuzu Sauce, Shiitake Nitsuke, Umeboshi.

☐ Miso soup ingredients: wakame, potatoes*, daikon, Chinese cabbage, green leafy vegetables, dried daikon, eggplant.

☐ Beverages: Brown Rice Tea, Bancha Tea, Kuzu Bancha Tea, Grain Milk.

☐ Avoid especially: all animal food including fish and shellfish, dairy foods (including ice cream), sweet foods and drinks, tomatoes, peanuts, corn on the cob, hot spices, black tea.

Note: The potato is used as a curative in this special circumstance, and its inclusion is not meant as an endorsement for continued use.

ARRHYTHMIA

See HEART-RHYTHM IRREGULARITY.

ARTERIOSCLEROSIS

Heart disease is the number one cause of death in the United States. In addition, hardening of the arteries contributes to over 70 percent of the deaths in this country. Therefore, it is important to monitor any abnormal heart condition with proper medical attention. Medications and drugs have a strong effect on the body, and the advice of a professional experienced in the effects of dietary change is recommended if medications or drugs are being used. Still, it is important that you understand as much as you can about your condition and the underlying causes of heart diseases.

Arteriosclerosis refers to a group of diseases characterized by the thickening and loss of elasticity of arterial walls. A common form of arteriosclerosis is atherosclerosis in which a narrowing of the arteries is caused by deposits of yellow plaques containing cholesterol materials. The most important symptom of all these diseases is a decrease in the internal diameter of the arteries so that the blood supply to the organs concerned is reduced; as a result, the organs start to malfunction. For example, coronary arteriosclerosis is the hardening and degeneration of the coronary arteries that provide the blood supply to the heart. There are two main coronary arteries. When they become narrowed, they can no longer provide adequate oxygen for heart cells. Often there are no symptoms until sudden pain (angina pectoris) or a heart attack occurs. If arteriosclerosis or atherosclerosis involves the blood vessels to the heart, a heart attack results. Muscle cramps result if it involves blood vessels in the legs; stroke or a deficiency of blood to the brain results if the condition involves vessels to the neck and brain. Because of the blockage of blood flow, arteriosclerosis may lead to kidney damage.

According to our macrobiotic understanding, the primary cause of arteriosclerosis is eating too much fatty, animal food, resulting in a yang type of arteriosclerosis. Eating too much sugary food, which produces fat by way of the liver, will result in a yin type of arteriosclerosis. A cholesterol-rich diet is the most important cause of atherosclerosis.

A yang heart condition is indicated by stagnated, thick blood, causing the heart to contract. The thick blood has a darker color and is usually overly acidic. When someone has an extreme yang heart condition, the fists are clenched, and the face and ears are red. However, if you touch the person's hands, they won't feel hot because all the heat goes to the heart area.

In the case of a yin heart condition, the heart is overly expanded. The blood is very thin, the person is generally anemic, and the pulse is very weak.

Helpful Suggestions

FOR EITHER THE YIN OR YANG TYPE

Don't take hot baths if you have either yin or yang types of any heart disease. Short, warm showers are okay. However, the use of a FAR-INFRARED SAUNA is recommended because the sauna will eliminate (melt away) deep deposits of fats and crystalized salt. Perspiring and elimination of fat are especially good for atherosclerosis and high blood pressure. When fat inside of the capillaries and arteries melts and is eliminated through blood circulation, the blood pressure goes down. This can also be achieved by sweating. However, in order to sweat enough to eliminate fat from the arteries and capillaries, a person must run about two to three miles. This is almost impossible for someone who has heart and circulatory troubles. And a normal sauna is too hot for people with heart trouble. Therefore, a far-infrared sauna, which is much safer for persons with heart problems, is preferable.

OBJECTIVE	REMEDY
	FOR THE YANG TYPE
To quiet a too-strong pulse	Every 4 hours, try drinking SOUR APPLE JUICE made from 1 small apple. A large person may use 2 to 3 apples. The grated apple juice goes to the intestines to help take away the heat, and the lemon juice goes to the kidneys to activate urination.
	and
	A DAIKON PLASTER over the heart area is helpful. If you are really in pain, change the plaster every 5 minutes. The daikon will become hot even in such a short time. If you have no daikon, use an APPLE PLASTER. Use the plaster for only 1 hour because grated daikon or apple reduces the heart's heat and can make the heart too cold (yin). The Daikon (or Apple) Plaster is used only to relieve the symptoms.
To alleviate palpitations	Try drinking ½ to 1 cup of SHO-BAN TEA 2 to 3 times per day.
	and
	Use a DAIKON or APPLE PLASTER on the heart (see Figure 3.8 on page 176) for no

more than an hour, changing it every 20 minutes. If this treatment is not effective, try a TOFU PLASTER applied to the heart area for 1 hour.

To relieve chest pain	Apply an ALBI PLASTER on the painful area, changing it every 4 hours.
To alleviate constipation	Eat ½ cup of AZUKI BEANS WITH KOMBU 2 times per day and use less salt than usual.

	FOR THE YIN TYPE
To strengthen a weak pulse	Drink the RANSHO DRINK prepared from 1 egg once a day for 3 days before going to sleep. If once a day is not enough, drink a second 1-egg preparation of ransho per day until the heart becomes stronger (shows a stronger pulse).
	and/or
	Eat 1 teaspoon of TEKKA MISO at each meal for 1 week.
To improve circulation	Apply a MUSTARD PLASTER to the heart (see Figure 3.8 on page 176) until the skin turns a red color (about 15 minutes), then apply an ALBI PLASTER for up to 4 hours. Apply these plasters for 1 week.
	and
	Eat ½ teaspoon of EGG OIL 3 times per day for 1 week to help make the heart stronger.
To relieve chest pain	Apply an ALBI PLASTER on the painful area, changing it every 4 hours as needed.
To alleviate constipation	Eat ½ cup of AZUKI BEANS WITH KOMBU once a day for 1 week, and use less salt than usual.

Dietary Recommendations

The following dietary suggestions may be used until your heart condition improves or for about one month. Sea vegetables help make the blood vessels flexible and are helpful at every meal (about one-fourth cup) for a few weeks. Then use sea vegetables as a regular part of a macrobiotic dietary approach (see page 11).

FOR THE YANG TYPE

☐ Main foods: Brown Rice (or any whole grains) served with Gomashio, Brown Rice Mochi.
☐ Side dishes (one-third of the main foods): Tekka Miso, Hijiki Nitsuke, Nori Nitsuke, Shio Kombu, Vegetable Tempura, Azuki Beans with Kombu and Winter Squash, Burdock Carrot Nitsuke. Use less salt than usual in the cooking of side dishes.
☐ Miso soup ingredients: wakame, tororo kombu, daikon, burdock.

☐ Beverages: Brown Rice Tea, Bancha Tea, Grain Coffee.

☐ Avoid especially: all animal foods including fish and shellfish, all sweet foods and drinks, ice cream, all fruit, all alcohol.

FOR THE YIN TYPE

☐ Main foods: Brown Rice, Azuki Rice served with Gomashio, Fried Rice, Brown Rice Mochi. Chew each mouthful more than 100 times.

☐ Side dishes (one-fourth of main foods): Tekka Miso, Oily Miso, Hijiki Lotus Root Nitsuke, Burdock Carrot Nitsuke, Carp Soup, Vegetable Tempura, Nori Roasted with Oil, Miso Pickles. Slowly increase the amount of salt, measured by taste, in side dishes.

☐ Miso soup ingredients: wakame, scallions, onions, Brown Rice Mochi, tororo kombu.

☐ Beverages: Brown Rice Bancha Tea, Sho-Ban Tea, Kombu Tea, Mu Tea. Drink less than usual.

☐ Avoid especially: all animal foods including fish, shellfish, dairy foods (especially ice cream), and eggs; all fruit; sweet foods; alcoholic drinks; vinegar; mushrooms; melons; all beans except azuki beans.

ARTHRITIS

Arthritis is an inflammation of the joints. There are many forms of arthritis but here we discuss three of the more common types: rheumatoid arthritis, osteoarthritis, and infectious arthritis.

Rheumatoid arthritis is a chronic disease that involves the muscles and membrane linings of the joints and cartilage. It occurs in any or all of the active joints in the hands, wrists, elbows, shoulders, feet, and ankles and is characterized by the slow or sudden onset of tenderness, pain, and redness. The cause is unknown but autoimmune-system disorders and viral infection have been suggested, and physical or emotional stress often accompany the first symptoms. Women are affected three times more than men. The juvenile form is troublesome since it can lead to impaired growth and development; it appears four times more frequently in girls than in boys. Symptoms include a rapid rise in temperature, usually in the evening; pain, swelling, and stiffness in the joints; anemia; poor appetite; weight loss; irritability; and swollen lymph glands.

Osteoarthritis is a degenerative joint disease occurring mostly in adults over forty-five. It may occur in any joint but is most common in the fingers, spine, hips, knees, and feet. Symptoms include stiff and painful joints—especially after prolonged activity and/or in cold,

damp weather—resulting in a loss of movement in the affected joints. Swelling is often present, especially in finger joints. At times, with movement, there is a cracking sound in the joint.

Infectious arthritis is an infection caused by bacteria or fungi entering a joint. Symptoms include swelling and pain in the affected joints along with chills and fever. The pain worsens with movement and is most likely to occur in the larger joints.

According to our macrobiotic understanding, the basic cause of arthritis is an imbalanced diet containing a predominance of acid-forming foods; in particular, a diet high in protein, simple carbohydrates, and fat. In other words, the long-term overconsumption of dairy foods (especially milk with vitamin D added), eggs, animal foods (including chicken and fish), sugary cakes and candy, and refined grains causes an overly acidic condition that leads to greater risk of arthritis and other joint and bone diseases such as osteoporosis. High amounts of protein supply bacteria or fungi with building materials, and simple sugars and fat supply energy for them to grow. This microorganism growth inflames the cartilage between the joints. The inflammation presses against the nerves in the joint, which causes pain. Furthermore, a predominance of acid-forming foods, especially when coupled with a low- or no-salt diet, causes the synovial fluid (fluid between the cartilage in the joints) to become overly acidic. If there are not enough alkaline-forming elements (calcium, sodium, potassium, and magnesium) in the bodily fluids or in the diet, then calcium is dissolved from bones to alkalize the synovial fluid, and a calcium deposit results. Since this deposit has sharp edges, it causes pain when the joint moves. These calcium deposits can deform the joint over a period of time.

A predominance of animal foods causes a yang type of arthritis, while a predominance of simple sugars causes a yin type of arthritis. Arthritis pain can also result from a lack of good-quality oil in the diet. Good-quality vegetable oil in the diet is needed to maintain the lubricating quality of the synovial fluid and to help prevent contractures.

Helpful Suggestions

The following suggestions are provided for times of active flare-up.

OBJECTIVE	REMEDY
To preserve strength and joint mobility	Bed rest is most important during periods of active flare-up. When you have gotten past that, remaining active and keeping a positive self-image are important so that strength and joint mobility are preserved. However, from a

macrobiotic perspective, it is important to realize that activity and stress are acid-forming. Thus, it is wise to include periods of rest during the day and to get plenty of sleep, up to 12 hours, at night.

and

Passive exercises are useful for painful joints to help prevent contractures. In other words, massage the muscles around the painful joints rather than massaging the painful joint itself.

To relieve pain	Try a GINGER COMPRESS on the affected area 4 times a day for 20 minutes at a time, then follow the last compress with an ALBI PLASTER for 4 hours.
	or
	An UMEBOSHI PLASTER for 30 minutes to 1 hour 3 or 4 times a day is also effective and may be tried in place of the ginger compresses and albi plaster.
To relieve mild pain	A GINGER COMPRESS for 20 minutes or a GINGER SESAME OIL MASSAGE on the area can relieve mild discomfort.
To reduce high fever while relieving bodily pain	Use a TOFU PLASTER on the forehead and, at the same time, a GREEN LEAFY VEGETABLES APPLICATION on the painful places. Tie the vegetables on with a bandage and change both the plaster and the green leafy vegetables every hour.
	or
	Instead of the application of green leafy vegetables, use a BUCKWHEAT PLASTER WITH SALT, changing it every 2 hours. Place a ROASTED SALT PACK on top of the buckwheat plaster to keep it warm.
To cool skin and improve blood circulation	Placing a 1/8-inch-thick slice of any raw red meat on the crippled area every day or overnight may be helpful. Change the application every 4 hours.

Dietary Recommendations

Use the following dietary suggestions until there is no pain or for about one month. Then widen your food choices based on a macrobiotic dietary approach (see page 11). If your arthritis comes from overindulgence in both yang and yin foods, try the suggestions for the yin type first.

FOR THE YANG TYPE

☐ Main foods: Brown Rice, Azuki Rice, Brown Rice with Barley, Brown Rice Mochi, Brown Rice Cream with Oil.

☐ Side dishes (one-third of main foods cooked with less salt than usual): Sesame Miso, Ginger Miso, Hijiki Burdock Nitsuke, Carp Soup, Grated Daikon with Soy Sauce, Vegetable Stew, Vegetable Stew with Fish, Okara Nitsuke, Deep-Fried Kombu, Nori Nitsuke, Eggplant Nitsuke with Miso, Sour Cabbage, Takuan Pickles. Use a natural sesame oil in your cooking.

☐ Miso soup ingredients: daikon, sweet potatoes, tofu, spinach, eggplant, cucumber, Chinese cabbage, green leafy vegetables, Homemade Agé, Brown Rice Mochi.

☐ Beverages: Brown Rice Tea, Brown Rice Bancha Tea, Bancha Tea, Grain Coffee. Drink 2½ cups maximum per day.

☐ Avoid especially: all animal food, fish, shellfish, eggs, dairy foods, meat-based soups, sweet foods, hot spices, alcohol.

FOR THE YIN TYPE

☐ Main foods: Brown Rice, Azuki Rice, Azuki Millet Rice, Vegetable Fried Rice, Brown Rice Mochi, all served with Gomashio.

☐ Side dishes (one-fourth of main foods): Scallion Miso, Shio Kombu, Carp Soup, Hijiki Nitsuke, Burdock Carrot Nitsuke, Vegetable Stew with Fish, Vegetable Tempura, Nori Roasted with Oil, Deep-Fried Chuba Iriko, Takuan Pickles, Miso Pickles. Eating less side dishes is better. Eating less in general is better. Use a natural sesame oil in your cooking.

☐ Miso soup ingredients: wakame, tororo kombu, burdock, onions, scallions, dried seitan, Brown Rice Mochi.

☐ Beverages: Brown Rice Tea, Brown Rice Bancha Tea, Sho-Ban Tea, Bancha Tea, Kombu Tea, Grain Milk.

☐ Avoid especially: all animal foods, fish, shellfish, eggs, all dairy foods (including ice cream), sweet foods and drinks, fruit, black tea, tomatoes, eggplant, potatoes, melons, hot spices, peanuts.

ASTHMA

The many forms of asthma can be broken down into two main categories. One is extrinsic and is thought to be caused by environmental agents such as pollen, feathers, dust, insecticides, mold, and so on. The other one is called intrinsic and is said to be caused by an infection within the respiratory system. Asthma often affects children, but most commonly it affects young adults. Sometimes it doesn't begin until victims are in their forties. There is tightness in the throat or chest with a feeling of suffocation. Breathing is difficult, especially breathing out, and gasping in efforts to breathe can cause panic. The veins of the neck stand out; there is sweating, and one's face becomes flushed or sometimes pale. Attacks commonly come in the night or early morning and last from minutes to hours. After the severe gasping subsides, an asthma sufferer starts coughing and produces thick mucus. Eventually the violent coughing stops and the attack is over. However, if the mucus cannot pass down the throat, convulsions or spasms result. Without some form of treatment, severe attacks can be fatal.

According to our macrobiotic understanding, the primary cause of either category of bronchial asthma is basically eating too much yin food and not having enough sodium in the bodily fluids. Because of excessive consumption of sweet foods and fruit, the mucous membranes of the throat become expanded. In this case, the thick mucus cannot pass easily and convulsions or spasms follow. If the membrane is not expanded, the mucus will pass down easily and the attack is less severe. Mucus is a sign of too much protein, especially animal protein. Thus, people suffering from asthma should avoid animal protein in general and dairy foods in particular. Since the kidneys help determine the sodium levels in the bodily fluids, weak kidneys may lead to asthma as well. The kidneys, by cleaning up toxic acids and other toxic material in the blood, help prevent the buildup of mucus. Having enough sodium in the bodily fluids is important for proper functioning of the kidneys. When an attack starts (wheezing, difficulty in breathing, suffocating feeling), it is because the parasympathetic nerves are too active. When an asthma attack occurs, salt should be avoided because salt stimulates the parasympathetic nervous system, which in turn inhibits lung function, making breathing more difficult.

Helpful Suggestions

OBJECTIVE	REMEDY
To relieve severe asthma attack	Slowly sip 1 to 2 tablespoons of LOTUS ROOT JUICE with no salt, or drink ½ to 1 cup LOTUS ROOT TEA with no salt (the younger or more frail the person, the lesser the amount), 1 to 2 times during the attack.
	and/or
	Drinking 2 cups of BROWN RICE TEA WITH LOTUS ROOT AND SHISO LEAVES every day is very helpful.
	and/or
	You may use CHARCOALED KOMBU WITH LOTUS ROOT POWDER. Eating 1 teaspoon of this dry powder 2 times per day for 1 month is beneficial.
To relieve acute asthma attack	Try sipping 1 to 2 tablespoons of LOTUS ROOT JUICE with no salt each time an attack starts.
	or
	If you have no lotus root, drinking ¼ cup of DAIKON JUICE WITH RICE SYRUP at the beginning of each attack can be helpful.
To relieve less acute cases	Apply a GINGER COMPRESS WITH SAKÉ OR RUBBING ALCOHOL to the chest for 20 minutes every night. Then use a GINGER SESAME OIL MASSAGE on the chest after the ginger compress has been removed. One massage is usually enough.

Dietary Recommendations

The most important foods to eat are burdock, lotus root, sea vegetables (especially hijiki), mustard greens, daikon, and Carp Soup. One teaspoon of Tekka Miso once a day at meals is also beneficial. Dairy foods, fruit, nut butters, refined grians, and overeating promote the formation of mucus and should be avoided until your condition improves. Be judicious in your use of oil also. The following dietary suggestions may be used until the attacks become less severe or for about one month. Then, widen your food choices following a macrobiotic dietary approach (see page 11).

☐ Main foods: Brown Rice, Azuki Rice, Brown Rice Mochi, Fried Rice (use less oil than usual).

☐ Side dishes (less than one-third of main foods): Tekka Miso, Hijiki Lotus Root Nitsuke (eat 1 heaping tablespoon at every meal), Burdock Carrot Nitsuke, Green Leafy Vegetables (use mustard greens), Carp Soup, Miso Pickles, Dried Daikon Pickles.

☐ Miso soup ingredients: wakame, onions, scallions, Homemade Agé, Brown Rice Mochi.

☐ Beverages: Brown Rice Tea or Brown Rice Tea with lotus root (use the part of the lotus root that joins the segments together), Sho-Ban Tea, Kombu Tea, Mu Tea, Grain Milk.

☐ Avoid especially: all animal protein, fish, eggs, dairy (including ice cream), shellfish, all sweet foods, all fruit, potatoes, melons, tomatoes, eggplant, hot spices, mushrooms, fresh soybeans, vinegar, sushi, nut butters, refined grain products.

ASTIGMATISM

An astigmatism is a vision condition in which a ray of light is not sharply focused on the retina but is spread over a diffuse area, making objects appear blurred in either the vertical or horizontal line of focus.

According to medical thinking, an astigmatism results from an irregular curvature of the cornea. According to our macrobiotic understanding, the fundamental cause of this condition is an unbalanced diet that causes the radius of curvature in one plane to be longer or shorter than that of the radius at right angles to it. The common remedy for this condition is the use of eyeglasses with cylindrical lenses in the proper axis to make objects appear in focus. However, this is not a cure but rather a symptomatic treatment.

Helpful Suggestions

OBJECTIVE	REMEDY
To improve blood circulation	Try a SALT BANCHA EYE BATH 3 times per day and a SESAME OIL EYE TREATMENT in each eye at bedtime until eyesight improves.

Dietary Recommendations

Follow a macrobiotic dietary approach (see page 11), avoiding both extreme yin and yang foods.

ATHEROSCLEROSIS

See ARTERIOSCLEROSIS.

ATHLETE'S FOOT

According to *Webster's Dictionary*, athlete's foot is ringworm of the feet caused by fungi found in gyms and on shower floors. Symptoms include scaling on the feet, especially between the toes; itching; inflammation; damp, musty foot odor; dead skin between the toes; and small blisters. Athlete's foot is thought to be caused by fungi because sufferers often frequent warm, damp places such as public showers or live in hot, humid climates. Not changing your socks and shoes often enough and not washing your feet often contribute to the problem. Antibiotics and drugs that destroy beneficial bacteria allow the fungus to spread more rapidly. But, this does not explain why some people are affected by the fungi and others are not.

According to our macrobiotic understanding, the cause of athlete's foot is eating too much yin food such as watery or sweet foods, especially fruit.

Helpful Suggestions

OBJECTIVE	REMEDY
To alkalize infected area	Lightly rub *UME EXTRACT* on the feet and between the toes 3 or 4 times per day for several days. This is very helpful.
	and
	You might want to try placing an 1/8-inch-thick slice of fresh garlic (organic is best) on the sole of the foot near the toes with the cut part touching the skin. Attach with a bandage and walk on it. Change periodically.
	and
	Bathing your feet daily and changing your socks and shoes daily is also beneficial. Make sure to dry your feet thoroughly. Dust with garlic powder to absorb excess moisture.
	and
	Using socks made only of natural fibers such as cotton or wool will also help this condition as will going barefoot when possible—in places other than warm, damp ones, of course.
To prevent the spread of infection	Avoid using the same towel on other areas, especially the groin area, and avoid reusing it on the feet. You might try using a hair dryer on the feet instead of a towel.

Dietary Recommendations

Balancing your dietary selections on the basis of macrobiotic principles is most important. Follow a macrobiotic dietary approach (see page 11) with no fruit.

According to our macrobiotic understanding, all skin problems are related to the condition of the kidneys. If there is any pain in the kidneys, use less or no salt in your cooking and reduce your liquid intake to a minimum. If your kidneys are in good condition or as they improve, increase the amount of salt in your cooking little by little. It is a good idea to continue to drink less until the athlete's foot is gone.

BACKACHES

Common causes of backaches are thought to be poor posture (such as slouching when sitting), recent strenuous exercise, improper lifting, or sleeping on a mattress that is overly soft. Deep-seated emotional or stress-related problems may also cause lower back problems. A recent fall or injury may lead to a damaged spinal cord or muscle injury resulting in back pain. Any number of disorders such as osteoporosis, acute kidney infection, osteoarthritis, rheumatism, or a ruptured disk may lead to lower back pain.

While these are all valid causes of back pain, according to our macrobiotic understanding, the fundamental cause is improper diet, especially eating too much meat and other animal foods. These foods are high in protein and fat. Too much protein makes the bodily fluids more acidic and overworks and weakens the kidneys. Eating too much fatty food causes the capillaries in the lower back to narrow, which results in less blood and therefore less oxygen to the kidneys. When the kidneys do not get enough oxygen, the nerves surrounding the kidneys do not get enough oxygen and pain results. Eating acid-forming food (protein and fat), either yin or yang, causes the kidneys to be overworked. In this case, the kidneys consume too much oxygen, creating an oxygen deficiency in the nerves around the kidneys, which results in pain.

Helpful Suggestions

OBJECTIVE	REMEDY
To relieve pain	Try applying a GINGER COMPRESS on the affected area for 20 minutes.
To improve kidneys	Apply a GINGER COMPRESS over the kidneys (see Figure 3.8 on page 176) every day for 20 minutes.
	and
	Several times a week, take a 1 percent SALT BATH and/or a SAUNA at 100° to 115°F until sweat appears.
To avoid further back pain	Until your condition improves, avoid heavy lifting and strenuous exercise. Moderate activity such as walking, gardening, or swimming is recommended because a lack of exercise can lead to back pain.
	and
	Make sure your chairs and tables are at a comfortable height and that your mattress is firm.

Dietary Recommendations

Following a macrobiotic dietary approach (see page 11) with plenty of vegetables and sea vegetables is most beneficial. If you are in a weak condition, eat four to six small dried fish in miso soup each day. Drinking less than usual is also helpful.

BAD BREATH (HALITOSIS)

Bad breath may be caused by gum infection, decayed teeth, decaying material such as food particles within the teeth or surrounding tissue, or the residue from dead bacteria. The normal flow of saliva is reduced during sleep so that the cleansing action is less than during waking hours or when chewing food. Therefore food particles that remain in the mouth at bedtime may lead to bad breath in the morning. Other possible causes of bad breath are infections in the nasal cavity, sinuses, or upper respiratory tract, or infected tonsils and adenoids.

Overall, however, bad breath is a signal of poor health and may indicate intestinal or stomach disease, liver malfunction, or weak kidneys. If you are constipated and eat large amounts of animal food, putrefaction that occurs in the intestines creates gas that manifests itself as bad breath in the mouth. Fasting and excessive smoking can create bad breath as well.

Helpful Suggestions

Suggestions for eliminating the causes of bad breath can be found under the names of the disorder(s) you have.

OBJECTIVE	REMEDY
To eliminate mouth odor	Chewing 1 teaspoon of organic bancha tea or green tea leaves can help eliminate odor.
	and
	Always clean your teeth and tongue thoroughly after eating.

Dietary Recommendations

Observe a macrobiotic dietary approach (see page 11), chew well, and use plenty of kuzu in your cooking. Eat plenty of vegetables and don't overcook them.

BED-WETTING

The involuntary passage of urine while sleeping is not considered significant until a child is older than 6; 10 percent of children have this problem at age 6. By age 12, the rate of occurrence is down to 3 percent. The most common causes of bed-wetting are a small or weak bladder, an underlying illness, psychological problems such as stress resulting from separation from the mother, or nutritional disorders such as food allergies.

According to our macrobiotic understanding, there are two types of bed-wetting, yang and yin. Yang bed-wetting results from eating too much animal food and causes frequent urination in small amounts. Yin bed-wetting results from not enough salt in the diet, from eating too much yin food such as sugary cakes or fruit, or from drinking too much. Adult bed-wetting may indicate an organ defect or illness such as a bladder problem, tuberculosis, diabetes, or urinary tract infection.

Helpful Suggestions

OBJECTIVE	REMEDY
To improve blood circulation in the bladder	Until bed-wetting stops, use a DAIKON or ARAME HIP BATH WITH GRATED GINGER every night just before going to bed.
To control the bladder	Do a MOXA TREATMENT. Apply on top of the foot at the base of the large toe where the toe meets the foot. Do this once a day for 2 to 3 weeks. Apply 3 to 5 times per treatment depending on the age of the child (younger children should be given the lesser amount).
To avoid placing stress on a child	Instead of scolding the child for accidents, give praise for successful nights. Perhaps a calendar with gold stars or other stickers can be used. Avoid using candy as an award, of course. *and* Letting the child know that others have the same problem can also help relieve stress. Realize that the bed-wetting is usually out of the child's control and punishing, blaming, or criticizing can only lead to further emotional problems. *and* Have the child urinate before going to bed and let him or her know it's okay to get up during the night. Provide adequate lighting. You can awaken the child to urinate during the night until the child is old enough to use an alarm clock. *and* Making every effort to allow the child to take care of the problem without your help can have positive results. For example, make sure children know where extra night clothes are and where to sleep after an accident without having to awaken you.

Dietary Recommendations

A macrobiotic dietary approach (see page 11) should help bed-wetting caused by food allergies. In general, try eating and drinking less and in extreme cases try to refrain from eating or drinking after 3 P.M. For the yang type, eat less animal food and salt. White vegetables or any white noodles such as udon noodles are beneficial. For the yin type, Hijiki Nitsuke is particularly beneficial. Use the following suggestions until the bed-wetting stops or for about one month.

☐ Main foods: Brown Rice, Brown Rice Mochi, Baked Mochi with Soy Sauce (once a day), Brown Rice Gruel with miso.

☐ Side dishes (one-fourth of main foods): Tekka Miso, Carp Soup, Vegetable Stew, Vegetable Stew with Fish, Vegetable Tempura, Burdock Carrot Nitsuke, Hijiki Nitsuke, Organic Pheasant, Takuan Pickles, Miso Pickles.

☐ Miso soup ingredients: wakame, tororo kombu, dried daikon, scallions, onions, dried seitan, Homemade Agé, Brown Rice Mochi.

☐ Beverages: Brown Rice Tea, Brown Rice Bancha Tea, Bancha Tea, Sho-Ban Tea, Amasake Drink, Grain Coffee.

☐ Avoid especially: milk, fruit, all sweet foods including refined sugar and honey, sweet drinks, ice cream, wine, beer, sake, coffee, cocoa, mushrooms.

BERIBERI

According to Western medicine, the cause of beriberi is a diet deficient in B vitamins, especially B_1 (thiamine). The early symptoms of beriberi are numbness in legs and feet, no reflex response of knee caps, difficulty in walking, and a faster heartbeat. Later, there is diarrhea, fatigue, and swelling of the legs, feet, and the whole body. These secondary symptoms may eventually lead to weight loss, pale complexion, difficult breathing, vomiting, paralysis, and finally death.

According to our macrobiotic understanding, beriberi is caused by a shortage of B vitamins. Eating refined grains rather than whole grains can cause such a shortage since the B vitamins are contained in the outer layers of whole grains and are removed during the milling process. There are yin and yang types of beriberi. The yang type is caused by eating too much animal food such as red meat, shellfish, fish, chicken, pork, and cheese. These supply little or no B vitamins. The yin type of beriberi is caused by eating too much sugar and too many sweet foods that use many B vitamins for their metabolism, thus causing a general shortage of B vitamins.

Helpful Suggestions

Many people have a history of excess of both yin and yang foods. In this case, use the suggestions for the yin type first.

OBJECTIVE	REMEDY
FOR THE YANG TYPE	
To clean out toxins	Drink 1 cup HABUCHA TEA 3 times per day for 2 to 3 weeks.
To draw out excess salt	Try hot baths twice a day until you feel better. *and* Eating seasonal fruit once a day plus ½ to 1 tablespoon of GRATED DAIKON WITH SOY SAUCE for 1 to 2 weeks can be helpful.
To reduce swelling	Once a day until swelling subsides, eat ½ cup of AZUKI BEANS WITH KOMBU AND WINTER SQUASH, using less salt than usual.
To calm a faster heartbeat	Try drinking 2 to 3 cups of DAIKON GINGER TEA per day until it becomes normal. *and* Eat 2 to 3 tablespoons of natural sesame oil to help induce diarrhea (do this only once).
To relieve numbness	Use a GINGER COMPRESS on the affected area for 20 minutes 3 times a day.
FOR THE YIN TYPE	
To clean out toxins	Drink 1 cup HABUCHA TEA 3 times per day for 1 to 2 weeks. In this case, avoid taking hot baths and eating seasonal fruit.
To reduce swelling	Once a day, eat ½ cup of AZUKI BEANS WITH KOMBU AND WINTER SQUASH, cooked to a less salty taste than usual.
To reduce swelling and remove toxins	Drink 1 cup of DAIKON GINGER TEA, 2 times a day.
To relieve numbness	Use a GINGER COMPRESS on the affected area for 20 minutes 2 to 3 times a day.

Dietary Recommendations

The following dietary suggestions may be used until the symptoms disappear, or for about one month. Then widen your food choices using a macrobiotic dietary approach (see page 11). In either case, it is best not to drink with meals because most of the B vitamins are washed out by liquids consumed at the same time as the foods containing B vitamins. Again, for a history of excess of both yin and yang foods, use the dietary suggestions for the yin type first.

FOR THE YANG TYPE

☐ Main foods: Brown Rice, Brown Rice with Barley, Azuki Rice, Brown Rice Cream. Chew each mouthful 200 times and have Gomashio with each meal.
☐ Side dishes (one-fourth of main foods): Vegetable Stew, Carp Soup, Natto with Soy Sauce and Scallions served with Grated Daikon, Azuki Beans with Kombu and Winter Squash, Burdock Carrot Nitsuke, Green Leafy Vegetables with Homemade Agé, Tofu with Kuzu Sauce, Cucumber Salad with Rice Vinegar, Eggplant Pressed Salad, Grated Daikon.
☐ Miso soup ingredients: daikon, green leafy vegetables, Chinese cabbage, spinach, sweet potatoes, tofu, eggplant, winter squash, celery.
☐ Beverages: Brown Rice Tea, Brown Rice Bancha Tea, Bancha Tea, Vegetable Broth, Grain Coffee. Drink a maximum of 2½ cups of beverages per day.
☐ Avoid especially: all animal foods, meat-based soups, fish, dairy foods, sweet foods, and alcohol.

FOR THE YIN TYPE

☐ Main foods: Brown Rice, Azuki Rice, Brown Rice Mochi all served with Gomashio.
☐ Side dishes (one-fourth of main foods): Tekka Miso, Scallion Miso, Shio Kombu, Hijiki Nitsuke, Burdock Carrot Nitsuke, Vegetable Stew, Vegetable Stew with Fish, Carp Soup, Azuki Beans with Kombu, Takuan Pickles, Miso Pickles.
☐ Miso soup ingredients: wakame, tororo kombu, onions, scallions, Brown Rice Mochi.
☐ Beverages: Brown Rice Tea, Brown Rice Bancha Tea, Bancha Tea, Sho-Ban Tea, Kombu Tea, Grain Milk. Drink less; this is best.
☐ Avoid especially: animal protein, fish (except carp and fish in vegetable stew), shellfish, eggs, all dairy foods (including ice cream), all fruit, sweet foods, all sweet drinks, tomatoes, eggplant, potatoes, melons, black tea, green tea, peanuts, hot spices, mushrooms, pressed salads.

BIRTHMARKS

A birthmark is a mark or blemish that developed before birth and is confined to a limited space. Many of these marks are so common that they are considered to be normal and will disappear after a given length of time. Others are not of the common variety and require some remedy.

In Western medicine, birthmarks are not considered to be caused by external factors. However, according to our macrobiotic understanding, birthmarks result from a mother's unbalanced diet during pregnancy and may even result from an emotional shock during pregnancy. If the mother's diet during pregnancy is too yin, then the baby may be born with a blue (yin) birthmark. If the mother's diet is too yang, then a red (yang) mark may occur.

Helpful Suggestions

If you use an albi plaster every day, the birthmark should disappear in about one month. It is easier to remove birthmarks when a child is young.

OBJECTIVE	REMEDY
	FOR RED MARKS
To neutralize toxins	Try an EGGPLANT SULFUR MASSAGE or VINEGAR MASSAGE 2 to 3 times per day. *and* After each treatment, a GINGER SESAME OIL MASSAGE on the area helps stop air from going into the skin.
To eliminate toxins	After the massage, apply an ALBI PLASTER; change the plaster every 4 hours and apply a plaster just before going to bed and leave on overnight. Do this until the mark disappears or for 2 to 3 weeks.
	FOR BLUE MARKS
To open skin pores and break up excess proteins	Try applying a GINGER COMPRESS for 20 minutes followed by an ALBI PLASTER for up to 4 hours. Repeat both the compress and the plaster as needed. Apply a new albi plaster just before going to bed and leave the plaster on overnight.
To stop air from going into the skin	Use a GINGER SESAME OIL MASSAGE on the affected area in the morning.

Dietary Recommendations

It goes without saying that an expectant mother should be careful with her diet. After the birth, continue following a macrobiotic dietary approach (see page 11), especially if you are breastfeeding the baby. In the case of a blue birthmark, breastfeeding mothers should eat slightly more yang foods, cook foods a longer time, and use more salt. In the case of a red birthmark, breastfeeding mothers should eat slightly more yin foods and use more yin preparations such as boiling and steaming.

Bites and Stings

Insect bites and stings usually result in skin eruptions that may be painful and/or itchy. Bites from small animals may produce similar results. The symptoms usually disappear within days; scratching the site may prolong the symptoms. There are many home remedies for bites and stings of all kinds and here we have included a few more.

CORNELLIA'S NATURAL HEALING AT WORK

If a bee or an insect is attracted to your ear, then it is likely that you smell sweet, like honey. This happens when you eat too much fruit or sugar and your body becomes sweet smelling. You may soon become diabetic. If you stop eating sugar, fruit, or honey completely, the insects will not come to you. Your blood is no longer sweet smelling so you do not attract insects.

Once at our annual French Meadows Summer Camp, hornets attacked two children because they were sweeter smelling than the other campers. I healed the stings by applying chewed bancha tea leaves to the sites. The children stopped crying quickly. The bancha tea and the saliva alkalized the acid poison of the stings. If you have no bancha tea, then use dark green vegetable leaves, rub with saliva, and apply. The acid is then neutralized. ∎

BITES AND STINGS

According to our thinking, there is a relationship between an overly yin condition brought about by excessive consumption of yin foods (sugar, fruit, and honey), the number of bites or stings, and the severity of the reaction to them. For serious symptoms or a severe allergic reaction, consult with your health-care advisor.

Helpful Suggestions

OBJECTIVE	REMEDY
	FOR BITES IN GENERAL
To alleviate pain	Try a GINGER SESAME OIL APPLICATION directly on the bite.
To eliminate acid	Try applying an ALBI PLASTER, changing it every 4 hours as needed.
To relieve itchiness	Grind morning glory leaves, mugwort leaves, albi leaves, or coltsfoot leaves and squeeze out the juice. Apply juice directly on the bites.
	FOR SPECIFIC BITES AND STINGS
To relieve mosquito bites	Mix dentie powder with enough saliva or sesame oil to form a pastelike mixture. Apply directly on the bites. *and/or* Swim in warm ocean (salt) water or take a SALT BATH for 20 minutes.
To relieve bee and wasp stings	Use a BANCHA TEA LEAVES APPLICATION. *or* Finely grate burdock root and squeeze out the juice. Apply directly on any insect sting.

To relieve spider bites	Mix equal amounts of sesame oil and salt and apply to the bite and surrounding area.
To relieve non-rabid dog bites	Drink ½ cup of AZUKI BEAN DRINK 3 times per day for 2 days to help protect the intestines and kidneys from any dangerous toxins. Children should drink only ½ cup while adults can drink up to 1 cup.
	or
	Chop and grind wild scallions or chives in a suribachi or blender and squeeze out the juice. Drink ⅓ cup 2 times per day for 2 days.
To relieve non-poisonous snake bites	Keep the area cool by applying an UME EXTRACT COMPRESS.

FOR POISONOUS BITES OR STINGS, OR BITES OF RABID ANIMALS

To deal with bites from poisonous snakes or centipedes, rabid dogs, etc.	Seek emergency care immediately. If treatment is to be delayed for any reason, follow standard emergency first-aid procedure.
To protect the heart	Drink the RANSHO DRINK made with 1 egg once only to help protect the heart. Drinking a small amount of LEEK or SCALLION JUICE is helpful if you have no ransho.
	then
To neutralize acid (toxins)	Place the meat of an umeboshi directly on the bite.

Dietary Recommendations

Following a balanced macrobiotic dietary approach (see page 11), and especially avoiding overly yin foods and drinks, is recommended in all cases.

BLADDER INFECTIONS

Inflammation of the urinary bladder is called cystitis and symptoms include a burning or stinging sensation during urination; frequent urination, especially at night, although the amount may be small; lower back pain; blood in the urine; bad smelling urine; and pain around the bladder. The presence of blood in the urine may indicate a more serious problem, especially in men, and a medical practitioner should be consulted.

Although all ages and both sexes can be affected, females are more likely to develop bladder infections. Sometimes women have problems with bladder infections because carelessness in cleaning the vagina can lead to cystitis. This carelessness allows microbes or intestinal germs to come in from the outside and access

---

CORNELLIA'S NATURAL HEALING AT WORK

In the winter of 1960, I had a bladder infection. I had been stomping on a rug in the bathtub to wash it. My feet were wet and I walked barefoot on the wooden floors. My hips became cold and my bladder contracted, resulting in frequent and painful urination. The next day, George Ohsawa, who was then visiting, theorized that even though my bladder was contracted there was a yin cause of my bladder infection because I had been physically and mentally weak since an operation on my heart in 1958. For the yin bladder infection, Ohsawa advised me to cut out all yin foods such as honey, sugar, and fruit; to eliminate certain yang foods, especially cheese; and to stay on a macrobiotic dietary approach with plenty of burdock carrot nitsuke and hijiki nitsuke. He also suggested that I take a daikon hip bath every day for about ten days. I followed this advice, and my condition improved quickly; I was completely well in less than a month.

In November 1970, after moving to California, I was trying to make winter daikon pickles. I sat down outside on a straw mattress on a concrete floor. My hips again became cold even though I was wearing wool pants. I tried a daikon hip bath, which did help the pain, but the infection kept recurring for the next two years. Then Mr. Muramoto, the noted herbalist and author of *Healing Ourselves* and *Natural Immunity*, came and told me my bladder infection was of a yang type resulting from too much salt intake. The cause and type of infection were both different from my previous experience, even though my bladder was again contracted, resulting in painful urination. Mr. Muramoto suggested early-morning barefoot-walks on the wet grass for twenty minutes each morning for ten days or until I got better. Then a chiropractic doctor advised me to wash my vagina with cold water after taking a hot bath. Since then, I have been washing my vagina as well as my feet with cold water after my hot bath. This improves circulation and helps rid the area of infection. If you don't know what the cause of your bladder trouble is, try eating one salted plum, and if you have pain in the bladder, this is a sign of a yang bladder infection. ■

BLADDER INFECTIONS

---

the bladder or kidneys. Bacteria can also reach the bladder through the blood stream. Injury to the urethra and use of a urinary catheter to empty the bladder are other probable causes. The likelihood of cystitis increases with stress, excessive alcohol consumption, increased sexual activity, an infection in an adjoining area, or any illness causing lowered resistance.

Chronic urinary-tract infections may lead to kidney failure if they are not adequately treated. Although prompt medical treatment using antibiotics and analgesics can abate any flare-up, recurrence is very common. The macrobiotic approach does not recommend such procedures (unless a change in eating habits does not help) because these medications destroy beneficial bacteria along with the harmful ones. Also, these medications work only on the symptoms of cystitis.

According to our macrobiotic understanding, the underlying causes of cystitis are the overconsumption of yin foods and drinks, including dairy foods such as milk and ice cream; and the overconsumption of yang foods such as salt and salty cheeses. The yin type results in a chronic illness, long-lasting and often recurring, while the yang type is more acute, coming on suddenly and often more vehemently. The long-term overconsumption of yin foods and drinks results in an overall weakened condition and also creates an internal environment in which bacteria thrive. The yang type results in contraction of the urinary bladder, making urination painful.

Helpful Suggestions

OBJECTIVE	REMEDY
FOR THE YANG (ACUTE) TYPE	
To promote urination and alkalize the system	Try drinking 2 cups of DAIKON GINGER TEA plus 3 or 4 cups of BROWN RICE TEA or GRAIN COFFEE per day for 2 to 3 days.
To prevent a woman's recurring bladder infection	Try drinking 1 cup of DAIKON GINGER TEA followed 30 minutes later with 1 cup of DAIKON TEA. Do this once a day for 2 to 3 days and your condition should improve.
To improve bladder circulation	Take a DAIKON or ARAME HIP BATH, or sit in a daikon or arame bath every night for 1 to 2 weeks.
FOR THE YIN (CHRONIC) TYPE	
To relieve pain and pressure	Try using a BUCKWHEAT PLASTER 1 time over the bladder (see Figure 3.8 on page 176) for 2 hours or until the pain lessens. Place a ROASTED SALT PACK on top to keep the buckwheat plaster warm. This should improve your circulation. *and* Take a DAIKON or ARAME HIP BATH every night until pain stops.
To promote urination and alkalize the system	Try drinking 3 or 4 cups of GRAIN COFFEE per day for 2 to 3 days at the beginning of each flare-up.

FOR BOTH TYPES	
To avoid recurrence	Some common sense measures can be helpful in avoiding recurrence of this condition. Cleansing the body by showering with a natural soap is preferable to taking tub baths. Avoid douching and hygiene sprays until you no longer have chronic cystitis. Drinking water before sexual intercourse and urinating soon after is a good preventative as is using a water-soluble lubricant. Use a heating pad on the bladder area to improve circulation to the area. Cotton underwear breathes and is preferred over nylon or polyester. Keeping the genital area clean and dry is probably the best advice. Wipe yourself from front to back after urination or bowel movements. Empty your bladder frequently even though it may be painful each time. Avoid sexual intercourse.

Dietary Recommendations

The macrobiotic dietary approach strengthens the body so it can deal with all kinds of infections. Use the following suggestions until your condition improves or for about one month. Then, widen your food choices using a macrobiotic dietary approach (see page 11).

FOR THE YANG TYPE

☐ Main foods: Brown Rice, Azuki Rice, Brown Rice with Barley.
☐ Side dishes (one-third of main foods): Azuki Beans with Kombu and Winter Squash, Green Leafy Vegetables served with Sesame Miso Dressing, Turnip Albi Burdock Cooked with Homemade Agé, Boiled Daikon, Azuki Beans with Kombu. Use less salt than usual in these dishes.
☐ Miso soup ingredients: daikon, Chinese cabbage, tofu, wakame, winter squash.
☐ Beverages: Brown Rice Tea, Bancha Tea, Grain Coffee.
☐ Avoid especially: all meats and fish, meat-based soups, eggs, dairy foods, potatoes, fruit, sweet foods, coffee, hot spices, all alcohol.

FOR THE YIN TYPE

☐ Main foods: Brown Rice Balls, Brown Rice Mochi.
☐ Side dishes (one-third of main foods): Daikon Nitsuke, Lotus Root Nitsuke, Burdock Nitsuke, Green Leafy Vegetables with Homemade Agé, Green Leafy Vegetables served with Grated Daikon.
☐ Miso soup ingredients: wakame, tororo kombu, scallions, onions, Homemade Agé, Brown Rice Mochi.
☐ Beverages: Grain Coffee, Bancha Tea.
☐ Avoid especially: all fruit, sweet foods, dairy foods (including ice cream), all meats and fish, meat-based soups, eggs, potatoes, yams, sweet potatoes, ice water, coffee, hot spices, all alcohol.

Blood Poisoning (Septicemia)

Septicemia is a systemic disease associated with a bacterical infection (or the toxins from bacteria) in the blood. Symptoms include fever, rapid temperature rise, shaking, chills, fast heartbeat, lower blood pressure, general lack of mental clarity, and a general ill-feeling. Left unattended, septicemia can lead to shock and even death. According to Western medicine, the cause is a bacterial infection in any body part or area.

According to our macrobiotic understanding, the underlying cause is overeating of animal foods, especially red meat, because animal foods contain a higher percentage of protein than do vegetable foods. This higher mass of protein provides growing materials for bacteria or viruses. Red meat is more easily contaminated by disease-causing bacteria than are vegetable foods. For example, meat may be contaminated through feeds and fertilizers, by heat and humidity, during transport, or during processing. Meat may also become contaminated during storage in the market or the home, or during cooking.

Helpful Suggestions

OBJECTIVE	REMEDY
To relieve pain	Try applying a GINGER COMPRESS to the affected area for 20 minutes. Follow with an ALBI PLASTER for up to 4 hours. Repeat both the compress and the Albi Plaster as often as necessary until the symptoms have disappeared.
To reduce a high fever	Try using a TOFU PLASTER on the forehead along with a hot water bottle on the feet. (Remember, fever is the body's attempt to mobilize its defenses against the infection. Fevers under 104°F are not dangerous and should be left alone.) Change the plaster every hour until the fever goes down.

Dietary Recommendations

The only true remedy is to change to a diet that does not rely on animal foods and that results in strengthening the overall condition of the blood and of the body. The following dietary suggestions may be used until the symptoms improve or for about one month. Then widen your food choices using a macrobiotic dietary approach (see page 11).

☐ Main foods: Brown Rice Gruel, Brown Rice Cream (Special), Brown Rice with a little Gomashio as condiment. Chew each mouthful 200 times.

☐ Side dishes (one-fourth of main foods cooked to a less salty taste than usual): Okara Nitsuke, Eggplant Nitsuke with Miso, Carp Soup, Grated Daikon, Rice Bran Pickles, pressed salads, Sour Cabbage, Umeboshi, raw organic apples and pears.

☐ Miso soup ingredients: daikon, Chinese cabbage, eggplant, burdock, tofu, cabbage, scallions.

☐ Beverages: Vegetable Broth, Bancha Tea, Barley Tea, Habucha Tea, Grain Coffee, Grain Milk.

☐ Avoid especially: all animal foods, fish, shellfish, all dairy foods (including ice cream), sweet foods and drinks, vinegar, tomatoes, eggs, alcohol.

Blood Pressure, High

Normal young adult blood pressure is 120/80 mm of mercury. The top number is the systolic pressure (exerted by the blood while the heart is pumping) and the bottom number is the diastolic pressure (exerted by the blood while the heart is at rest between beats). Generally, blood pressures measuring above 150/90 are regarded as high and those above 180/115 are considered severely elevated. However, blood pressure increases with age, especially the systolic value. For example, systolic pressures of 130 at forty years of age and of 145 at sixty are considered average.

Usually, high blood pressure shows no symptoms until it reaches an advanced stage. Headaches, drowsiness, numbness and tingling in the hands and feet, severe shortness of breath, buzzing in the ears, fatigue, or irritability may be indications of a crisis situation. Advanced cases of high blood pressure may be accompanied by arteriosclerosis, forgetfulness, irritability, disturbed vision, cerebral hemorrhage, angina pectoris, myocardial infarction (heart attack), or kidney failure.

The cause of high blood pressure is generally thought to be unknown although many contributing factors are known. Obesity, genetic factors, family history of heart disorders, smoking, stress, the use of stimulants such as caffeine, drug abuse, a high-fat (especially saturated fat) diet, and a sedentary life-style all increase your risk of developing high blood pressure. High sodium intake is often singled out as well.

However, according to our macrobiotic understanding, it is sodium intake along with too much fat in the diet that cause high blood pressure. Salt causes the heart to contract and, as a result, the blood is pushed faster through the arteries. When the arteries are clogged, the blood pressure goes up. On a low-fat diet, salt (sodium) does not create heart trouble although you must be careful with sodium intake if you already have clogged arteries and high blood pressure. A problem occurs among healthy individuals who decrease or stop the intake of salt because they fear getting high blood pressure. From our macrobiotic view, a lack of salt (sodium) is thought to weaken the heart, contribute to a feeling of tiredness, and result in lowered blood pressure. If the heart is strong and the arteries are not clogged, the blood pressure goes down with the intake of sodium since sodium stimulates the parasympathetic nervous system, which in turn inhibits heart action and all yang organs. In addition, salt is needed in making white blood cells, one of the principal constituents of the immune system. On the other hand, too much salt can overwork and damage the kidneys. Thus, the proper amount and use of salt is one of the most critical issues in our lives.

Helpful Suggestions

OBJECTIVE	REMEDY
To control blood pressure	Don't take hot baths if you have high blood pressure. Short, warm showers are okay. Exercising moderately in a nonstressful way, maintaining a normal body weight, avoiding stressful situations, giving up smoking, and avoiding nonprescription cold and sinus remedies that elevate blood pressure are also recommended.
To quiet a too-strong pulse	Every 4 hours, try drinking SOUR APPLE JUICE made from one small apple. A large person may use 2 to 3 apples. The grated apple juice goes to the intestines to help take away the heat, and the lemon juice goes to the kidneys to activate urination.
	and
	A DAIKON PLASTER over the heart area is helpful. If you are really in pain, change the plaster every 5 minutes. The daikon will become hot even in such a short time. If you have no daikon, use an APPLE PLASTER. Use the plaster for only 1 hour because grated daikon or apple reduces the heart's heat and can make the heart too cold (yin). The Daikon (or Apple) Plaster is used only to relieve the symptoms.
To alleviate palpitations	Try drinking ½ to 1 cup SHO-BAN TEA 2 to 3 times per day.
	and
	Use a DAIKON or APPLE PLASTER on the heart (see Figure 3.8 on page 176) for no more than an hour, changing it every 20 minutes. If this treatment is not effective, try a TOFU PLASTER applied to the heart area for 1 hour.

OBJECTIVE	REMEDY
To lower blood pressure	Take a SAUNA (FAR-INFRARED) several times a week. When fat inside of the capillaries and arteries melts and is eliminated through blood circulation, the blood pressure goes down.

Dietary Reccomendations

The following dietary suggestions may be used until your heart condition improves or for about one month. Then, widen your food choices based on a macrobiotic dietary approach (see page 11).

☐ Main foods: Brown Rice (or any whole grains) served with Gomashio, Brown Rice Mochi.

☐ Side dishes (one-third of main foods): Tekka Miso, Hijiki Nitsuke, Nori Nitsuke, Shio Kombu, Vegetable Tempura, Azuki Beans with Kombu and Winter Squash, Burdock Carrot Nitsuke. Use less salt than usual in the cooking of side dishes.

☐ Miso soup ingredients: wakame, tororo kombu, daikon, burdock.

☐ Beverages: Brown Rice Tea, Bancha Tea, Grain Coffee.

☐ Avoid especially: all animal foods including fish and shellfish, all sweet foods and drinks, ice cream, all fruit, all alcohol.

BODY ODOR

Primarily, body odor is produced by the putrefaction of protein, particularly protein of animal origin. Putrefaction is caused by anaerobic (without oxygen) decomposition of protein, which is the result of eating too much fatty, animal food, especially red meat. Fatty foods cause red cells to stick to each other, disturbing blood flow and causing an oxygen shortage that creates the anaerobic decomposition. This anaerobic decomposition of protein produces foul-smelling compounds such as ammonia or hydrogen sulfide. The result is excessive body odor.

Helpful Suggestions

OBJECTIVE	REMEDY
To absorb body odor	Try applying a GINGER COMPRESS under the armpits for 20 minutes once a day.
	or
	Finely grate an apple or daikon and squeeze out the juice. If using an apple, add an equal amount of freshly squeezed lemon juice. Or, finely chop several scallions,

grind in a suribachi or blender, and squeeze out the juice. Wet your hands with whichever juice you choose and rub some of it into the armpits every day for as long as body odor continues to be a problem.

and/or

Use a hot RICE PLASTER under the armpits for 3 to 4 hours once a day.

Dietary Recommendations

This problem should be eliminated by adopting a primarily vegetarian macrobiotic dietary approach (see page 11).

BONE MARROW AND TISSUE DISORDERS

See OSTEOMYELITIS *and* PERIOSTITIS.

BREAST CANCER

Breast cancer is indicated by malignant growth of breast-tissue cells that is characterized by swelling or a lump in the breast, vague discomfort in the breast without true pain, and enlarged nodes under the arms. Breast cancers are divided into many types and all are considered fatal if left untreated, the major problem being a spreading of the cancer to vital organs. Once a cancerous growth is discovered, some form of surgical removal is often recommended by the medical community. The earlier breast cancer is detected, the less radical the surgery and the better your chances of survival. You are considered to be at risk if you are female, have a family history of breast cancer or a personal history of benign tumors of the breast, have never had children or conceived after age thirty-five, or you are more than fifty years old, although this age is constantly being lowered as dietary and life-style habits become worse. Men can also get breast cancer, although it is much more rare. Because the incidence increases in women after menopause, high estrogen levels have been suggested as contributing to breast cancer.

It is encouraging to see science now recognizing the role of a high-fat diet in the development of many diseases including breast cancer. For many years, those who have followed a macrobiotic approach have recommended a diet low in fat (20 percent of caloric intake as opposed to the typical American diet of 40 percent or more). Thus, a change in diet and life-style is the most important step in reducing your risk of breast cancer. According to our macrobiotic understanding, there are two types of breast cancer. One type, yang breast cancer, is caused by the long-time overconsumption of yang animal foods that are also high in fat such as meat, poultry, fish, and eggs and from insufficient consumption of vegetables. Yin breast cancer is caused by a history of overconsuming alcohol, fruit, sugary foods, and vinegar, along with not eating enough salt to balance the sweet foods in the diet.

Helpful Suggestions

OBJECTIVE	REMEDY
To monitor yourself	Monthly self examination of the breasts is especially recommended because the macrobiotic approach is based on each person's need to more fully understand his or her own body.
To remove toxins and pain	Apply an ALBI PLASTER wherever there is pain, changing it every 4 hours. Apply a new one before going to bed and leave it on overnight. If the area feels hot or a red color appears after using an albi plaster, it is normal and no cause for concern as long as your appetite is good. Adequate nourishment is very important when you use albi plasters to remove toxins and old fat; lack of eating will leave you too weak to combat the cancer. Even if you have no appetite, eat something such as *BROWN RICE CREAM* or *BUCKWHEAT CREAM* rather than discontinue the plasters. *and* Do not use a Ginger Compress. With other cancerous conditions, a Ginger Compress is usually suggested before an Albi Plaster; however, for some people the Ginger Compress has caused a spreading of breast cancer, so we have stopped recommending ginger compresses on the chest area for persons with breast cancer.
To relieve severe pain	Try a TOFU PLASTER instead of an Albi Plaster, changing it every hour. Return to using albi plasters when the severe pain is gone or for use overnight.
To combat cancer	Regular exercise is helpful in preventing illness, especially cancer. Thus, a change from a sedentary life-style is helpful. However, if you already have cancer, avoid rigorous or strenuous exercises because these are generally too acid-forming for a cancerous condition. Cancer thrives in an overly acidic environment. Engage in walking and gardening.

Dietary Recommendations

A macrobiotic dietary approach has been helpful to many people. However, there is one danger. Once they begin to feel better and tests show the cancer is gone, the people tend to go back to the high-fat diet that created the cancer in the first place. The question is whether the cancer is cured or only in remission. It is wiser to consider that the cancer is still present since a recurrence can be very difficult to deal with and the results are not so promising. The following dietary suggestions may be used for about one month. Then widen your choices based on a macrobiotic dietary approach (see page 11). If you have been eating a diet high in both yin and yang foods, use the suggestons for the yin type first.

FOR THE YANG TYPE

☐ Main foods: Brown Rice Balls, Azuki Rice Balls. Chew each mouthful 200 times. Use a little Gomashio as a condiment.

☐ Side dishes (one-half of main foods): Tekka Miso, Grated Daikon with Soy Sauce, Burdock Carrot Nitsuke, burdock dishes, Carp Soup, Eggplant Nitsuke with Miso, Soybeans with Kombu, Rice Bran Pickles, pressed salads, Sour Cabbage, Umeboshi.

☐ Miso soup ingredients: daikon, albi, green leafy vegetables, eggplant, spinach, tofu.

☐ Beverages: Brown Rice Tea, Brown Rice Bancha Tea, Bancha Tea, Vegetable Broth, Grain Coffee. Drink a maximum of 2½ cups of beverages per day.

☐ Avoid especially: all animal foods including eggs and meat-based soups.

FOR THE YIN TYPE

☐ Main foods: Brown Rice Balls, occasionally made out of sweet brown rice. Chew each mouthful 200 times. Eat these with a little Gomashio as a condiment.

☐ Side dishes (one-third of main foods): Tekka Miso, Hijiki Lotus Root Nitsuke, Burdock Lotus Root Nitsuke, Shio Kombu, azuki kombu dishes, Carp Soup, Miso Pickles, and Dried Daikon Pickles. Choose one or two side dishes per meal.

☐ Miso soup ingredients: wakame, tororo kombu, burdock, onions, scallions, Homemade Agé.

☐ Beverages: Brown Rice Tea, Brown Rice Bancha Tea, Sho-Ban Tea, Mu Tea. Drink a maximum of 2 cups of beverages per day.

☐ Avoid especially: all meats, fish, eggs, dairy foods (including ice cream), soy milk, sweet drinks, sweet foods, fruit, hot spices, mushrooms, tomatoes, potatoes, eggplant, melons, peanuts, rice bran pickles, sour cabbage, pressed salads.

BREAST INFECTION

Here we discuss a breast infection or mastitis related to breastfeeding. Breastfeeding has many benefits for both the mother and the child and is highly recommended if at all possible. There are a few problems that may occur and one of these is an infection. The infected breast swells, becomes sore and red, and may feel hot. Fever and other flu-like symptoms are very likely. This condition may occur anytime while nursing but usually begins three to four weeks after delivery.

The problem really begins with a plugged duct, which may be the result of the baby's incomplete emptying of the milk or of some physical cause such as a bra that is too tight. Yang fatty foods contribute to the duct's clogging and encourage the infection. According to our macrobiotic understanding then, the underlying cause of breast infection is eating too much yang, fatty food such as meat, chicken, eggs, red meat fish, and shrimp.

Helpful Suggestions

OBJECTIVE	REMEDY
To relieve pain	Try a GINGER COMPRESS for 20 minutes followed by an ALBI PLASTER over the entire breast area. Change the plaster every 4 hours.
To relieve severe pain	Use a TOFU PLASTER only, changing it every hour until the severe pain diminishes. Then, apply a GINGER COMPRESS for 20 minutes followed by an ALBI PLASTER as explained above.
To deal with pus resulting from an Albi Plaster	In rare cases, the Albi Plaster may draw out pus (from an abscess) making an open sore. George Ohsawa said this was not necessarily a bad sign and recommended rubbing the area around the sore with good-quality sesame oil. But if this condition persists, seek advice from a health-care practitioner. *and* If nursing is painful, you can still feed your baby with breast milk by expressing the milk into a bottle. However, if your breast is abscessed, express and *discard* the milk.
To relieve constipation	Try eating ½ cup of AZUKI BEANS WITH KOMBU 2 times per day until you have a bowel movement. Prepare this dish slightly salty.

Dietary Recommendations

The following dietary suggestions are to be used until the infection is over or for two to three weeks. Then, widen your food choices using a macrobiotic dietary approach (see page 11). Try the special suggestions for extreme pain only until the extreme pain diminishes. If it does not diminish, consult a health-care practitioner.

☐ Main foods: Brown Rice, Azuki Rice, with a little Gomashio as a condiment.

☐ Side dishes (one-third of main foods): Tekka Miso, Scallion Miso, Hijiki Nitsuke, Shio Kombu, Burdock Carrot Nitsuke, and sea vegetable dishes.

☐ Miso soup ingredients: wakame, tororo kombu, onions, and scallions.

☐ Beverages: Brown Rice Bancha Tea, Bancha Tea, Kombu Tea.

☐ Avoid especially: meats, red-meat fish, and shellfish including shrimp.

SPECIAL DIETARY SUGGESTIONS FOR EXTREME PAIN

☐ Main foods: Brown Rice Balls or Azuki Rice Balls served with Gomashio, Buckwheat Noodles with Tempura.

☐ Side dishes (one-third of main foods): Tekka Miso, Oily Miso, Hijiki Lotus Root Nitsuke, Shio Kombu, Deep-Fried Kombu, Burdock Carrot Nitsuke, Oyster Tempura, Vegetable Tempura, Miso Pickles. Eat 1 to 2 side dishes per meal.

☐ Miso soup ingredients: wakame, tororo kombu, onions, scallions, and Brown Rice Mochi.

☐ Beverages: Brown Rice Tea, Brown Rice Bancha Tea, Bancha Tea with Gomashio, Sho-Ban Tea, Kombu Tea. Drink a maximum of 2 cups beverages per day.

☐ Avoid especially: all meats, fish (especially red-meat fish), shellfish, eggs, all dairy foods, all overly yin foods including fruit and sugar.

BREAST MILK FLOW, INHIBITED

Inhibited breast-milk flow occurs when the ducts in the nipple are closed. Fatty foods such as meat, fish, chicken, turkey, tuna, salmon, mackerel, shellfish, clams, and shrimp are considered to be the cause and should be avoided. This condition may lead to a breast infection as previously discussed.

Helpful Suggestions

OBJECTIVE	REMEDY
To remove excess fat and relieve pain	Apply a GINGER COMPRESS over the breast for 20 minutes followed by an ALBI PLASTER; change the plaster every 4 hours until milk flow returns. If you do not have albi, try a GREEN PLASTER to relieve pain, changing it every 4 hours.
To relieve severe pain	If the pain is too severe for the Green Plaster, try a TOFU PLASTER, changing it every hour. When there is less pain, try the Albi or Green Plaster again.
To replace mother's milk when necessary	RICE MILK may be used as a temporary substitute for mother's milk, if needed.

Dietary Recommendations

Follow a macrobiotic dietary approach (see page 11). If you eat yang animal food, be sure to balance it with plenty of vegetables, salads, and/or Grated Daikon (especially useful for fatty food). For balance, persons in good health may want to eat some fruit after meals containing yang animal food. Of course, persons with cancer or other illnesses should not eat animal foods or fruit until their condition improves. If you have an open sore, fever, or any flu-like symptoms, see the section on Breast Infection.

CORNELLIA'S NATURAL HEALING AT WORK

I had this problem once on the left breast; the nipple was closed. I remembered I had eaten salted salmon (yang), and this along with eating other fatty foods was probably the reason the nipple became clogged. The salty salmon caused the stimulation of the parasympathetic nervous system, which in turn caused the nipple muscles to contract and the flow of milk to stop. After I used a ginger compress, the milk started to flow again because the ginger (yin vegetable) stimulated the sympathetic nervous system, causing the nipple muscles to relax.

My friend also experienced a clogged nipple after eating too much tempura. In this case, the underlying cause was too much fat. However, tempura is quite yang because, during cooking, the vegetables absorb much heat (yang). Eating too much tempura stimulated the parasympathetic nervous system as in my case. After my friend ate an orange (yin fruit), the nipple opened. I should point out that eating salty animal or other fatty food one time does not clog the nipple. It is the overconsupmtion of these foods that leads to a clogged nipple.   ■

BREAST MILK FLOW, INHIBITED

BRONCHITIS

Bronchitis is an inflammation of the air passages of the lungs. The acute form of bronchitis is thought to be caused by a viral infection and often follows a cold in the nose and throat. Breathing air that contains irritants such as cigarette smoke can also lead to lung inflammation. Symptoms include a low fever, an unproductive cough (one that produces little or no sputum), and chest discomfort. Recurrent episodes can result in chronic bronchitis, a non-contagious and non-cancerous degeneration of the bronchial tubes. The cause is thought to be repeated irritation from air pollution, allergens, and cigarette smoke or repeated infections that cause the air passages to thicken, thus narrowing the passages and resulting in a loss of elasticity. Symptoms include shortness of breath and frequent coughing spasms with or without thick sputum, depending on the presence of an infection at the time of the cough. It should be pointed out that this disease is difficult at best to self-diagnose because of the symptoms' similarity to many lung and heart disorders.

According to our macrobiotic understanding, the underlying cause of acute bronchitis is a diet high in yang animal foods that are also high in fat. These foods make the air passages narrower and also clog the passages with excess fat. The long-term effect of such a diet coupled with the overconsumption of yin foods such as refined sugar, alcohol, and fruit results in the chronic form of bronchitis. The long-term effect of overly yin foods is to weaken the body's condition in general and the bronchial tubes in particular.

Helpful Suggestions

The single most helpful thing you can do is stop smoking and encourage those around you to stop because passive smoking is very detrimental as well. The following remedial suggestions are broken into yang and yin types. If you are uncertain which suggestions to use because of years of a diet high in both extreme yin and yang foods, consider your present condition. If you are weak, use the suggestions for the yin type; if you are strong, use those for the yang type. Deal with your symptoms in the following order:

OBJECTIVE	REMEDY
FOR THE YANG TYPE	
To reduce high fever	Try drinking 1 cup of BROWN RICE TEA WITH LOTUS ROOT AND SHIITAKE MUSHROOM, omitting the salt, 2 to 3 times per day until the high fever goes down.
To relieve severe coughing	Try drinking 1 cup of LOTUS ROOT TEA, using dried lotus root, 3 to 4 times per day until coughing stops.
	and
	A GINGER COMPRESS WITH SAKE applied to the chest for 20 minutes followed by an ALBI PLASTER for up to 4 hours is helpful. Repeat both the compress and the plasters as needed.
To relieve chest pain	Try applying an ALBI PLASTER to the chest, changing it every 4 hours. Afterwards use a GINGER SESAME OIL MASSAGE on the chest.

	FOR THE YIN TYPE
To reduce high fever	Try drinking 1 cup of BROWN RICE TEA WITH DRIED PERSIMMON AND TANGERINE SKIN with a pinch of salt added 2 to 3 times per day until the high fever goes down.
	and
	Using a GINGER SESAME OIL MASSAGE on the scalp is helpful.
To relieve chest pain	Use a GINGER SESAME OIL MASSAGE on the chest and then apply an ALBI PLASTER, changing the plaster every 4 hours.
To relieve cough	Try drinking 1 cup of LOTUS ROOT TEA or KUZU BANCHA TEA WITH GINGER 3 to 4 times per day until coughing stops.

Dietary Recommendations

The most important dietary recommendation is to eat locally grown foods in season to strengthen your whole body and its general resistance. To correct loss of appetite, try Brown Rice Cream (thick) served with a little Gomashio or hijiki (or other sea vegetables), and Lotus Root Nitsuke. Use the following dietary suggestions until your condition improves or for about one month. Then widen your dietary choices using a macrobiotic dietary approach (see page 11). For a persistent chronic condition, try using the same dietary suggestions given in the Asthma section.

FOR THE YANG TYPE

☐ Main foods: Brown Rice Cream, Brown Rice Gruel with Mochi.

☐ Side dishes (less than one-third of main foods): Ginger Miso, Burdock Carrot Nitsuke, Carp Soup, Vegetable Tempura served with Grated Daikon, Daikon Nitsuke served with Homemade Agé, steamed vegetables, Umeboshi.

☐ Miso soup ingredients: daikon, Chinese cabbage, tofu, Homemade Agé, Brown Rice Mochi.

☐ Beverages: Brown Rice Bancha Tea, Grain Coffee.

☐ Avoid especially: all meats, all fish (except carp) and shellfish, all dairy foods, eggs, meat-based soups, all sweet foods, and hot spices.

FOR THE YIN TYPE

☐ Main foods: Brown Rice, Azuki Rice served with Gomashio, Brown Rice Cream, Brown Rice Gruel with Mochi.

☐ Side dishes (less than one-fourth of main foods) Tekka Miso, Hijiki Lotus Root Nitsuke, Oysters Cooked with Miso, Burdock Carrot Nitsuke, Vegetable Tempura, Azuki Beans with Kombu and Winter Squash, Miso Pickles, Umeboshi.

☐ Miso soup ingredients: wakame, scallions, onions, Homemade Agé, Brown Rice Mochi.

☐ Beverages: Sho-Ban Tea, Brown Rice Tea, Bancha Tea, Kombu Tea, Grain Milk, Mu Tea.

☐ Avoid especially: all meats, fish and shellfish (except oysters), dairy foods, eggs, fruit, sweet foods, potatoes, tomatoes, eggplant, mushrooms, melons, vinegar dishes, alcohol, ice cream, soft drinks.

BRUISES

Helpful Suggestions

OBJECTIVE	REMEDY
To remove coagulated blood	Any of the following may be applied on a bruise one at a time: ALBI PLASTER, TOFU PLASTER, or RICE PLASTER. Whichever plaster is chosen should be changed every 4 hours and used for 1 or 2 days. Tofu plasters are most commonly used on head bruises while the albi plaster is the strongest one for body bruises.
	or
	Mix buckwheat flour with sesame oil or mix egg whites with any kind of flour to form a pastelike mixture. Apply directly on the bruise, changing it every 4 hours, for 1 to 2 days.
	and/or
	Lightly rubbing the bruise with a ¼-inch-thick round piece of daikon may be helpful. Use as often as needed.

BURNS

Burns refer to an injury of the skin caused by a heat source, chemicals, or radiation, including sunlight. Burns are divided into three categories, depending on the severity of the burn. First-degree burns affect only the upper layer of the skin and are characterized by redness, pain (tenderness), swelling, and sometimes a slight fever. Second-degree burns affect deeper layers of the skin with more severe manifestations of first-degree symptoms plus the formation of blisters. Third-degree burns affect all layers of skin and sometimes the underlying muscle. Most second-degree burns and all third-degree burns require a doctor's treatment and possible hospitalization depending on the severity, location, and extent of the burn. First-degree burns and some second-degree burns may be cared for at home. The following suggestions are

---

> **CORNELLIA'S NATURAL HEALING AT WORK**
>
> I had a car accident a number of years ago. I was hit in the right cheekbone, the right arm, right chest, and both knees as well as my spine. There was no bleeding, only black bruises. This was two days before summer camp, so I didn't go to the hospital. I just used tofu plasters.
>
> On a Saturday night in Oroville, California, it was impossible to get enough tofu, so I was only able to apply a plaster once on my knees and twice on my eye, two hours apart. I had no time to squeeze out the tofu thoroughly on a board, so I just quickly wrung it out with a cotton cloth and applied it. I usually have a good appetite but not during this time. I only drank kuzu and ate a little bit of soba. Mr. Otake, a Japanese chiropractor who was a guest at camp, taught me how to make a rice plaster. This was a great help because I could not get any tofu at summer camp. I used these plasters, and my bruises healed very quickly.　　　　■
>
> BRUISES

offered for these cases and in the event that no hospital or doctor is immediately available.

Helpful Suggestions

OBJECTIVE	REMEDY
	FOR FIRST-DEGREE BURNS
To relieve pain	As quickly as possible, immerse first-degree burns that cover a small area in a cool SALT WATER BATH for 30 minutes.
	then
	Soak a towel in the salt water and cover the burn with this towel to keep the burn cool. Exposure to air may result in increased pain or blisters may appear.
	and
	Place a thin layer of good-quality sesame oil on the burn area and cover with a towel dipped in sesame oil. Wrap or secure the towel, changing it every 6 hours for 1 week or more until the skin has healed.
	FOR SECOND-DEGREE BURNS TREATABLE AT HOME
To relieve pain	Try an OIL COMPRESS as soon as possible, reapplying every 4 hours for up to 1 month. This helps reduce the pain and keeps the body from scarring.
	or
	If you don't have the materials for an oil compress, the important thing is to shut off the air supply to the burn area. This can be done quickly by applying any good-quality

raw miso or honey; finely grated albi, potatoes, or yams; or a TOFU APPLICATION directly on the burn area. Secure with bandages. Reapply every 4 hours for a couple of days to about 1 week.

or

Mix egg whites with enough flour to make a pastelike material. Apply directly on the burn area, changing it every 4 hours, for a couple of days to about 1 week.

Dietary Recommendations

Follow a macrobiotic dietary approach (see page 11), especially avoiding animal protein. Drinking less liquid is also helpful. Large amounts of calories in general and protein in particular are usually advised for rebuilding tissues and muscle in cases of more severe burns. According to our macrobiotic understanding, the protein should not be taken from animal sources because animal protein is directly related to infections.

It is theorized that too much liquid intake is responsible for weak kidneys and further that the health of the skin is directly related to the health of the kidneys. Therefore, the advice to drink less. If animal sources of protein were to be used, then more liquid would be needed. If vegetable sources that contain large amounts of water are used, then less liquids are needed, the kidneys remain strong, and the skin is allowed to repair itself naturally.

CORNELLIA'S NATURAL HEALING AT WORK

I remember my friend's baby was burned (first degree) on the thigh by boiling water. Of course, the baby felt pain and started crying. After I applied grated potato on the burn, the baby stopped crying; no blisters formed, and the burn healed quickly.

A burn causes much pain because after the nerve cells' exposure to oxygen, oxidation becomes more rapid, resulting in a shortage of oxygen in the nerve cells. The sensation of pain results from a shortage of oxygen in the nerve cells. However, more oxygen to the area increases the pain because it fuels the oxidation process. When the baby cries, more and more oxygen is inhaled causing more burning or pain. Putting grated potato (or sesame oil) on the burn shuts the area off from oxygen and reduces the pain. Then the baby stops crying, less oxidation occurs, and pain is further reduced. In other words, when the pain goes away, the baby forgets its own trouble and the body's natural healing system takes over. As long as the baby continues to cry, the healing process will take a longer time.   ■

BURNS

CANCER

See BREAST CANCER, COLON CANCER, ESOPHAGEAL STRICTURE, LEUKEMIA, LIVER CANCER, LUNG CANCER, SMALL INTESTINE CANCER, SKIN CANCER, STOMACH CANCER.

CANDIDIASIS

Candidiasis is an infection by a yeast-like fungus of the genus *Candida*, most generally affecting the moist skin areas of the body, oral mucous membranes, respiratory tract, and vagina. This fungus normally lives in the body without any ill effects. However, if the number of fungi increase disproportionately to other bacteria and yeast in the body, an infection and an overall weakening of the immune system can result. As *Candida* increases in its numbers and strength in the gastrointestinal tract, it enters the blood stream and can pass through cell walls into various organs, including the brain. Candidiasis can result when friendly bacteria that keep the normally friendly *Candida* in check are destroyed by antibiotics and/or chlorinated water. Among the sources of antibiotics we ingest are prescription drugs and the meat of animals that have been given antibiotics. The bacteria killed by antibiotics or chlorination decompose and become proteins that feed *Candida* and cause it to grow. Candidiasis can also result from kidney weakness. Weak kidneys cannot maintain the proper amount of sodium in the bodily fluids. As a result, *Candida* proliferate. See the section on Kidney Failure for causes of and suggestions for kidney weakness.

Some of the many possible symptoms of candidiasis are acne; tingling sensations; numbness in hands, legs, or face; canker sores; sore throat; nagging cough; congestion; fatigue; depression; mood swings; hyperactivity; muscle and joint pain; arthritis; muscle weakness; allergies to foods, yeasts, molds, and/or chemicals; hypothyroidism; heartburn; abdominal pain; kidney and bladder infections; vaginitis; constipation or diarrhea; colitis; and diabetes.

Helpful Suggestions

Improve the condition of your kidneys through the daily practice of one or more of the following remedies. These remedies make the kidneys stronger because they improve blood circulation and increase the amount of oxygen available to the kidneys.

OBJECTIVE	REMEDY
To improve kidneys	Apply a GINGER COMPRESS over the kidneys (see Figure 3.8 on page 176) for 20 minutes. *and/or* Walk barefoot for 20 minutes in the early morning dew. *and/or* Take a SAUNA until you break into a sweat. *and/or* Take a 1 percent SALT BATH for 30 minutes. *also*
To alkalinize the system	Eat a soybean-sized portion of *UME EXTRACT* 1 to 2 times per day.

Dietary Recommendations

Follow a macrobiotic dietary approach (see page 11) using less salt than usual until the kidneys begin to improve. Then, gradually increase the amount of salt in your cooking. Chew very well since the lack of enzymes in a *Candida*-filled gastrointestinal tract will make it more difficult to digest foods. Drink less than usual and only when thirsty.

☐ Avoid especially: fruits (even though these are alkaline forming), sweeteners of any kind, salted snacks, salt or soy sauce added at the table or after cooking. *Candida* love a sugary environment, so avoid simple carbohydrates and refined grains.

CANKER SORES

Canker sores are painful ulcerations that occur in the mouth and adjacent areas. They can appear on the tongue, inner cheeks, lips, gums, palate, and throat. Canker sores are thought to result from emotional or physical stress; poor dental hygiene; allergies to chocolate and other foods; anxiety or fatigue; injury to the mouth lining caused by rough dentures, dental work, or hot food; and viral infection. Canker sores have white centers covered by a gray membrane and are surrounded by an intense red border. Sores can range from the size of a pinhead to that of a quarter.

According to our macrobiotic understanding, the cause of canker sores is the overconsumption of yin foods such as milk, yogurt, candy, cakes, and fruit and the eating of too much yang food such as animal protein. This type of diet may cause infections and allergic reactions thus increasing the risk of canker sores.

Helpful Suggestions

The suggestions for improving the kidneys make them stronger because they improve blood circulation and increase the amount of oxygen available to them.

OBJECTIVE	REMEDY
To relieve pain	Use a WOOD ASH WATER TREATMENT twice a day on the canker sore for pain relief. *or* Use a DENTIE POWDER TREATMENT twice a day on the sores. *also* Drinking ½ cup *UME EXTRACT TEA* 1 to 2 times per day is helpful.
To improve kidneys	Do one of the following daily to improve the condition of the kidneys: Apply a GINGER COMPRESS over the kidneys (see Figure 3.8 on page 176) for 20 minutes. *or* Walk barefoot for 20 minutes in the early morning dew. *or* Take a SAUNA until you break into a sweat. *or* Take a 1 percent SALT BATH for 30 minutes.

Dietary Recommendations

Follow a macrobiotic dietary approach (see page 11) with less emphasis on protein foods (including beans) and simple carbohydrates such as fruit. Chew well and drink less fluids than usual until the canker sores and the kidneys improve.

See also ALLERGIES.

CATARACTS

Cataracts are the most common eye problem for older men and women. A cataract is a slowly growing opaqueness in the lens of the eye resulting finally in the loss of vision. The lens is made of a clear protein substance that can, just like the white of an egg, become less flexible and less clear if the fluid (aqueous humor) temperature goes up. In my opinion, it is the increased number of microbes (infection) in this fluid that makes the temperature go up. Furthermore, the lens has no blood supply and it is the fluid that surrounds the lens that nourishes it. If the fluid is not properly nourished, a condition that can occur with hardening of the arteries, then the lens loses its nourishment also, becomes less flexible, and develops cataracts. This is the reason that adults over sixty are most often affected.

According to our macrobiotic understanding, hardening of the arteries is not a normal result of aging; aging is a result of hardening of the arteries. The incidence of both infections and hardening of the arteries increases with a diet high in animal foods that are also high in fat and cholesterol such as red meats, fish, dairy products, and eggs. Any injury to the eye, exposure to radiation, or consumption of drugs that interfere with the supply of nutrients to the fluid surrounding the eye can greatly increase the risk of cataracts. There are some similarities between chronic simple glaucoma and cataracts because diminishing vision is gradual in both cases and sometimes glaucoma appears without pain as is characteristic of cataracts.

Helpful Suggestions

You may continue the following remedies until the cataracts show improvement.

OBJECTIVE	REMEDY
To reduce bacterial infection	Try using a SALT BANCHA EYE BATH at a warm to hot temperature 4 to 5 times a day for about 2 weeks.
To lower eye temperature	You may wish to take a 1 percent SALT BATH for 30 minutes every day or every other day until the cataracts improve.
	and/or
	A SESAME OIL EYE TREATMENT in each eye before bedtime every night during the same 2 weeks is helpful.
	or
	Apply an ALBI PLASTER on each temple and leave it on all night.

Dietary Recommendations

The following dietary suggestions may be used until the cataracts improve or for about one month. Then, widen your food choices using a macrobiotic dietary approach (see page 11).

☐ Main foods: Brown Rice, Azuki Rice, Brown Rice Balls, Brown Rice Mochi; use Gomashio as a condiment.
☐ Side dishes (one-third of main foods): Tekka Miso, Hijiki Nitsuke, Burdock Carrot Nitsuke, Azuki Beans with Kombu and Winter Squash; use sesame oil and have sea vegetables every day.
☐ Miso soup ingredients: wakame, onions, carrots, scallions.
☐ Beverages: Bancha Tea, Brown Rice Tea, Grain

Coffee. Beverage consumption should be limited to 1 cup per day maximum if your overall condition allows it.
☐ Avoid especially: all meat, fish, shellfish, fruit, tomatoes, potatoes, eggplant, refined sugar, sweet foods and drinks, vinegar, dairy foods including cheese and butter, coffee, alcohol, fruit drinks.

See also GLAUCOMA.

CHAPPED LIPS

Chapped or cracked lips that do not result from exposure to cold, wind, or sun are caused by overeating and overdrinking. According to our macrobiotic understanding, the upper lip mirrors the condition of the stomach and the lower lip indicates the intestine's condition. Thus, if the lips develop an abscess or crack, this shows that you are overeating.

Helpful Suggestions

OBJECTIVE	REMEDY
To improve health of cells	FAST for 1 day if your condition allows and you will be amazed by the results.
	and
	Organic honey applied on cracked lips may be helpful.

Dietary Recommendations

Follow a macrobiotic dietary approach (see page 11) with an emphasis on foods that are easy to digest such as Brown Rice Kayu or whole-grain noodles.

CHICKENPOX

Chickenpox is a very contagious but mild disease caused by the herpes zoster virus. It is mostly a childhood disease, but adults can also be affected. Symptoms appear after a seven- to twenty-one-day incubation period, and include fever, abdominal pain lasting for a couple of days, and red rashes that develop all over the body, but mainly on the face and trunk. The rashes change to water blisters that are about the size of red beans. The blisters collapse within twenty-four hours, forming scabs. New blisters erupt every three to four days. Adults who get chickenpox have flulike symptoms in addition to those listed above. Those who take anticancer or immunosuppressive drugs have a higher risk of contracting this disease.

Once a person has had chickenpox, he or she is supposed to have an immunity against contracting it again. However, the same virus can cause shingles in adults. Thus, it is commonly recommended that children with chickenpox be kept away from adults until all the blisters have formed scabs. According to our macrobiotic understanding, chickenpox is the result of overeating animal protein, which causes putrefaction in the intestines and suppresses the immune system. Thus, avoiding large quantities of animal proteins and keeping the immune system strong are good preventatives for both chickenpox and shingles.

Helpful Suggestions

OBJECTIVE	REMEDY
To relieve itchiness	Try drinking 1/3 to 1/2 cup of DAIKON GINGER TEA twice per day depending on the age of the person (younger or more frail persons use the lesser amount).
	and/or
	Take a RICE BRAN BATH every day.
	and/or
	A DAIKON GINGER COMPRESS or RICE BRAN COMPRESS may be applied to the itchy area for 20 minutes once a day. After removing the compress, use a SESAME OIL or GINGER SESAME OIL MASSAGE on the area.
	and
	Try not to scratch the blisters as this can lead to scarring and further infections; rub the area instead with a slice of daikon.
	and
	Try placing a thin straw mat on top of your sheet at night; this helps keep you cooler and you will be less itchy. Use linen pajamas.
	and
	Before bed every night, apply a WOOD ASH WATER TREATMENT until itching stops.
To cleanse the skin	Avoid the use of soap; wash with a RICE BRAN BAG (see BATHS, page 173) instead.

Dietary Recommendations

Following a macrobiotic dietary approach (see page 11) is most helpful.

☐ Avoid especially: all animal food especially red meat and fish such as tuna, bonita, salmon, sardines, mackerel, shellfish, and abalone. Also avoid eggs, alcohol, milk, ice cream, cocoa, coffee, black tea, all fruit, sweet foods, hot spices, vinegar dishes, eggplant, tomatoes, potatoes.

CHOLERA

According to Western medicine, cholera is an acute infectious disease caused by bacteria and, in the form common in Asia, is spread by water and food contamination. It is characterized by severe and constant diarrhea resulting in extreme fluid depletion, up to 20 quarts per day. Other symptoms include vomiting, stomach and leg cramps, intense thirst, chills, and extreme exhaustion. Sodium absorption is blocked by a toxin in the cholera bacteria and the excretion of water and electrolytes is promoted. This leads to severe dehydration that may end in shock, renal failure, and death.

According to our macrobiotic understanding, the underlying cause of cholera is eating too much extreme yang food such as animal foods along with too much yin food such as sugary foods and fruit. Animal and sugary foods produce acidity, which in excess leads to a weakened immune system and a greater susceptibility to cholera bacteria. Fruits are alkaline-forming in the body, but, in excess, they help the growth of bacteria because of their high fruit-sugar content and because bacteria thrive in a sugary (yin) environment. A strong immune system that can deal with the bacteria and avoiding food that helps the bacteria grow are the best preventatives.

Helpful Suggestions

If an outbreak of cholera is announced in your area, eat one to two umeboshi with soy sauce every morning. This will help protect you from getting cholera because umeboshi is very effective in killing cholera and helps protect against putrefaction inside the body; it has a sterilizing power. If there is an infection, consult a medical professional immediately. The following suggestions are complementary.

OBJECTIVE	REMEDY
To remove toxins	Try drinking 1 cup of UMEBOSHI TEA several times a day to help flush out the system.
To relieve leg cramps	Take a DAIKON or ARAME HIP BATH WITH MUSTARD POWDER until the skin turns a red color.

Dietary Recommendations

Follow a macrobiotic dietary approach (see page 11), avoiding both extreme yin and yang foods, to keep the immune system strong.

CIRRHOSIS OF THE LIVER

Cirrhosis of the liver is a chronic disease in which the liver is congested, distorted, and scarred, leading to a loss of normal liver function. Some of the first signs of cirrhosis of the liver are fatigue, poor appetite, nausea, enlarged liver, and red palms. Later-stage symptoms include jaundice, dark yellow or brown urine, fluid accumulation in the abdomen and legs, enlarged spleen, hair loss, and diarrhea. Cirrhosis of the liver is preceded by excessive alcohol consumption, but viral hepatitis, poor nutritional habits, and exposure to toxic chemicals can also impair liver function.

The underlying cause of cirrhosis of the liver is anything that causes or continues a liver inflammation that is accompanied by a destruction of liver cells and a scarring of regenerated cells. According to our macrobiotic understanding, inflammations result from eating too much animal food such as meat, fish, dairy foods, poultry, and eggs. Because the liver has strong regenerative power, even the most damaged liver can be rebuilt by eating well, as with a macrobiotic approach.

Helpful Suggestions

OBJECTIVE	REMEDY
To test for an enlarged liver	Lie down on your back and bend your knees. Push in with your third and fourth fingers under the center of your right ribs. You should be able to push the fingers in to the second finger joint (two full finger sections from the tip). If the liver is enlarged, you will not be able to do this. You will not experience any pain or tenderness if your liver is in a healthy condition.
To reduce an enlarged liver	Try applying a GINGER COMPRESS over the liver area (see Figure 3.8 on page 176) for 20 minutes followed by an ALBI PLASTER for up to 4 hours. Continue both a compress and the plaster each day for 2 to 3 weeks until the liver is no longer enlarged.
To relieve pain	Put a ROASTED SALT PACK on the stomach (see Figure 3.8 on page 176) to keep the abdomen warm and help increase circulation.
To reduce bloating in stomach or spleen	A GINGER COMPRESS applied to the swollen organ for 20 minutes may be helpful. Follow this with a BUCKWHEAT PLASTER once a day for 4 hours with a ROASTED SALT PACK on top of the Buckwheat Plaster to keep it warm. Do this for up to 10 days.
To relieve nausea	Eat 1 or 2 BROWN RICE BALLS WITH GOMASHIO, chewing very well.

Dietary Recommendations

Use a macrobiotic dietary approach (see page 11) with less oil and eat less for three days to one week, especially if the illness is in the later stages.

☐ Beverages: Brown Rice Tea, Brown Rice Bancha Tea, Bancha Tea, and Grain Coffee.
☐ Avoid especially: all animal foods and overly yin foods, especially alcohol.

See also JAUNDICE, HAIR LOSS, *and* DIARRHEA *if you have these symptoms.*

COLD SORES, FEVER BLISTERS

Cold sores and fever blisters are eruptions of small, painful blisters with local tenderness. The blisters are grouped together and surrounded by a red ring. They fill with fluid and sometimes pus oozes from the blisters. These sores occur most often around the mouth, but sometimes on the genital organs. Although herpes simplex virus I is cited by medical authorities as the cause, there are many contributing factors such as physical or emotional stress, sunburn, skin abrasions, fever, the common cold, or the use of immunosuppressive drugs.

According to our macrobiotic understanding, infection by this virus is the result of an excessively yin diet. Thus, the reason that the infection becomes active is too much yin food or a lack of salt in the diet, and weak kidneys, which are hampered in retaining sodium in the bodily fluids. Without sodium in the bodily fluids, there is a loss of natural immunity against viruses. It should be noted that the herpes simplex virus I remains in the body for life, but is usually dormant until the conditions mentioned above present themselves.

Helpful Suggestions

The suggestions for improving the kidneys make the kidneys stronger because they improve blood circulation and increase the amount of oxygen available to them.

OBJECTIVE	REMEDY
To relieve pain in the mouth	Try using a WOOD ASH WATER TREATMENT 2 times per day or a DENTIE POWDER TREATMENT on the sores 2 or 3 times per day.
To improve overall condition	Drink ½ cup of UME EXTRACT TEA twice a day.

To improve kidneys	Do one of the following daily:
	Apply a GINGER COMPRESS over the kidneys (see Figure 3.8 on page 176) for 20 minutes
	or
	Walk barefoot in the grass every day in the early morning for 20 minutes
	or
	Take a SAUNA until you break into a sweat.
	or
	Take a 1 percent SALT BATH for 30 minutes.

Dietary Recommendations

This condition is much more difficult to remedy than canker sores because the virus is very yin. Therefore, one should maintain a limited macrobiotic dietary approach, mostly whole grains and seasonal vegetables, until the symptoms disappear and a normal macrobiotic dietary approach (see page 11) for at least one year after the symptoms disappear. Most importantly, avoid sugar, molasses, honey, yinnie syrup, milk, soft drinks, candy, cakes, fruits, and fruit juice.

COLDS

According to modern medicine, the common cold is a contagious infection of the upper respiratory tract caused by as many as 200 different viruses. A cold usually comes on suddenly: the throat is frequently irritated and the nose runs; there is some sneezing, a general feeling of discomfort, and moderate headaches. Other symptoms may include a nonproductive cough (one that produces little or no sputum), a low fever, appetite loss, fatigue, and a stuffy nose with a clear discharge at first followed by a thick, greenish yellow discharge.

A virus is thought to be the cause of colds, although many factors—such as overwork, stress, lack of sleep, smoking, poor nutritional habits, and living in unsanitary conditions—add to one's susceptibility to viruses. According to our macrobiotic understanding, however, the most common underlying cause of a common cold is overeating and/or overdrinking of any kind. Why do overeating and overdrinking cause colds? Overeating weakens the stomach, which then reduces the production of antibodies, leaving one vulnerable to a viral attack. Overdrinking weakens the kidneys so that they cannot maintain the proper amount of sodium in the bodily fluids. This condition causes one to be infection-prone. Proper practice of a macrobiotic dietary approach is the best preventative for colds.

There is no known cure for the common cold and each occurrence takes about seven to fourteen days to run its course. Colds can lead to bacterial infections, so some care needs to be taken. Many diseases such as measles, diphtheria, whooping cough, strep throat, and meningitis begin with symptoms similar to the common cold. Check with your health-care advisor if the symptoms progress beyond those listed here, if the symptoms do not go away, or if you have frequently recurring colds.

Helpful Suggestions

If fever persists after trying the following remedies, consult a health-care advisor. Usually, the fever will go away in a day or two. Three days is the limit before seeking the opinion of a health-care advisor since this is one indication that you have more than a common cold.

OBJECTIVE	REMEDY
To reduce fever	Apply a TOFU PLASTER to the forehead, changing it every hour
	and
	Place a GREEN LEAVES APPLICATION on the back of the neck; change leaves every 2 hours.
	and/or
	Any of several teas may be helpful. Try drinking 2 to 3 cups of DAIKON GINGER TEA once a day for up to 3 days.
	or
	If you are weak, use ½ to 1 cup of BROWN RICE TEA WITH DRIED PERSIMMON AND TANGERINE SKIN 2 to 3 times per day for up to 3 days
	or
	Use 1 cup of BURDOCK BONITA TEA, SCALLION BANCHA TEA, or CHARCOALED UMEBOSHI TEA 2 to 3 times per day for up to 3 days. These teas help alkalize the body and promote sweating.
To ease the discomfort of colds with fever	Try drinking 1 cup of SCALLION MISO TEA as often as desired.
To relieve headache	MASSAGE the entire head with GINGER SESAME OIL.
To quiet a cough	Try drinking 1 cup of LOTUS ROOT TEA 2 to 3 times per day for 3 days.
	or
	Sip 1 tablespoon of DAIKON JUICE WITH RICE SYRUP 2 to 3 times per day.
To quiet a persistent cough	If after 3 days Lotus Root Tea has not worked, apply a slightly warmed ½-inch-thick ALBI PLASTER mixture to the chest over the breasts and another plaster to the spinal region of the upper back opposite the chest. Use two 6-inch square plasters on the chest, changing every 4 hours.
	or
	Take ½ cup of DAIKON SEED COUGH DRINK 2 to 3 times per day.

CORNELLIA'S NATURAL HEALING AT WORK

Once in a while, I feel a cold coming on and my spine feels cold. In such cases, for twenty-four hours I don't drink any-thing—no liquids, no soups. Then, usually, the cold doesn't develop. If you avoid overdrinking, the body will be more yang. If this doesn't work, I work in the garden until I start to sweat. This usually protects me from getting a cold.

Sweating occurs as a result of an increase in body tem-perature. The result is a partial burning of fat in the blood vessels. This improves blood circulation so that body cells, organs, the nervous system, etc., receive a good supply of oxygen and other nutrients. At the same time, waste prod-ucts are eliminated more quickly so that the body's heal-ing power is increased and a healthy condition is achieved and maintained more easily.

Sweating also helps because it reduces the amount of bodily fluids. This, in turn, reduces the body's heat loss because with a greater amount of bodily fluids there is a greater need for heat energy to maintain a constant body temperature. Reduced bodily fluids also reduce the num-ber of bacteria in the system because bacteria thrive in a moist environment. Also, reduced bodily fluids reduce the work of the kidneys and lead to stronger kidneys. Stronger kidneys are better able to maintain a slightly alkaline (healthy) condition. This improves the body's healing power. ■

COLDS

Dietary Recommendations

The following dietary suggestions may be used until the symptoms disappear or for one month. Then, widen your food choices using a macrobiotic dietary approach (see page 11).

☐ Main foods: warm-to-hot Brown Rice Gruel served with scallions, Brown Rice Gruel with Grated Daikon and Homemade Agé, Brown Rice Gruel with Mochi (add shiitake mushroom if the person is strong).

☐ Side dishes (less than one-fourth of main foods): Tekka Miso, Shio Kombu, Scallion Miso, Hijiki Lotus Root Nitsuke, Burdock Carrot Nitsuke, Tororo Kombu Soup, Oysters Cooked with Miso, boiled vegetables, Vegetable Tempura, Umeboshi, Miso Pickles.

☐ Miso soup ingredients: wakame, scallions, daikon, Homemade Agé, Brown Rice Mochi.

☐ Beverages: Brown Rice Tea, Brown Rice Bancha Tea, Sho-Ban Tea, Bancha Tea, Mu Tea, Grain Coffee, Grain Milk, Kombu Tea, Amasake Drink. Drink a maximum of 2 cups of beverages per day after the first days of car-ing for a fever or cough.

☐ Avoid especially: all meat, fish, shellfish, dairy (includ-ing ice cream), fruit, sweet foods, salads, melons, vine-gar, sweet drinks, hot spices, tomatoes, potatoes, eggplant, alcohol, coffee, cocoa.

COLON CANCER

Colon (or colorectal) cancer refers to an uncontrolled growth of malignant cells in the rectum or colon. According to modern medicine, the cause of colon can-cer is unknown. Bloody or black stools; cramping abdom-inal pain and/or rectal pain; changes in stool condition, sometimes diarrhea and other times constipation; unex-plained weight loss; or an anemic condition may be warning signs of colon cancer, although there are often no symptoms in the early stages. As with all cancers, the major problem is uncontrolled growth of malignant cells, resulting in death. The success rate for colon cancer surgery is high compared to other types of cancer surgery. A colostomy or other surgery is not recommended unless absolutely necessary and requires special instructions for care from your doctor. The macrobiotic approach is to find and control the underlying causes of the cancerous growth rather than to remove the tumors.

According to our macrobiotic understanding, the underlying cause of colon cancer is a diet high in fatty foods, especially yang animal foods such as meat, poul-try, and eggs; a lack of dietary fiber; and the overcon-sumption of yin drinks such as alcohol, sugary drinks, and milk. If there is a predominance of yang animal foods, yang cancer results, while a predominance of yin drinks or refined fiberless foods results in a yin colon cancer. Your overall condition reflects the type of can-cer you have. People with a more yang condition are more aggressive, have a tendency to get angry, and are stronger overall. A yin type is indicated by a more pas-sive nature, a tendency to complain, and a weaker over-all condition.

Helpful Suggestions

OBJECTIVE	REMEDY
To relieve pain	Use a GINGER COMPRESS on the abdomen (see Figure 3.8 on page 176) for 20 minutes fol-lowed by an ALBI PLASTER for up to 4 hours. Continue with a Ginger Compress followed by an Albi Plaster as often as needed each day until pain stops.
To alkalize blood	You may use a UME EXTRACT ENEMA every other day for 2 to 3 weeks. Ume extract is a very strong alkalizing agent and since can-cer cells thrive in an acidic environment, it is thought that alkalizing the blood will weaken the cancer cells.
	or
	You may try drinking ½ cup of UME EXTRACT TEA 3 times a day, 30 minutes before eating for 1 to 2 weeks.

To remove excess acids	Taking a daily SAUNA until you break into a sweat is effective; however, if you have a weak heart, the temperature must be lower than 200°F. For those with a weak heart, a SAUNA (FAR-INFRARED) can then be ideal, as it is for those with a strong heart.
To prevent an overly acidic condition	Exercise is very important in the prevention of cancer. However, avoid vigorous and strenuous exercises since these can produce an overly acidic condition. Gardening and brisk walking are good daily exercises. Avoiding stress is also wise.

Dietary Recommendations

The following dietary suggestions are to be used for the first month. Then, widen your food choices based on a macrobiotic dietary approach (see page 11). This is most important since a return to a high-fat, low-fiber diet usually results in a recurrence of cancer. If you are uncertain as to which type of colon cancer you have, try the suggestions for the yin type first.

FOR THE YANG TYPE

☐ Main foods: Brown Rice or Azuki Rice served with a little Gomashio. Chew each mouthful 200 times.

☐ Side dishes (one-third to one-half of main foods cooked to a less salty taste than usual): a little Tekka Miso, Ginger Miso, Grated Daikon (raw, about 2 tablespoons) with Soy Sauce, Burdock Carrot Nitsuke, Carp Soup, Rice Bran Pickles, Umeboshi.

☐ Miso soup ingredients: daikon, albi, green leafy vegetables, Chinese cabbage, spinach, nigari tofu, eggplant.

☐ Beverages: Brown Rice Tea, Brown Rice Bancha Tea, Bancha Tea, Grain Coffee, Vegetable Broth. Drink a maximum of 2½ cups of beverages per day.

☐ Avoid especially: all animal foods including fish, shellfish, eggs, meat-based soups; all alcohol; all sweet foods and drinks; fruit; and ice cream.

FOR THE YIN TYPE

☐ Main foods: Brown Rice Balls and Brown Rice Mochi. Use a little Gomashio at each meal. Chew each mouthful 200 times.

☐ Side dishes (one-third of main foods cooked to a salty taste): Tekka Miso, Hijiki Nitsuke, Burdock Carrot Nitsuke, Shio Kombu, Carp Soup, Natural Caviar, Takuan Pickles, Miso Pickles.

☐ Miso soup ingredients: wakame, tororo kombu, onions, scallions, Homemade Agé, Brown Rice Mochi.

☐ Beverages: Sho-Ban Tea, Brown Rice Tea, Brown Rice Bancha Tea, Bancha Tea, Mu Tea. Drink a maximum of 2 cups of beverages per day.

☐ Avoid especially: all animal foods, dairy foods (including ice cream), soy milk, eggs, all alcohol, fruit, sweet foods, vinegar, hot spices, tomatoes, mushrooms, melons, peanuts, Rice Bran Pickles (except Takuan Pickles), rice gruel.

CONSTIPATION

Constipation is indicated when there are infrequent bowel movements, hard feces, or straining during bowel movements. Constipation is thought to have many possible causes, but insufficient fiber in the diet, inadequate fluid intake, and a lack of exercise are the most common causes. Many diseases, such as chronic kidney failure, colon cancer, depression, and hypothyroidism to name a few, also result in constipation. And constipation can lead to many adverse conditions from hemorrhoids, appendicitis, and hernias to bad breath, insomnia, and obesity. Your likelihood of experiencing constipation is increased with any illness requiring complete bed rest, added stress from any source, and the use of certain medications.

According to our macrobiotic understanding, constipation can have a yin or a yang cause. Yang constipation is caused by the overconsumption of animal foods with an accompanying lack of fiber in one's diet. Fiber increases the number of intestinal microbes that help to digest food and determine the bulkiness of the stool, making it easier for the stool to move through the colon. Yang foods cause the colon to contract, restricting the passage of feces. Yin constipation is caused by eating too much yin food such as sugary foods and fruit, and by drinking too many sugary and/or alcoholic drinks. In this case, the colon becomes too expanded, peristaltic action is reduced, and waste material doesn't move properly through the colon.

Helpful Suggestions

If you are uncertain which type of constipation you have, try the suggestions for the yin type first.

OBJECTIVE	REMEDY
	FOR THE YANG TYPE
To relieve constipation	Each day, on an empty stomach, drink ⅓ to ½ cup of the liquid in which sour cabbage has been prepared (see page 225) or the liquid from natural dill pickles. Use only the liquid from good-quality natural sour cabbage or dill pickles. *and* The STOMACH MASSAGE is very effective.

FOR THE YIN TYPE

To relieve constipation	Apply a GINGER COMPRESS just below the belly button for 20 minutes followed by a MISO PLASTER below the belly button for 4 hours once per day. Do not place a Miso Plaster directly on the belly button. *also* Try the STOMACH MASSAGE.

Dietary Recommendations

The following dietary suggestions are for remedial use until the constipation is over. Then, widen your food choices based on a macrobiotic dietary approach (see page 11).

FOR THE YANG TYPE

☐ Main foods: Brown Rice, Azuki Rice served with a little Gomashio.

☐ Side dishes (one-third of main foods cooked with less salt): Sesame Miso, Natto with Soy Sauce and Scallions or Grated Daikon with Soy Sauce, Burdock Carrot Nitsuke, Eggplant Pressed Salad, Carp Soup, Vegetable Tempura, Azuki Beans with Kombu (for an occasional snack, a little rice syrup can be added to the beans as a sweetener).

☐ Miso soup ingredients: daikon, scallions, string beans, eggplant.

☐ Beverages: Brown Rice Tea, Brown Rice Bancha Tea, Bancha Tea, Vegetable Broth, Grain Coffee.

☐ Avoid especially: all animal protein including fish (except carp) and shellfish, dairy foods, eggs, meat-based soups, all alcohol, all sweet foods (except rice syrup as described above), coffee.

FOR THE YIN TYPE

☐ Main foods: Brown Rice, Azuki Rice. Use Gomashio at each meal.

CORNELLIA'S NATURAL HEALING AT WORK

Sometimes people have constipation when beginning a macrobiotic diet. Don't worry even if it lasts for one week as long as your energy level is good. At the Vega Study Center, one student was constipated for two weeks after beginning the diet. She was very heavy, over 200 pounds, and her intestines were very expanded. I showed her a stomach massage technique (see page 185) and gave her hijiki carrot nitsuke to eat and sour cabbage juice to drink. She started bowel movements again after two days. ■

CONSTIPATION

☐ Side dishes (one-third of main foods): Tekka Miso, Sesame Miso, Hijiki Nitsuke, Vegetable Stew, Azuki Beans with Kombu, Shio Kombu, Vegetable Tempura, Burdock Carrot Nitsuke, Takuan Pickles, Miso Pickles.

☐ Miso soup ingredients: wakame, onions, scallions, string beans, Homemade Agé, winter squash, Brown Rice Mochi.

☐ Beverages: Brown Rice Tea, Umesho Bancha Tea, Brown Rice Bancha Tea, Grain Milk, Bancha Tea.

☐ Avoid especially: all animal foods, red fish, shellfish, dairy foods, eggs, all fruit, all sweet foods, sweet drinks, tomatoes, eggplant, potatoes, vinegar, hot spices, Rice Bran Pickles.

CONVULSIONS, CHILDREN'S

Convulsions are violent involuntary contractions or a series of uncontrolled muscle spasms. According to Western medicine, the cause of children's convulsions is unknown. It is thought that the cause may be a malfunction of the central nervous system. Children's convulsions are indicated by insomnia, teeth grinding, body stiffness, cramps, skin pallor, and foaming from the mouth. Children's convulsions may result in coma.

Another type of convulsion, known as a febrile convulsion, results from a seizure triggered by fever. Symptoms include fever; infection; jerking and twitching of arms, legs, or face for two to three minutes; loss of bladder or bowel control; irritability; and unconsciousness. Febrile convulsions primarily affect children six months to four years of age. Repeated infections may lead to febrile convulsions; thus, reducing the fever of a child who has had convulsions in the past is recommended as a preventative for febrile convulsions.

According to our macrobiotic understanding, the underlying cause of a convulsion is the excessively yin diet of either a mother or a child. A mother may be consuming an excessively yin diet (too many sugary foods and fruits with not enough salt) at the beginning of pregnancy or while she is nursing; a child may also be consuming a diet that is too yin (too many sugary foods, fruits, and cow's milk without enough salt or other yang foods). In the case of convulsions, the symptoms (all yin) lead us to the conclusion that an overly yin diet is the real cause. Insomnia indicates a lack of salt in the diet and therefore a lowered amount of sodium in the blood. A higher proportion of potassium to sodium stimulates the sympathetic nervous system, resulting in muscle tension such as teeth grinding and body stiffness. When the body is overacidic from taking in too much acid-forming food (sugary foods are acid-forming), weakened kid-

---

CORNELLIA'S NATURAL HEALING AT WORK

On June 22nd, 1979, my last day at the Moniteau Farm Summer Camp in Missouri, I was helping in the kitchen when a girl called me to an emergency. A baby, one and a half years old, was having convulsions. The baby had vomited oatmeal from her nose and mouth. Her eyes were blank-looking and her body was limp. I thought this was caused by some trouble in the brain, so I placed my hand on the baby's head. Her head was very hot. We sucked mucus from the baby's nose and she went to sleep. An hour later, the baby had another convulsion. This time the baby's cheeks were trembling and her breathing was very shallow, almost nonexistent. The baby's lips were cut where she had bitten them. I put a couple of drops of fresh ginger juice in the baby's mouth and a hot salt pack on the baby's abdomen to keep her warm. Then Herman arrived and held his cold hand on her head. The convulsions stopped.

The previous day we had had fresh melon for brunch and strawberry shortcake for dinner at the full-moon party. Also, the baby had gone swimming. These three yin factors along with an absence of salt had made the baby's blood too yin (less hemoglobin) and reduced the circulation. These conditions made her unable to stand (see Epilepsy) and, therefore, she could only turn over.

The baby's mother explained that her baby often had convulsions at home. The cause of such convulsions, it seems to me, was that the mother was afraid to give salt to the baby. At one time, I had spoken about how much salt to feed children. I said they need less salt than adults, but I don't recommend a salt-free diet for babies or children. You must think about how much salt your baby needs. Many mothers have a fear of feeding salt to their children.

The mother of this sick baby had smoked marijuana during her pregnancy and stopped when the baby was one year old. If you eat a macrobiotic diet and also smoke marijuana, you cannot make a balance. You will become too yinnized. The mother's marijuana smoking made the baby more yin. In addition, this baby was fed no miso, soy sauce, or salt in any form. So when the baby ate fruit, she became too yin and couldn't stand up. If a proper macrobiotic diet is followed, a child should never have convulsions. ■

CONVULSIONS

---

neys may result, leading to a loss of calcium in order to balance the excess acidity; the end result is cramps. A pale face (skin pallor) signals an anemic condition and the overconsumption of sugary foods. Foaming from the mouth indicates that even the saliva is overly rich in potassium; it is oxidizing in the mouth rather than further on down the alimentary canal. A coma shows an overly acidic condition of brain cells and the intercellular fluid of the brain.

In the case of a febrile convulsion, the fever demonstrates that there is an overgrowth of microbial activity (chemical reactions) caused by an infection. The infection is caused by eating too many yin protein foods such as cow's milk, beans, tofu, and mushrooms along with simple carbohydrates such as sugar, molasses, honey, amasake, fruits, and alcohol. This leads to a higher proportion of potassium to sodium in the blood and muscles. Jerking and twitching occur because the higher proportion of potassium to sodium stimulates the sympathetic nervous system, resulting in muscle contractions. Unconsciousness results from a lack of oxygen in the brain cells because increased muscle contractions use more oxygen. If yang foods, including yang animal foods, are eaten, the amount of sodium in brain cells and muscles increases. This suppresses nerve activities and there is no convulsion or seizure. Thus, this is a condition that results from too much yin, potassium-rich food and not enough yang, sodium-rich food.

Helpful Suggestions

Convulsions caused by fever only are usually not serious. However, the underlying cause should be found and a health-care advisor consulted. The following suggestions are complementary or for when there is no doctor available.

OBJECTIVE	REMEDY
To improve blood circulation	Quietly lay the baby or child on its back. Put a GINGER COMPRESS on the abdomen (see Figure 3.8 on page 176) for 20 minutes, changing towels often to keep the compress warm.
To keep the brain cool	The brain is weakened by the convulsion, so use a cold, wet towel on the head to keep it cool. Place a cool, wet towel on the heart as well to protect it.
To move blood circulation away from the head	Put hot water bottles on the feet and apply a MUSTARD PLASTER to the calves and/or to the bottom of both feet to bring circulation to the lower extremities. Apply once only at the start of the convulsion, removing the plaster after the skin becomes red.
To bring some blood circulation back to the head	Massage and push gently at the base of the skull (see Figure X on page xxx) for 30 minutes.

IF THE CHILD REMAINS UNCONSCIOUS
AND HELP IS STILL UNAVAILABLE

To wake an unconscious child (shock method)	Try squeezing 2 or 3 drops of fresh ginger juice (finely grate ginger and squeeze out the juice) onto a cotton cloth and dabbing the child's tongue with this. Hold a cotton handkerchief between the child's teeth so the child will not bite its tongue. If the child doesn't wake up, it is imperative that medical attention be found immediately. Use the ginger shock method only once.

AFTER THE CONVULSION	
To increase strength	Give 1/3 cup SHO-BAN TEA 1 to 2 times per day for 1 week.
To relieve constipation	Give an ENEMA, but only once.

Dietary Recommendations

Changing your child's dietary choices or yours if you are breastfeeding is a way to achieve lasting results. Cut down on all yin foods while following a macrobiotic dietary approach (see page 11). Especially cut down on all sweet foods including milk, dairy foods, fruit, fruit products, etc. Season food with good-quality miso and soy sauce, and sauté with sesame oil. Eating small dried fish is very helpful. Teach children to chew well.

CORNEAL INFLAMMATION

Inflammation of the cornea is one of the most common corneal diseases. A corneal ulcer refers to any open sore in the thin transparent layers that cover the eye. When the ulcer is accompanied by an acute viral infection, it is called *herpetic keratitis*. Like cold sores in the mouth, these corneal infections tend to recur once the virus has become established. The infection is dangerous in that it can erode the cornea and produce dense scars that impair vision. Symptoms of corneal ulcers and *herpetic keratitis* include: sensitivity to bright light, blurred vision, pain, redness, a feeling of heat behind the eyes, green mucus in the eyes, tearing, and itchiness.

According to modern medicine, corneal ulcers are caused by an injury to the eye, infections that often follow injury but that can occur without injury, and a defective closure of the eyelid. *Herpetic keratitis* is thought to be caused by the herpes simplex virus, although there are many precipitating factors.

According to our macrobiotic understanding, there is both a yin type and a yang type of corneal and eyelid disease. Generally, eating too much fatty animal food overly activates the liver and creates yang eye diseases. The yang condition usually comes on suddenly and is characterized by redness, pain, and a feeling of heat behind the eyes. Sometimes there is fever, as well.

The yin condition is characterized by green mucus in the eyes, no pain, and sometimes tearing of itchy eyes. The yin condition usually develops more gradually and is caused by the intake of too much yin food such as sweets, soft drinks, and chemicalized foods. Many eye problems are a result of overeating fruit and a lack of

---

CORNELLIA'S NATURAL HEALING AT WORK

During the 1981 French Meadows summer camp, a fire spark flew into and burned a friend's eye. I looked for and found a mother who was nursing at that time. She was kind enough to supply some of her breast milk to apply into my friend's eye. I put a cabbage leaf over the eye and a triangle bandage over that to hold the leaf in place. By the next morning, the eye was completely normal. If no breast milk is available, use your finger to put one drop of sterilized sesame oil in the corner of your eye before going to sleep.   ■

CORNEAL INFLAMATION

---

good-quality vegetable oil in the diet. Macrobiotic theory recommends that you stop eating fruit and use good-quality sesame oil in cooking if you have any eye problem.

Helpful Suggestions

The following suggestions are useful for both yin and yang types of corneal inflammation or other eye problems.

OBJECTIVE	REMEDY
To relieve mild pain	Try using a BANCHA TEA EYE COMPRESS 4 times per day for 10 minutes at a time until the pain stops. *also* Until you have recovered, you can use a SESAME OIL EYE TREATMENT before going to sleep every night.
To relieve severe pain and eye infection	You can use an ALBI PLASTER with the albi on the outside of the cloth (not touching the skin of the eyelid) or use an UMEBOSHI EYE PLASTER for 4 hours or overnight until pain stops. This treatment is also effective for bloodshot eyes.
To reduce heat behind the eyes	Place a small ALBI PLASTER on both temples and a TOFU PLASTER on both eyes. Change the tofu every hour and the albi every 4 hours. *or* If you have no tofu, you can place a 1/4-inch-thick piece of any red meat on the eyelids. Change this 3 to 4 times a day.
To reduce high fever	Place a TOFU PLASTER on the forehead and change this every 2 hours. *and* Between Tofu Plaster changes, lightly rub good-quality sesame oil onto the eyelids and then reapply the tofu plaster.
To improve circulation	Use a GINGER COMPRESS for 20 minutes on the shoulders, and the eye trouble will be helped by the improved blood circulation.

Dietary Recommendations

Use the following dietary suggestions until the eyes have recovered or for two to three weeks. Then, widen your food choices using a macrobiotic dietary approach (see page 11).

FOR THE YANG TYPE

☐ Main foods: Brown Rice, Brown Rice with Barley in 3 to 1 proportion, Azuki Rice, and a little Gomashio.

☐ Side dishes (one-third of main foods and less salty): Ginger Miso, Miso Soup, Okara Nitsuke, natto served with Grated Daikon, Boiled Daikon served with Lemon Miso, Vegetable Tempura, Tofu with Kuzu Sauce, Pressed Salad.

☐ Miso soup ingredients: tofu, daikon, daikon greens, spinach, string beans, sweet potatoes or yams, burdock, other seasonal vegetables, Homemade Agé.

☐ Beverages: Bancha Tea, Brown Rice Tea, Grain Coffee, Vegetable Broth. Drink a maximum of 3 cups of beverages per day.

☐ Avoid especially: all meat, chicken, pork, eggs, cheese, fish, shellfish, all dairy foods including ice cream, all sweet foods and drinks, coffee, and hot spices.

FOR THE YIN TYPE

☐ Main foods: Brown Rice, Azuki Rice, a little Gomashio as a condiment.

☐ Side dishes (one-fourth of main foods with a little more salt than used for yang eye troubles): Tekka Miso, Oily Miso, Hijiki Burdock Nitsuke, Hijiki Lotus Root Nitsuke, Hijiki Carrot Nitsuke, Carp Soup, Burdock Carrot Nitsuke, Deep-Fried Kombu, Nori Roasted with Oil, Vegetable Tempura, Miso Pickles, and Rice Bran Pickles.

☐ Miso soup ingredients: wakame, tororo kombu, scallions, onions, burdock, Brown Rice Mochi.

☐ Beverages: Sho-Ban Tea, Kombu Tea, Bancha Tea with Gomashio, Grain Milk. Drink a maximum of 2 cups of beverages per day.

☐ Avoid especially: all animal foods, fish (except in carp soup), shellfish, all dairy foods, eggs, fruit, sweet foods including honey, molasses, coffee, potatoes, melons, tomatoes, mushrooms, eggplant, alcoholic drinks, hot spices.

CORNS AND CALLUSES

Corns are thickening of the skin, usually over bony areas such as toe joints. Corns may be painful, irritated, and swollen. A callus is a thickening of the skin that is caused by repeated irritation or pressure. Usually a callus is not painful. Corns are usually confined to the feet, while calluses can occur on any part of the body that experiences repeated pressure or irritation. The hands, feet, and knees are the most likely places. Pain in other body areas such as the back, hips, knees, or ankles may result from a change in the way you walk due to the uncomfortable feeling of the corn or callus.

According to our macrobiotic understanding, corns and calluses are much more likely if one is eating too much protein and cholesterol-rich foods, especially eggs and fish. When an area is subjected to repeated irritation, corns and calluses are formed by the body to help protect the skin from injury. Excess protein and cholesterol give the body an excess of building materials, and corns and calluses tend to form in order to rid the body of this excess when it is not necessary for the body to protect itself. Pressure in the area results in the faster growth rate of cells and eventually in an overgrowth of cells. Again, if the body has an excess of material, more corns and calluses tend to form.

Helpful Suggestions

Corns and calluses may take three to four weeks to heal once the source of the pressure or irritation is removed. However, if the underlying cause of too much protein and cholesterol foods is not controlled, recurrence is very likely.

OBJECTIVE	REMEDY
To dissolve the corn or callus	Try lightly rubbing it each day with the fleshy side of a cross-section cut off the bottom of an eggplant or with a piece of orange rind (peel) each day until the corn or callus is dissolved.
	and
	Drinking 1 cup of *HATOMUGI TEA* 2 to 3 times per day, eating 1 serving of *HATOMUGI* (pressure-cooked or boiled) every other day, or eating 1 serving of *BROWN RICE WITH HATOMUGI* every day until the corn or callus is smooth may be helpful.

Dietary Recommendations

Follow a macrobiotic dietary approach (see page 11) with an emphasis on low-protein foods until your condition is more balanced.

☐ Avoid especially: high-cholesterol foods such as eggs.

DANDRUFF

Dandruff refers to small, flaking, white snowlike particles from the scalp due to abnormal secretion of the sebaceous (oil) glands. These particles may cause itching and a burning sensation. According to our macrobiotic understanding, people with hot heads are more likely to have dandruff. A normal healthy condition is a cool head and warm feet. This means the blood circulation is good. If the head is hot and the feet are cold, the blood circulation is bad. The main cause of the bad circulation is eating too much fatty or oily food. Thus, a diet with more beans and animal foods such as meat, dairy products, and fish than whole grains contributes to dandruff.

Helpful Suggestions

Avoid shampoos that contain chemicals. Exposure to the sun helps some people and aggravates the condition in others.

OBJECTIVE	REMEDY
To alkalize the scalp	Try washing your hair with the water from a BATH of PEACH LEAVES, PINE NEEDLES, or CHESTNUT LEAVES every day until you have no more dandruff.

Dietary Recommendations

Follow a macrobiotic dietary approach (see page 11) with plenty of sea vegetables and less fatty or oily foods. Side dishes should be in smaller amounts than whole grains.

DENTAL CARIES (TOOTH DECAY)

Dental caries (cavities) refer to a disintegration of tooth enamel, allowing injury to the layers beneath the surface. Tooth decay is one of the most common disorders in humans. Symptoms include tooth discomfort, especially after eating refined sugar; tooth sensitivity to heat and cold; unpleasant taste in the mouth; and a darkening on the tooth or between the teeth. Eventually, the pulp of the tooth, which contains nerves and blood vessels, becomes involved and persistent tooth pain results. If left untreated, the death of the tooth is the final outcome. The cause of cavities is acid that is produced by bacteria in the mouth. Thus, good dental habits go a long way toward prevention of dental caries. However, a proper diet is also needed.

According to our macrobiotic understanding, the underlying cause of dental caries is the overconsumption of refined sugar and sweet foods. Such foods create a mineral imbalance in the body, and calcium is leached out of the teeth to restore balance. The leaching of calcium leads to the disintegration of enamel layers beneath the surface. Calcium is the most abundant alkaline-forming mineral in the body; when an overly acidic condition from eating too much acid-forming food such as meat and sugar is perpetuated, calcium loss occurs in both bone and teeth. A common cold and bad blood circulation can also cause tooth pain.

Helpful Suggestions

If you have a cavity, go to the dentist. If that makes you nervous, drink one cup of UMEBOSHI TEA before going to help you feel more relaxed. The following suggestions are supplemental for tooth pain and should not replace proper care of dental caries.

OBJECTIVE	REMEDY
To relieve pain	Try using a WOOD ASH WATER TREATMENT 3 times per day.
	and/or
	Apply CHARCOALED KOMBU directly to the tooth or cavity.
	or
	You can try a MUSTARD POWDER APPLICATION for 5 to 7 minutes and the pain should stop.
	or
	Gently rubbing dentie powder into the gums 3 times per day using your index finger may be helpful for pain.
To relieve a child's pain from a cavity	Finely grate an onion and squeeze out the juice. Soak a cotton ball in the onion juice and place the cotton ball on the cavity. Use new cotton balls as often as needed.

Dietary Recommendations

To help prevent future cavities, follow a macrobiotic dietary approach (see page 11), eating more sea vegetables than usual. Avoid simple sugars, especially refined sugar and fresh fruit.

DEPRESSION

Depression is a feeling of continuing sadness or hope-lessness and usually results in a lowering or decrease of functional ability. Some signs of depression include chronic fatigue, insomnia or excessive sleeping, loss of appetite or overeating, loss of sex drive, headaches, loss of interest in life, social isolation, irritability, colon dis-orders, feelings of worthlessness and inadequacy, and difficulty concentrating and making decisions. Oftentimes there are intense guilt feelings over minor mistakes or unexplained bouts of crying. The recovery rate is high, even though it is hard to realize this fact while you are depressed. Still, recurrence is common, especially if the underlying condtions are not dealt with and changed.

According to our macrobiotic understanding, depres-sion is an extremely yin condition. Depression is more likely in winter months when the nights are longer and the days are darker and colder (all yin conditions). Psychologically, the causes of an extreme yin condition such as depression are loss of a loved one, divorce, fail-ure in business, loss of something important in life, exces-sive stress, and worry over a major illness or disability. Physically, the cause is an overly acidic condition of nerve and brain cells, leading to a malfunction of enzymes and finally a lack of glucose and/or oxygen supply to the brain. An overly acidic condition results from the long-term reliance on a diet high in refined sugar and fat, such as a fast-food diet. This poor diet can lead to nutrition-al deficiencies, upset stomach, tension headaches, thy-roid disorders, endometriosis, or allergies all resulting, finally, in depression. Depression itself, along with any of the psychological events listed above, adds to the acidic condition of nerve cells, making depression very diffi-cult to remedy.

Helpful Suggestions

If these suggestions and a change in dietary habits don't relieve the depression or if you have a severe case, con-sult a medical practitioner.

OBJECTIVE	REMEDY
To rectify a mineral imbalance	Taking a 1 percent SALT BATH once a day can help restore mineral balance.
To relieve depression	Take a vacation or trip, or find a hobby or activity that interests you. Try to maintain good communication with family and friends and keep active; attend social func-tions even though you may not feel like it.

Regular strenuous, aerobic exercise helps to relieve depression. Try to avoid situations that are overly stressful for you.

Dietary Recommendations

A change to a macrobiotic dietary approach (see page 11) will be most helpful. Avoid sugar, sugary foods, fruits, fruit juices, and fatty foods. Eat 4 to 5 small dried fish every day. This will aid blood formation and, in turn, supply glucose and oxygen to the blood and brain.

DIABETES, INSULIN-DEPENDENT

Diabetes is a general term referring to metabolic disor-ders characterized by excessive urine excretion. Insulin-dependent diabetes mellitus is a chronic pancreatic disease in which the pancreas cannot produce enough insulin to efficiently process carbohydrates, fat, and protein. Although insulin-dependent diabetes usually begins before the age of thirty, it may appear at any age. If it begins in childhood, it is known as juvenile diabetes. A person with insulin-dependent diabetes may exhibit the following conditions: fatigue; excessive thirst; excessive or frequent urination; passing sugar in the urine; exces-sive hunger and weight loss even though one eats a lot of food; increased susceptibility to infections, especially urinary-tract infections and yeast infections of the vagi-na, skin, or mouth; and a deterioration of vision in the advanced stages.

Although one cause of diabetes is thought to be an insufficient production of insulin, the reason for this is unknown. A second cause is interference with the use of insulin in the body cells, again for unknown reasons. A viral infection in the pancreas can result in the symp-toms of diabetes. The usual approach to diabetes is the prescription of insulin injections and a carefully con-trolled special diet. This enables one to control the symp-toms and progress of the diabetes, but does nothing to cure the underlying causes. Diabetes is the third leading cause of death in the United States and the possibilities of many life-threatening complications, such as various cardiovascular diseases, kidney failure, hypoglycemia, and very high blood sugar (ketoacidosis), should be con-sidered and understood.

According to our macrobiotic understanding, insulin-dependent diabetes results from the long-term overcon-sumption of simple carbohydrate (sugary) foods and drinks along with the overconsumption of fatty foods.

The overconsumption of simple carbohydrates as opposed to complex carbohydrates such as whole grains leads to chaotic blood sugar levels and weakens the pancreas' ability to produce insulin. Without insulin, the body cannot utilize glucose properly, and the result is a high level of glucose in the blood with a low level of glucose absorption by the tissues. The overconsumption of fatty foods results in too much fat in the blood stream. In this case, there may be enough insulin but the glucose gets covered by the excess fat and is unable to pass through the membranes of the blood vessels and cells.

Dietary Recommendations

The macrobiotic approach emphasizes a diet that is low in fat, protein, and simple carbohydrates while high in complex carbohydrates. In fact, the macrobiotic dietary approach results in a fat intake of 20 percent of caloric intake as opposed to the 40 percent intake of a typical American meat-and-sugar diet. The following dietary suggestions may be used until the symptoms improve or for about one month. Then, widen your food choices using a macrobiotic dietary approach (see page 11). Consult your health-care advisor if you are already taking insulin or if you are already in the advanced stages of disease.

☐ Main foods: Brown Rice, Millet Rice, Azuki Rice, Sweet Brown Rice, Brown Rice Mochi, and Gomashio every meal. Chew each mouthful 200 times.

☐ Side dishes (one-third of main foods): Tekka Miso, Scallion Miso, Shio Kombu, Hijiki Nitsuke, Carp Soup, Vegetable Stew with Fish, Baked White Fish, Poached Fish, Azuki Beans with Kombu and Winter Squash, Vegetable Tempura, Deep-Fried Kombu, Burdock Carrot Nitsuke, Takuan Pickles, Miso Pickles.

☐ Miso soup ingredients: wakame, tororo kombu, scallions, onions, dried daikon, Homemade Agé, Brown Rice Mochi.

☐ Beverages: Brown Rice Tea, Brown Rice Bancha Tea, Bancha Tea, Kombu Tea, Mu Tea. Drink a maximum of 2 cups of beverages per day.

☐ Avoid especially: all animal foods, shellfish, red-meat fish, all dairy foods (including ice cream), all sweet foods and drinks, all fruit, vinegar, hot spices, tomatoes, potatoes, eggplant, melons, all mushrooms. Be sure to avoid vinegar and vinegar salad dressings as they are very bad for this condition.

DIABETES, NON-INSULIN-DEPENDENT

Non-insulin-dependent diabetes is a type of diabetes mellitus characterized by the inability of the body to produce enough insulin to efficiently process carbohydrates, fat, and protein. While the causes, possible complications, and symptoms are very similar to insulin-dependent diabetes, the major differences are that non-insulin-dependent diabetes begins in adulthood, mostly occurs in obese adults, and sometimes does not require insulin injections. Weight loss, exercise, and diet can often control this form of diabetes. However, this is often difficult because one of the symptoms is increased appetite.

Read the entire section entitled Diabetes, Insulin-Dependent for a full explanation of our macrobiotic understanding and suggestions. In the case of non-insulin-dependent diabetes, however, it is the overconsumption of fatty foods that is the primary cause since eating fatty foods is directly related to obesity. If you have eaten large quantities of simple carbohydrates and small amounts of fatty foods, you are more likely to have insulin-dependent diabetes.

Dietary Recommendations

Use the following dietary suggestions until your condition improves or for about one month. Then, widen your food choices based on a macrobiotic dietary approach (see page 11). The macrobiotic approach is generally successful when used to help control one's weight. If it doesn't work for you, find some manner of exercise and life-style change to control your weight.

☐ Main foods: Brown Rice, Azuki Rice, Brown Rice with Barley, Udon Noodles. Chew each mouthful 200 times.

☐ Side dishes (one-fourth of main foods cooked with less salt than usual): Sesame Miso, Ginger Miso, Okara Nitsuke, Soybean Soup, Carp Soup, Hijiki Burdock Nitsuke, Burdock Carrot Nitsuke, Azuki Beans with Kombu and Winter Squash, Vegetable Tempura, Eggplant Nitsuke with Miso, Cucumber Pressed Salad, Shiitake Nitsuke.

☐ Miso soup ingredients: daikon, string beans, summer and winter squash, tofu, eggplant.

☐ Beverages: Vegetable Broth, Brown Rice Broth, Brown Rice Bancha Tea, Bancha Tea, Grain Coffee. Drink a maximum of 2½ cups of beverages per day.

☐ Avoid especially: all animal foods including fish, shellfish, dairy foods (including ice cream), eggs, meat-based soups; all alcohol; sweet foods and drinks; vinegar; black tea; coffee.

DIARRHEA

Diarrhea is an abnormally frequent evacuation of watery feces. Diarrhea is not a disease but rather a symptom associated with many diseases. Oftentimes diarrhea is the body's way of ridding itself of toxins and shouldn't be stopped unless it lasts longer than forty-eight hours. If your eliminations have a green color, bad smell, and mucus, it means your stomach is weak and is not digesting food properly. A high fever; mucus, blood, or worms in the stool; severe pain; and dehydration are signs that more is involved and a health-care advisor should be contacted. Young children may have a chronic, nonspecific diarrhea whereby they have more than five watery or loose stools per day. If they are healthy and maintaining normal growth and development patterns, this is nothing to worry about; it may take a couple of years before bowel movements become normal. Any signs of disease, listlessness, lack of appetite, or abnormal growth and development need to be carefully watched, however.

According to our macrobiotic understanding, there are two types of diarrhea, yang and yin. If you have diarrhea and also have a good appetite and energy, this is a yang type of diarrhea and there is no need to worry. If you have no energy, then it is more serious. This is yin diarrhea. If the diarrhea lasts longer than two days, a disease of the yin type is indicated; see the Enteritis section in addition to the suggestions below.

Helpful Suggestions

If a mother is nursing a baby, she should avoid extreme yin or yang foods and drinks.

OBJECTIVE	REMEDY
FOR THE YANG TYPE	
To contract large intestine	Try eating ½ of a sour apple and drinking ½ cup of SOUR APPLE JUICE 2 or 3 times for 1 day.
	and
	If diarrhea continues a second day, eat a baked apple that day. Avoid hot baths.
FOR THE YIN TYPE	
To improve poor eliminations that have a green color, bad smell, and/or mucus	Drink 1 cup of KUZU BANCHA TEA WITH GINGER 2 to 3 times per day until elimination improves.
	and
	If poor elimination continues, add ½ teaspoon of CHARCOALED UMEBOSHI to the tea.

or

	Ume extract is good; eat a soybean-sized ball either plain or mixed in ⅓ cup of warm water. Take this 30 minutes before meals until elimination improves.
To warm cold feet associated with diarrhea	Use a FOOT BATH as often as desired.
	and
	Try using a GINGER COMPRESS on the stomach (see Figure 3.8 on page 176) for 20 minutes once a day to keep warm. This is most helpful.
To increase appetite	Eat 1 cup of thick KUZU SOUP 2 to 3 times per day until diarrhea stops.
	and
	If desired, 2 to 3 times per day, try eating 1 to 2 cups of BROWN RICE (cooked to a very soft consistency) or BROWN RICE CREAM WITH UMEBOSHI cooked for at least 1 hour.
	and
	Drink 1 cup of BROWN RICE TEA 2 to 3 times per day.
	and
	Apply a GINGER COMPRESS to the intestines (see Figure 3.8 on page 176) for 20 minutes 1 or 2 times per day.
FOR CHILDREN'S DIARRHEA	
To contract large intestine	Give 1 tablespoon of SWEET UMEBOSHI JUICE 2 to 3 times per day.

Dietary Recommendations

Use the following dietary suggestions during periods of diarrhea; in the case of the yang type, this is a two-day maximum. Then, widen your food choices using a macrobiotic dietary approach (see page 11).

FOR THE YIN TYPE

☐ Main foods: Brown Rice Gruel with Miso, Brown Rice Gruel with Mochi and Scallions, Brown Rice Balls with Gomashio, Azuki Rice Balls with Gomashio (use 1 teaspoon of Gomashio for each rice ball). Chew each mouthful 200 times. Gradually increase the amount of salt in your cooking.

☐ Side dishes (one-fourth of main foods): Shio Kombu, Umeboshi, Takuan Pickles, Miso Pickles.

☐ Miso soup ingredients: wakame, scallions, onions, Homemade Agé, Brown Rice Mochi.

☐ Beverages: Brown Rice Tea with Umeboshi, Umesho Bancha, Sho-Ban Tea, Brown Rice Bancha Tea, Kuzu Bancha Tea, Grain Coffee.

☐ Avoid especially: all animal foods, fish, shellfish, dairy foods, meat-based soups, black teas, all fruit and sweet foods, alcohol, mushrooms, melons, vinegar, tomatoes, hot spices, Rice Bran Pickles.

FOR THE YANG TYPE

☐ Main foods: Brown Rice Cream, Brown Rice Kayu, Brown Rice Gruel with Mochi served with a little soy sauce. Use less salt in your cooking.

☐ Side dishes (one-fourth of the main foods): Grated Daikon with Soy Sauce, Dried Daikon Nitsuke, Daikon Nit-suke, Eggplant Mustard Pickles, Pressed Salad, Sour Cabbage, Takuan Pickles.

☐ Miso soup ingredients: daikon, daikon greens, cabbage and other white vegetables, green leafy vegetables, scallions, Homemade Agé, Brown Rice Mochi.

☐ Beverages: Umesho Bancha Tea, Brown Rice Tea, Grain Coffee, Kuzu Bancha Tea. Drink a maximum of 2½ cups of beverages per day.

☐ Avoid especially: all animal protein including fish, shellfish, milk, all dairy, meat-based soups, alcohol, all sweet foods.

DIPHTHERIA

Diphtheria is a highly contagious throat infection caused by the diphtheria bacteria *(Corynebacterium diphtheriae)*, which produces toxins that destroy tissue and poisons that may spread to the heart, central nervous system, and other organs. This bacteria attacks the mucous membranes, primarily of the nose, throat, or larynx. Diphtheria may begin with a sore throat, followed by fever, headaches, vomiting, and bad mouth odor. The voice is husky, swallowing is difficult, and the throat is swollen. There is usually pain and loss of voice; respiratory obstruction can occur when the membranes of the larynx are affected. In late stages, breathing is blocked and difficult and shock may result. A delay in treatment may result in long-term heart disease or death.

There are, however, many children who do not suffer from diphtheria even though they contract the diphtheria bacteria. According to our macrobiotic understanding, the underlying cause of susceptibility to this bacteria is in one's eating habits, especially in the overconsumption of sweet foods, including fruit, along with eating too much animal food. This kind of diet provides excess protein (building materials) and an environment in which bacteria (microbes) thrive and grow.

Helpful Suggestions

Diphtheria is a medical emergency and hospitalization is usually required. The suggestions given here are supplemental to the instructions of your doctor and local health department.

OBJECTIVE	REMEDY
To reduce swelling in the throat	GARGLE with *BANCHA TEA WITH SALT* 3 times per day.
To lower fever	Try drinking 1 cup of *DAIKON GINGER TEA* 3 times per day, or for a weak child, use ½ cup of *BROWN RICE TEA WITH DRIED PERSIMMON AND TANGERINE SKIN* 3 times per day.

Dietary Recommendations

Use the following suggestions until the symptoms subside or for about one month. Then, widen your food choices using a macrobiotic dietary approach (see page 11).

☐ Main foods: Brown Rice Cream, Mochi Soup with Miso, Azuki Rice, vegetable soup with miso.

☐ Side dishes (one-third of main foods): daikon, turnips, or burdock (see Waterless Cooked Vegetables), or Green Leafy Vegetables with Mock Goose served with Grated Daikon with Soy Sauce.

☐ Miso soup ingredients: wakame, tororo kombu, daikon.

☐ Beverages: Bancha Tea, Sho-Ban Tea, Brown Rice Bancha Tea, Brown Rice Tea, Brown Rice Broth.

☐ Avoid especially: all sweet foods and drinks, all animal foods including eggs.

DIVERTICULAR DISEASE

Diverticulosis is the presence of variable-sized pouches or saclike swellings (diverticula) in the wall of the large intestines. The number of diverticula in the large intestine increases with age. They are present in 30 to 40 percent of persons over the age of fifty. Although the cause is considered to be unknown, recent evidence shows that a diet high in refined foods and lacking in dietary fiber contributes to the formation of diverticula. There are usually no symptoms or indications of the presence of diverticula. However, there may be a mild cramping in the left side of the abdomen that is relieved with bowel movements or passing gas, constipation, or occasionally bright red blood in the stool.

Diverticulitis is the inflammation of diverticula characterized by intermittent cramping, abdominal pain that becomes constant, nausea, fever, chills, and tenderness over the left side of the large intestine. A poor diet lacking in fiber, family history of the disease, gallbladder disease, obesity, and coronary artery disease increase the possibility of developing diverticular disease.

A macrobiotic dietary approach is high in fiber and low in fat so the long-term effect is a greatly reduced risk of diverticular disease. Keeping active—which helps ensure good cardiovascular fitness—also is important. A diet high in fat, especially from animal foods, contributes to blood-vessel disorders and may also contribute to diverticular disease. Excessive amounts of animal foods contribute to the possibility of infections. Once the diverticula become infected, they may erode the intestinal wall and cause greater damage.

Helpful Suggestions

Try to have a bowel movement at the same time each day and avoid straining. If you notice blood in your stool or it is black, take a portion of it to your health-care advisor for analysis.

OBJECTIVE	REMEDY
To relieve pain	Apply a GINGER COMPRESS over the left side of the abdomen (see Figure 3.8 on page 176) for 20 minutes or a CASTOR OIL COMPRESS for 30 minutes whenever you have pain. *and* Give yourself a STOMACH MASSAGE, paying particular attention to the left side of the abdomen.

Dietary Recommendations

The best remedy for diverticular disease is an improved diet with plenty of fiber. Follow a macrobiotic dietary approach (see page 11) with an emphasis on more yang foods such as miso and tekka. If your case is advanced, use rice cream or very soft cooked grains along with plenty of vegetables. Eating less or fasting may be beneficial if your condition allows it.

☐ Avoid especially meats and other animal products including dairy foods, sugary foods, and refined foods.

DYSENTERY, ADULTS'

Dysentery is a term used for a number of disorders characterized by inflammation of the intestines and caused by chemical irritants, bacteria, protozoa, or parasitic worms. The two specific varieties are amebic and bacillary. While our discussion here concerns bacillary dysentery, the suggestions are helpful for any type. Dysentery results in a loss of water from the body along with diarrhea, watery bowel movements up to 20 or more times

per day; blood, mucus, or pus in the stool; nausea; vomiting; and abdominal cramps.

The Western medical view identifies the bacteria *Shigella bacillus* as the cause of bacillary dysentery. While this bacteria may be involved in the infection, according to our macrobiotic understanding, the infection occurs when a person's blood is too yin from eating too much sugary food and fruit, and has lost its natural immunity to the bacteria. The long-term effect of such a diet makes one susceptible to all forms of dysentery.

Helpful Suggestions

Bed rest is important until the symptoms have been gone for about three days. Exercise your legs while in bed. Seek medical attention if you become dangerously dehydrated or severely ill.

OBJECTIVE	REMEDY
To weaken bacteria	Try drinking 1 cup of UMESHO BANCHA TEA 3 times per day until the bacteria are weakened and symptoms subside.
To alleviate diarrhea	After eating and until the diarrhea stops, eat a soybean-sized ball of UME EXTRACT. (Ume Extract can be used to reduce a high fever that results from weak intestines.)
To stop vomiting and cramps	A DAIKON or ARAME HIP BATH WITH MUSTARD POWDER is helpful. Stay in this bath for 7 to 8 minutes. Then, after the bath, place a ROASTED SALT PACK on the abdomen (see Figure 3.8 on page 176) for 10 minutes and keep warm.

Dietary Recommendations

Use the following dietary suggestions until the symptoms have been gone for several days. Then, follow a macrobiotic dietary approach (see page 11).

☐ Main foods: Brown Rice Balls, Brown Rice Gruel with Grated Daikon, Homemade Agé (cooked with less salt than usual), Brown Rice Gruel with Mochi, Brown Rice Gruel with Miso, Brown Rice Mochi. To improve appetite serve Brown Rice Cream (thick) only.
☐ Side dishes (less than one-fourth of main foods): Grated Daikon with Soy Sauce, Ginger Miso, Umeboshi, Eggplant Mustard Pickles, Takuan Pickles.
☐ Miso soup ingredients: daikon, Homemade Agé, scallions.
☐ Beverages: Brown Rice Tea, Brown Rice Bancha Tea, Bancha Tea, Grain Coffee.
☐ Avoid especially: overly yin or yang foods (especially sugars or meats).

DYSENTERY, CHILDREN'S

Children also may suffer from dysentery. It develops very quickly and can be fatal because of severe dehydration. Similar to adult dysentery, it is caused by eating too much fruit and/or sugary foods combined with eating too much animal food. Symptoms include dehydration; diarrhea, watery bowel movements up to 20 or more times per day; blood, mucus, or pus in the stool; nausea; vomiting; and abdominal cramps.

Helpful Suggestions

OBJECTIVE	REMEDY
To reduce fever	Try placing a TOFU PLASTER on the forehead and one on the chest, changing each every hour.
To relieve stomachache and diarrhea	Use a MUSTARD POWDER or GINGER WATER HIP BATH for 20 minutes once a day.
To alleviate dry mouth	Give the child 1/3 to 1/2 cup of UMEBOSHI JUICE TEA depending on age (younger or more frail children use the lesser amount), or you can substitute UMESHO BANCHA TEA.
To relieve a cold belly due to dehydration	Use a ROASTED SALT PACK on the belly and a hot water bottle on the feet.
To improve overall condition	Drink 1/3 to 1/2 cup of UME EXTRACT TEA 2 to 3 times per day.

CORNELLIA'S NATURAL HEALING AT WORK

A friend from Seattle once told me that a three-year-old boy in her community had died. After hearing his symptoms, I said I thought that maybe the cause was dysentery. At that time, a spiritual leader from India was staying with the community in Seattle, and the families were serving dairy and fruit since he was accustomed to having these things. I think this might have been the reason dysentery started. My friend was involved with a macrobiotic kindergarten at the time, and I recommended that she give all the children ume extract every day to prevent this disease. No other children got dysentery.

If a child has dysentery, it may indicate that the whole family has a weakened condition, especially if they are sharing the same diet. In such a case, I recommend that all the family members take umeboshi or ume extract, and that they always have a bottle of the extract in their house. Umeboshi plums are too salty for children, but they can take ume extract.   ■

DYSENTERY, CHILDREN'S

Dietary Recommendations

To protect a child from dysentery, avoid all raw fruit. When starting the child on solid foods, take care of the quality and the quantity of the food given to the child. Give small amounts and teach your child to chew well. To control dysentery, fasting is best if the child's condition allows it. If the child is hungry, give Brown Rice Cream or Mochi Soup to eat or Kuzu Bancha Tea to drink. Slowly change to a macrobiotic dietary approach as the condition improves.

If fasting is not desired, use the following suggstions until several days after the dysentery symptoms have subsided. Then, slowly change to a macrobiotic dietary approach (see page 11). Follow these suggestions yourself if you are breastfeeding a baby with dysentery.

☐ Main foods: Brown Rice, Azuki Rice, Mochi Soup, Baked Mochi with Soy Sauce.
☐ Side dishes (one-fourth of main foods): Tekka Miso, kombu, Nori Nitsuke, Shio Kombu, Hijiki Nitsuke, Burdock Carrot Nitsuke served with Umeboshi.
☐ Miso soup ingredients: wakame, tororo kombu, onions, scallions, Homemade Agé, Brown Rice Mochi.
☐ Beverages: Brown Rice Cream, Brown Rice Tea, Grain Milk.
☐ Avoid especially: all animal food including dairy foods (ice cream), all baby formulas, sweet foods, all fruit, melons, tomatoes, eggplant, potatoes, all beans, vinegar, cocoa.

See also DYSENTERY, ADULTS'.

EAR INFECTIONS

Inflammations and infections may occur in the middle or outer ear canals. Middle-ear infections are most common among infants and children but all ages may be affected. Symptoms include an earache, a feeling of fullness or pressure in the ear, some hearing loss, discharge from the ear, diarrhea (sometimes), and a fever of 103°F or more. Middle-ear infections are commonly thought to be caused by bacteria or viruses in the nose and throat, blockage caused by allergies or enlarged adenoids, or a ruptured eardrum. Chronic middle-ear infections may result from repeated infections that cause the adenoids to become enlarged.

Outer-ear infections are characterized by ear pain that worsens when the earlobe is pulled, slight fever, discharge of pus from the ear, and temporary loss of hearing. The Western medical view suggests that outer-ear infections are caused by swimming in dirty water, polluted by bacteria or fungi; excessive swimming in chlorinated pools; or excessive moisture.

However, according to our macrobiotic understanding, the fundamental cause is eating too much sugary food such as ice cream and fruits, which create an environment conducive to microorganism growth in the body. For most of my American friends, ear trouble in general is caused by consuming too much chemically processed dairy food. These foods not only make the body more susceptible to bacteria, fungi, and viruses, but also damage the kidneys. From a macrobiotic perspective, all ear trouble is connected with weak kidneys. To me, if a child has mucus or wax running out of his or her ears, this is a sign of kidney trouble. Ear problems may also be brought on by cold weather.

Helpful Suggestions

OBJECTIVE	REMEDY
To reduce general pain in ears	Try using a ROASTED SALT PACK over the ears. or If you have been eating meat and dairy products, a salt pack might be painful; in this instance use a TOFU PLASTER, changing it every hour until the pain stops.
To relieve adult ear trouble	The APPLICATION of a drop of GINGER SESAME OIL inside the ear 3 times per day is helpful for any ear trouble experienced by adults.
To relieve children's ear trouble	Avoid putting drops or cotton balls in the ears of children. You may use the packs and plasters, but it is best to consult a doctor for children's ear troubles especially if the packs and plasters do not work.
To control adult ear infection	Try a GINGER SESAME OIL EAR TREATMENT for 2 to 3 hours, 3 times per day. This is also beneficial for ringing in the ears.
To control infection with pain	Use a ROASTED SALT PACK or TOFU PLASTER as described above. then After the pain is gone, an ALBI PLASTER applied around the ear (not directly over the ear opening), changed every 4 hours during the day and left on through the night, helps remove any blockage.
To improve the kidneys	Apply a GINGER COMPRESS on top of the kidneys (see Figure 3.8 on page 176) for 10 to 20 minutes every day. and Take a 1 percent SALT BATH for 30 minutes several times a week.

CORNELLIA'S NATURAL HEALING AT WORK

I remember taking care of a three-year-old American girl for three months while she was away from her parents. When her father returned to stay with us, pus started running from the girl's ear. Her father thought my cooking was too salty, so he tried a salt-free diet with her. When her father went to work, she would try to open the cabinet to dip her fingers in the miso and salt bins. One night, I served three-year-old daikon miso pickles. She ate them. I told her they were too salty. She said, "No, Mommy," (she called me mommy) "they are not too salty, they are very sweet." She ate them again the next morning. After two weeks, her ears stopped running completely. Her father said that her mother often gave the child cow's milk.

The condition of the ear is connected to the health of the kidneys, so if the kidneys are weak and cannot clean up toxins, the excess comes out the ear. If your children want miso, soy sauce, or sea salt, give it to them. Children don't have a knowledge of yin and yang, but they have very important natural senses and instincts. Even if they crave water after eating miso or soy sauce, continue giving the miso or soy sauce and water to them because they need new salt to replace old salts, especially when the old salts are of lesser quality. ■

EAR INFECTIONS

Dietary Recommendations

See the section on Kidney Failure for specific dietary suggestions to improve the condition of the kidneys. Otherwise, follow a macrobiotic dietary approach (see page 11). In more severe or recurring cases, use the following dietary suggestions until the symptoms improve or for one month.

☐ Main foods: Brown Rice with Barley (3 to 1), Azuki Rice, Brown Rice Cream (thick), Gomashio. Chew each mouthful 100 times.
☐ Side dishes (one-third of main foods): Carp Soup 2 to 3 times every day, Burdock Lotus Root Nitsuke, Burdock Nitsuke, and Hijiki Nitsuke. Use sesame oil and cook foods for a long time. Always eat warm food, never cold, if you have ear problems.
☐ Miso soup ingredients: wakame, daikon, turnips.
☐ Beverages: Sho-Ban Tea, Bancha Tea, Kombu Tea.
☐ Avoid especially: all meat, red-meat fish, chicken, dairy, all sweet foods and drinks, all fruit. Eggs are especially bad.

EARDRUM, RUPTURED

The middle ear is separated from the outer ear by a thin membrane (tympanic membrane) known as the eardrum. When this membrane becomes perforated, it is known as a ruptured eardrum. Symptoms include sudden pain in the ear, partial hearing loss, discharge of pus about two days after rupture, ringing in the ear, and dizziness. The most common causes are sharp objects inserted into the ear, a sudden inward or outward pressure, or a severe middle-ear infection. Hearing is usually not affected permanently even if the ruptured eardrum becomes infected, although treatment may be necessary.

According to our macrobiotic understanding, the underlying cause of a ruptured eardrum that results from a middle-ear infection is eating an unbalanced diet of extreme yin and yang foods. This condition can also sometimes develop from a cold. However, even in a chronic case of middle-ear infection, a positive change of condition can occur within a couple of weeks after a dietary change.

Helpful Suggestions

Avoid blowing your nose, if possible. If you must, blow gently. It is also advisable to keep water out of the ear canal. Use cotton ear plugs or a bathing cap while bathing.

OBJECTIVE	REMEDY
To relieve pain	Try applying an ALBI PLASTER to the front and back of the ear (not directly over the ear opening). Use this overnight.
	or
	If you do not have any albi, you can use a GREEN PLASTER.
	and
	Adults may use a GINGER SESAME OIL EAR TREATMENT for 1 hour, 3 times per day.
To relieve children's pain	Use an ALBI or GREEN PLASTER as described above but do not use a ginger sesame oil ear treatment. It is best to consult a doctor for children's ear pain, especially if the plasters do not help.

Dietary Recommendations

Use the following dietary suggestions until the symptoms improve or for one month. Then, widen your food choices using a macrobiotic dietary approach (see page 11).

☐ Main foods: Brown Rice with Barley (3 to 1), Azuki Rice, Brown Rice Cream (thick), Gomashio. Chew each mouthful more than 100 times.
☐ Side dishes (one-third of main foods): Carp Soup 2 to 3 times every day, Burdock Lotus Root Nitsuke, Burdock Nitsuke, and Hijiki Nitsuke. Use sesame oil and cook foods for a long time. Always eat warm food, never cold, if you have ear problems.
☐ Miso soup ingredients: wakame, daikon, turnips.
☐ Beverages: Sho-Ban Tea, Bancha Tea, Kombu Tea.
☐ Avoid especially: all meat, red-meat fish, chicken, dairy, all sweet foods and drinks, all fruit. Eggs are especially bad.

EDEMA

Edema is excessive fluid accumulation in any area of the body, often in the feet and ankles. Symptoms include swelling and muscular aches and pains. Persistent edema may result from weak kidneys, and/or bladder, heart, or liver disorders and these possibilities should be checked. Also, allergies often cause fluid retention. See the appropriate sections for suggestions on underlying disorders and for improving your overall condition.

Helpful Suggestions

The remedies to improve the kidneys make the kidneys stronger because they improve blood circulation and increase the amount of oxygen available to the kidneys.

OBJECTIVE	REMEDY
To reduce swelling caused by weak kidneys, bladder, and/or liver	Try drinking 1 cup of DAIKON TEA 3 times per day until swelling goes down. However, if you have a weak heart, instead of using daikon tea, drink 1 cup of BROWN RICE CREAM TEA 2 times per day until swelling goes down.
	and
	Sweating daily is important. So, exercise daily and take hot baths or SAUNAS every day until swelling does down. Stay in a sauna at 120° to 150°F for 5 to 10 minutes after beginning to sweat.
To reduce swelling and pain in the feet or ankles	Immerse your feet in a CEDAR LEAVES BATH for 30 minutes every evening.
To improve the kidneys	Do one of the following each day: apply a GINGER COMPRESS to the kidneys (see Figure 3.8 on page 176) for 20 minutes.
	or

Walk barefoot on the dew in the early morning for 20 minutes.

or

Take a 1 percent SALT BATH for 30 minutes.

Dietary Recommendations

Following a macrobiotic dietary approach (see page 11) is very helpful. When beginning a macrobiotic diet, eat less salt, miso, and soy sauce than is usually recommended. When the swelling goes away, start adding more salt.

☐ Avoid especially: all animal products, white flour, refined sugar, alcohol, caffeine, and tobacco.

EMBOLISM

See STROKE.

ENDOMETRIOSIS

Endometriosis is a condition in which tissue resembling the lining of the uterus (the endometrium) grows outside the uterus in the pelvic cavity, usually on the ovaries. Symptoms include increased pain in the uterus, lower back, and pelvic cavity during menstruation; painful intercourse; nausea; vomiting; constipation; infertility; and blood in the urine and sometimes in the stool.

The cause of endometriosis is unknown although many, varied theories exist. In my opinion, one cause is the use of medication or mechanical devices for pregnancy control. These upset the body's natural rhythm, and tissue-lining materials that are normally expelled in the menstrual flow pass backward into the pelvic cavity, increase in number, and produce pain and other symptoms. Some women have been permanently cured of endometriosis by becoming pregnant, and women who give birth while young are less likely to develop endometriosis.

Helpful Suggestions

OBJECTIVE	REMEDY
To relieve pain	Try applying a GINGER COMPRESS on the skin over the uterus (see Figure 3.8 on page 176) for 20 minutes once a day until the pain stops. *and* Take a DAIKON HIP BATH for 20 minutes once a day. *and/or* Take a 1 percent SALT BATH for 30 minutes once a day until symptoms improve.
To improve overall condition	Stretching and moderate exercise such as cleaning house or garden work are helpful.
To protect the lining of the uterus	Finding a means of birth control other than medications or mechanical devices is recommended.

Dietary Recommendations

A change in dietary habits can be very helpful for dealing with endometriosis. Follow a strict diet of whole grains and fresh vegetables unitl your condition improves. Then, switch to a macrobiotic dietary approach (see page 11).

ENTERITIS

Enteritis refers to an inflammation of the intestine that occurs primarily in the small intestine. Symptoms include cramping, abdominal pain, diarrhea, fever, appetite loss, and sometimes bloody stool. The causes are thought to be many including viral, bacterial, or parasitic infection; the use of harsh laxatives or drugs; or a change in bacteria that normally inhabit the intestinal tract.

According to our macrobiotic understanding, there are both yin and yang acute types and yin and yang chronic types of enteritis. The yin acute type is caused by the overconsumption of sweet drinks, ice cream, fruits such as apples, and other yin foods that cause the body suddenly to become cooler and result in intestinal inflammation. In a yin chronic condition, the intestines weaken slowly over a period of time, usually from a excessively yin diet. The yang acute form is caused by the overconsumption of yang foods such as meat and fish over a short period of time. The overeating of yang animal foods over an extended period of time can weaken the intestines and cause a yang chronic condition. If you have overeaten both yin and yang foods, try the suggestions for the yin type first, especially if you are in a weakened condition.

Helpful Suggestions

Avoid taking hot baths except for treatment baths.

OBJECTIVE	REMEDY
	FOR THE YANG TYPE
To control diarrhea	Take a DAIKON or ARAME BATH for 20 minutes once a day. Keep warm. *and* Try eating 1 cup of *BROWN RICE CREAM WITH GRATED DAIKON* 1 or 2 times per day until diarrhea stops. *or* Eat 1 cup of *BROWN RICE GRUEL WITH UMEBOSHI* 1 or 2 times per day until recovered.
To control chronic conditions	Drink *UMESHO BANCHA TEA* 2 to 3 times per day for a total of 2 cups per day until diarrhea stops. *and* DAIKON or ARAME HIP BATHS WITH GRATED GINGER can be taken for 20 minutes once a day.
	FOR THE YIN TYPE
To control diarrhea	Try drinking 1 to 2 cups of *UMESHO BANCHA TEA* or *UMESHO KUZU TEA* once a day. *or* Try eating 1 cup of salty *MISO SOUP WITH MOCHI* served with 1 tablespoon grated daikon on top 1 or 2 times per day until diarrhea stops.
To relieve intestinal pains or severe diarrhea	Take a DAIKON HIP BATH WITH GRATED GINGER once a day for 20 minutes. *or* Take an ARAME or DAIKON HIP BATH WITH MUSTARD POWDER once a day for 7 to 8 minutes until the skin turns red. *or* Take a GINGER WATER HIP BATH once a day for 20 minutes until diarrhea stops.
To control persistent diarrhea	Drink 1 cup of *UMEBOSHI TEA* 2 times per day until diarrhea stops.
To alleviate dry mouth	Drink 1 cup of *UMESHO BANCHA TEA* whenever thirsty, up to 3 cups per day.
To control constipation	Try eating 2 tablespoons of good-quality sesame oil (raw) once only.

Dietary Recommendations

The following dietary suggestions may be used until the symptoms improve or for about one month. Then, widen your food choices using a macrobiotic dietary approach (see page 11).

FOR THE YANG TYPE

☐ Main foods: Brown Rice Cream, Brown Rice Kayu, Brown Rice Gruel with Mochi served with a little soy sauce. Use less salt than you usually do in your cooking.

☐ Side dishes (one-fourth of main foods): Grated Daikon with Soy Sauce, Dried Daikon Nitsuke, Daikon Nitsuke, Eggplant Mustard Pickles, Pressed Salad, Sour Cabbage, Takuan Pickles.

☐ Miso soup ingredients: daikon, daikon greens, green leafy vegetables, scallions, Homemade Agé, Brown Rice Mochi.

☐ Beverages: Umesho Bancha Tea, Brown Rice Tea, Grain Coffee, Kuzu Bancha Tea. Drink a maximum of 2½ cups of beverages per day.

☐ Avoid especially: all animal protein including fish, shellfish, milk, all dairy, meat-based soups, alcohol, all sweet foods.

FOR THE YIN TYPE

☐ Main foods: Brown Rice Gruel with Miso, Brown Rice Gruel with Mochi and Scallions, Brown Rice Balls with Gomashio, Azuki Rice Balls with Gomashio (1 teaspoon of Gomashio for each rice ball). Chew each mouthful 200 times. Gradually increase the amount of salt in your cooking.

☐ Side dishes (one-fourth of main foods): Shio Kombu, Umeboshi, Takuan Pickles, Miso Pickles.

☐ Miso soup ingredients: wakame, scallions, onions, Homemade Agé, Brown Rice Mochi.

☐ Beverages: Brown Rice Tea with Umeboshi, Umesho Bancha, Sho-Ban Tea, Brown Rice Bancha Tea, Kuzu Bancha Tea, Grain Coffee.

☐ Avoid especially: all animal foods, fish, shellfish, dairy foods, meat-based soups, black teas, all fruit and sweet foods, alcohol, mushrooms, melons, vinegar, tomatoes, hot spices, rice bran pickles.

See also DYSENTERY *and* GASTRITIS

EPILEPSY

Epilepsy is a noncontagious disorder of brain function characterized by sudden seizures, a change in one's state of consciousness, or brief attacks of inappropriate behavior or bizarre movements. There are more than fifty brain disorders that can cause epilepsy, the more common include severe head injury, brain damage at birth, alcoholic drug abuse, and brain infection. Although the cause is often unknown, the reason for epilepsy is thought to be overexcitement of the nerves in the brain. The common thinking is that a number of mechanisms may be responsible. Because the impulses of the brain are activated by precise and measured amounts of electricity, overexcitement of nerves is thought to result from overproduction of electricity in the brain. However, modern science doesn't know the cause of this overproduction of electricity.

The onset of epilepsy occurs most commonly before the age of five, often at puberty, and is more rare after age thirty. There are many types of epilepsy. Grand mal epilepsy is characterized by attacks of fits, convulsions, and falls in a forward or backward direction (never sideways), unconscious, deep sleep for about five minutes, foaming at the mouth, reddening of the face, and dilation of pupils. Petit mal epilepsy mostly affects children; attacks are slight and often happen suddenly in the middle of conversation. The face turns blank and pale, and the epileptic is unaware of this. Petit mal seizures can occur several times a day. Psychomotor or temporal-lobe epilepsy is indicated by brief attacks of inappropriate or suddenly-out-of-character behavior including bizarre body movements such as odd chewing motions. During focal epilepsy, the person does not lose consciousness. An attack begins with a small part of the body twitching uncontrollably. The twitching may spread until the whole body is involved. These are the major types of epilepsy.

In my opinion, the most important causes for epilepsy are the overexcitement of nerves in the brain resulting in a seizure, the overexcitement of nerves in the muscles resulting in a convulsion, and in either or both cases, a weakened or frail body that cannot stand the overexcitement of nerves or muscles. Grand mal epilepsy happens when all three factors are present. Petit mal epilepsy occurs when the nerves in the brain are overexcited and the body is weak or frail. If the nerves in the brain are not overexcited, then a convulsion results and not epilepsy. But what causes the nerves in the brain to become overexcited?

To me, the cause is an increase in potassium in the cells, which stimulates the sympathetic nervous system, thus exciting the nerves. This condition results from an injury to the brain, either internal or external, that causes a loss of sodium and an increase of potassium in relation to sodium. Too much potassium in the cells also can occur when a mother eats too much sweet food including fruit and/or not enough salt at the beginning of pregnancy, or when a baby or child is fed too much fruit and dairy food such as cow's milk without enough yang foods such as meat, fish, eggs, or salty condiments to make balance.

Helpful Suggestions

There is no known cure for epilepsy, especially when a brain injury is involved, but the seizures can be controlled. Improving the body's overall condition through a change in dietary habits can be most helpful (see below).

OBJECTIVE	REMEDY
To lessen the intensity of a seizure about to occur	Try drinking 1 cup of SHO-BAN TEA, 2/3 cup BANCHA TEA WITH SALT, or eating 1 teaspoon GOMASHIO. (Always carry Gomashio with you.) The seizure will be lessened.
To clear cloudy thinking after a seizure	Try a GINGER COMPRESS on the head for 10 minutes every 4 hours and keep warm.
To cool a head that is too hot	Use a TOFU PLASTER over the entire head, changing every hour, until your head feels cooler.
To relieve numbness or pain	Use a GINGER SESAME OIL MASSAGE on the affected area.

Dietary Recommendations

The best way to overcome epilepsy is to eat less and drink less, until urination comes only twice a day. FAST often if your condition allows. The following dietary suggestions are useful for improving your condition and may be used during times of seizures or for up to one month. Then, widen your food choices using a macrobiotic dietary approach (see page 11).

☐ Main foods: Brown Rice, Azuki Rice, Brown Rice Mochi served with a little Gomashio as a condiment. Chew each mouthful 200 times.
☐ Side dishes (less than one-third of main foods): Tekka Miso, Hijiki Carrot Nitsuke, Azuki Beans with Kombu, Azuki Beans with Kombu and Winter Squash, Umeboshi, Miso Pickles, Carp Soup.
☐ Miso soup ingredients: wakame, scallions, kombu, onions, Brown Rice Mochi.
☐ Beverages: Sho-Ban Tea, Bancha Tea, Kombu Tea, Grain Milk.
☐ Avoid especially: all animal foods including cheese, red-meat fish, shellfish, milk, ice cream, butter, eggs, fruit, sugar, honey, and any very yin foods such as potatoes, tomatoes, eggplant, peanuts, cucumbers, melons, hot spices, pressed salad, and vinegar.

ESOPHAGEAL STRICTURE

Esophageal stricture refers to any narrowing of the esophagus, the tube connecting the mouth to the stomach. Within the esophagus, a narrowing can occur anywhere; however, most strictures occur in the lower esophagus. Strictures can occur following inflammation or damage caused by chronic heartburn or hiatal hernia, tuberculosis, an enlarged thyroid gland, syphilis, cancer, or, as is often the case with children, burning the throat by drinking chemicals. Symptoms include a decrease in the ability to swallow, pain in the mouth or chest after eating, rapid breathing, increased salivation, and vomiting.

According to our macrobiotic understanding, if the esophagus is contracted due to tuberculosis or thyroid gland trouble, this is caused by overeating yin foods. A hiatal hernia also is caused by overeating yin foods. Chronic heartburn results from eating both extreme yin and yang foods. In the case of syphilis or cancer, the causes can be eating too many extreme foods, either yin or yang, poor living conditions, and other environmental factors.

Helpful Suggestions

OBJECTIVE	REMEDY
To open stricture	Apply a GINGER COMPRESS on the throat for 20 minutes followed by an ALBI PLASTER for up to 4 hours. Repeat both the compress and plaster as often as needed until the esophagus opens.
To relieve sore throat	Try drinking 1 cup of BROWN RICE TEA 3 times per day.
To reduce the size of a child's swollen glands	Try slowly sipping ½ cup of DAIKON JUICE WITH SPRING WATER.
To help control cancer of the esophagus	Apply a GINGER COMPRESS to the throat and sternum (see Figure 3.8 on page 176) for 20 minutes and then an ALBI PLASTER for up to 4 hours. Repeat both the compress and plaster as often as needed and leave the plaster on overnight each night until your condition improves.

Dietary Recommendations

More important than external remedies is a strict approach to your diet. If you have cancer of the esophagus, use Brown Rice Cream, Brown Rice Gruel with Miso, Brown Rice Kayu (soft brown rice), and Buckwheat Cream as main foods. These soft foods are useful for any esophageal stricture until normal swallowing is possible. Then, for solid food use Buckwheat Noodles, Fried Noodles, or Buckwheat Pancakes. It is important to eat slowly and to chew well. See also the dietary suggestions listed for thyroiditis, syphilis, or tuberculosis. Once your condition improves, widen your food choices based on a macrobiotic dietary approach (see page 11).

FAINTING

There are many causes of fainting, and fainting is associated with many illnesses. Both the acute and the chronic type of fainting covered here are caused by a sudden decrease in blood pressure that results in temporary blood deprivation in the brain. The acute type is due to a loss of blood resulting from an accident or from a severe mental shock. The chronic type may be caused by malnutrition, chronic constipation, low blood sugar, epilepsy, heartbeat irregularities, or heart diseases. Conditions associated with fainting include facial pallor, cold sweats, vomiting, headaches, ringing in the ears, dizziness (sudden lightheadedness), and, finally, a temporary loss of consciousness.

Helpful Suggestions

If someone faints, you need to act quickly. Check for breathing and a neck pulse; call for medical help if either is missing. If the person is breathing and has a pulse, do not attempt to move the person; elevate the feet to help return blood to the heart. Call for help if the person doesn't regain consciousness within a few minutes.

If no help is available:

OBJECTIVE	REMEDY
To aid an unconscious man when no medical help is available	Wash the head with warm water.
To aid an unconscious woman when no medical help is available	Place a HOT TOWEL COMPRESS on the head for up to 20 minutes.
To aid an unconscious man or woman when no medical help is available	Keep the person warm. If at all possible, do not move a person who has fainted until medical help arrives. and Try placing an APPLICATION of 2 to 3 GREEN LEAVES at the back of the person's neck, elevating the person's feet, and applying a TOFU PLASTER to the forehead, changing both the leaves and plaster every hour until consciousness is regained.

To aid in an emergency involving a concussion	Try washing the victim's head with hot water and applying a HOT TOWEL COMPRESS on the head for 20 minutes every hour until consciousness is regained. After regaining consciousness, the person should drink 1 cup of SHO-BAN TEA every morning for a week.
To combat dizziness at any time	Sit down, bend at the waist, and grasp the ankles so that blood rushes to the head.
To move stagnant blood	Drinking 1 cup of BANCHA TEA WITH GRATED DAIKON 2 times per day for 2 to 3 days is helpful.
To aid in chronic cases	Drink 1 cup of SHO-BAN TEA every morning until fainting spells stop.

Dietary Recommendations

The following dietary suggestions may be used until your condition improves or for one month. Then, widen your food choices based on a macrobiotic dietary approach (see page 11).

☐ Main foods: Brown Rice (or any whole grain dishes), Azuki Rice, Brown Rice Mochi, Fried Rice, and Gomashio as a condiment.

☐ Side dishes (one-third of main foods): Tekka Miso, Hijiki Burdock or Hijiki Carrot Nitsuke, Vegetable Stew with Fish, azuki kombu dishes, Vegetable Tempura served with Grated Daikon with Soy Sauce, Miso Pickles, Umeboshi, and Rice Bran Pickles.

☐ Miso soup ingredients: wakame, scallions, kombu, onions, Brown Rice Mochi.

☐ Beverages: Sho-Ban Tea, Brown Rice Tea, Bancha Tea.

☐ Avoid especially: all meat, red-meat fish, shellfish, potatoes, mushrooms, hot spices, salads, sweet drinks, eggplant, tomatoes, ice cream, coffee, and all very yin foods.

FATIGUE

Fatigue is not a disease; it is a symptom and one of the body's first signals that things are not well. Chronic fatigue may indicate or lead to a disease. A mysterious ailment called "Yuppie Disease" by *Time* magazine was first reported in the early '80s. It still lacks an official name because medical research can find neither its cause or cure. It is similar in its symptoms to a mononucleosis infection and can cause severe fatigue.

According to our macrobiotic understanding, the cause of fatigue is a lack of oxygen and insufficient glucose supply to the body cells. Also, too much acidity can

be the cause. A lack of oxygen and glucose in the body cells is caused by the overgrowth of yeast, bacteria, and mold since these microbes steal (use up) our normal oxygen and glucose supply. (They also create a more acidic condition.) The cause of the overgrowth of microbes is the shortage of sodium in the bodily fluids due to weak kidneys. The correct proportion of sodium in the bodily fluids keeps microorganism growth in check. A diet high in animal proteins and refined sugar contributes to an overly acidic condition and may also result in weakened kidneys.

Helpful Suggestions

The macrobiotic approach to fatigue is to stop the overgrowth of yeast or bacteria. Since sodium in the bodily fluids will stop the overgrowth of microbes, an increase in one's sodium (salt) intake is the solution. However, the kidneys are the organs that control the amount of sodium in our bodily fluids. If the kidneys are weak, the body cannot retain sodium even when one consumes a high amount. It is important then to make the kidneys strong if one has weak kidneys. The following remedies, except for the Azuki Bean Tea, make the kidneys stronger because they improve blood circulation and increase the amount of oxygen available to the kidneys.

OBJECTIVE	REMEDY
To strengthen kidneys	Take a SAUNA for 30 minutes every other day (set the temperature at 150° to 160°F). In winter, take a sauna every day if you are not tired. If you have a weak heart, take a shorter sauna.
	and/or
	Walk barefoot in the grass in the early morning. (Your feet will tell you when you've walked enough.)
	and/or
	Take a 1 percent SALT BATH once a day, just before going to bed. The bath can be cold, warm, or hot.
	and/or
	A GINGER COMPRESS applied to the kidneys (see Figure 3.8 on page 176) for 20 minutes each day is also very helpful.
	also
	Drink 1 cup of AZUKI BEAN TEA once a day until the kidneys become stronger. In general, however, drink only when thirsty.

Dietary Recommendations

Following a macrobiotic dietary approach (see page 11), excluding all animal foods and dairy foods of any kind, will be most helpful. In other words, eat a low-protein, low-fat, low-simple-carbohydrate and high-complex-carbohydrate diet. Eat a low- or no-salt diet, especially if you have back pain or swelling. However, as soon as the kidneys are stronger, add salt to the diet. Increase the amount little by little. If you overeat food that is itself not overly salty, you may still be getting too much salt. So be careful not to overeat. Use only moderate amounts of natural sea salt and well-fermented (at least one year) miso and soy sauce. Avoid foods with chemical additives and drugs of any kind since anesthesia, pain killers, or other medications may weaken the kidneys.

FATIGUE, EXCESSIVE (NEURASTHENIA)

Neurasthenia refers to excessive fatigue of nervous system origin. Depending on the area affected, there are different forms, ranging from mental and visual disturbances and other head symptoms to stomach complications and disorders of sexual function. According to our macrobiotic understanding, neurasthenia is caused by a diet that contains too much yin food such as sugary foods, fruits, and alcohol and not enough yang food such as salt. This kind of diet increases the proportion of potassium in relation to sodium and results in the excitabilty of the sympathetic nervous system, leading to continuous expansion and a loss of contracting power. The long-term effect is excessive fatigue from over-expansion.

Helpful Suggestions

OBJECTIVE	REMEDY
To alleviate head symptoms	Try applying a TOFU PLASTER on the head, changing it every hour.
To alleviate body symptoms	Apply a GINGER COMPRESS to the affected area for 20 minutes to improve the circulation, then MASSAGE the area with GINGER SESAME OIL. Then apply an ALBI PLASTER on the affected area for up to 4 hours. Repeat this process as often as needed and as time allows until recovered.

Dietary Recommendations

A change to a more balanced diet is most helpful. Use the following dietary suggestions until your condition improves or for about one month. Then, widen your food choices using a macrobiotic dietary approach (see page 11).

☐ Main foods: Brown Rice, Azuki Rice, Azuki Millet Rice, Brown Rice Balls, Vegetable Fried Rice, all served with Gomashio.

☐ Side dishes (one-third of main foods): Tekka Miso, Scallion Miso, Shio Kombu, Hijiki Nitsuke, Carp Soup, Vegetable Stew, Vegetable Stew with Fish, Burdock Carrot Nitsuke, Vegetable Tempura served with Grated Daikon, Nori Roasted with Oil, Azuki Beans with Kombu, Miso Pickles. Also eat Grated Daikon with Sesame Oil and Soy Sauce since it is easy for the body to take in oil this way.

☐ Miso soup ingredients: wakame, tororo kombu, onions, scallions, Homemade Agé, Brown Rice Mochi.

☐ Beverages: Brown Rice Tea, Brown Rice Bancha Tea, Bancha Tea, Kombu Tea, Mu Tea, Brown Rice Cream. Drink less, a maximum of 2 cups of beverages per day.

☐ Avoid especially: all animal foods, including meat-based soups, red-meat fish, shellfish, dairy foods and eggs, and all yin foods, including fruit, soy milk, vinegar, peanuts, and sweet foods and drinks.

FEVER

Fever is body temperature that is elevated above normal. Actually, a fever is a symptom and not a disease. According to our macrobiotic understanding, it indicates the presence of an illness in the body and is part of the body's defense mechanism because fever destroys foreign microbes and eliminates toxins. Generally, fevers can be classified into four types: fever caused by a cold; fever caused by tuberculosis; fever caused by another contagious disease; and fever caused by stomach trouble. In the cases of contagious diseases, the metabolism of the germs causes the fever; the germs will die because of the heat produced by the fever as long as medication is not used to reduce the fever (heat).

Most of the time it is better to let the fever run its course. However, there are reasons for concern. An extremely high fever (over 103°F) can damage the brain of a small child. In this case, you must act to reduce the temperature. Fevers over 102°F are cause for concern among adults. Consult your health-care advisor if natural methods do not work or if a high fever lasts longer than two days. In general, fevers over 103°F are caused by putrefaction from overeating animal foods such as meat, fish, or eggs. In this case, or if you have a fever from liver or kidney problems, it is important to restore the functions of the liver and kidneys since they help clean up all the body's toxins.

Helpful Suggestions

See the appropriate section for fever caused by a cold, stomach problem, tuberculosis, or other contagious disease.

OBJECTIVE	REMEDY
To reduce high fever of unknown origin	Apply a TOFU PLASTER on the forehead, changing it every hour. *and* At the same time, place a GREEN LEAVES APPLICATION on your pillow at the back of your neck; change the leaves every 2 hours. *and* Try drinking 1 cup of DAIKON GINGER TEA 3 to 4 times per day.
To reduce high fever in weak people, those with weak lungs, and old people	Drink 1 cup of BROWN RICE TEA WITH DRIED PERSIMMON AND TANGERINE SKIN 3 to 4 times per day instead of Daikon Ginger Tea.
To reduce high fever in children	Often children do not like Daikon Ginger Tea. In this case, finely grate an apple and squeeze out the juice. Give ½ cup of juice every three hours. *or* Try giving ½ cup of BROWN RICE TEA WITH DRIED PERSIMMON AND TANGERINE SKIN or SOUR APPLE JUICE every 3 hours.
To reduce a child's very high fever from constipation	Use an ENEMA once only to remove the stool. This should help the fever go down.
To reduce fever in general	Try drinking 1 cup of SHIITAKE TEA, or 1 cup of SCALLION MISO TEA, or 1 cup of ROASTED BROWN RICE TEA, or ½ cup of LOTUS ROOT TEA (for children). The same or different teas can be taken every 3 hours until the fever goes down.

FIBROCYSTIC DISEASE OF THE BREAST

Fibrocystic disease of the breast refers to nonmalignant lumps in female breasts. The breast is tender and painful; pain is usually most severe before menstruation when the lumps often enlarge. They appear in various sizes and multiple lumps are common. Large lumps near the surface may be moved around freely and often come and go. Cancerous growths usually don't move freely or go away. Most often there is no tenderness either. It can be difficult to tell the difference with lumps deep with-in the breast, and, in any case, a breast exam to test for possible cancer is recommended by medical authorities.

The cause of benign lumps is unknown but probable contributing factors are iodine deficiency, hormonal imbalances, and abnormal breast-milk production caused by high amounts of estrogen. According to recent studies, drinking coffee and smoking cigarettes are associated with higher incidences of fibrocystic disease. From a macrobiotic viewpoint, the underlying cause of fibrocystic disease of the breast is the overconsumption of protein foods from either animal or plant sources (meat, chicken, fish, eggs, tofu, and beans) along with the overconsumption of simple sugars. The long-term effect of a diet of excess protein provides the building materials for making the lumps and may lead to hormonal imbalances also. When the body has an excess, it must be stored somewhere. Smoking cigarettes brings energy to the breast (lung) area, and drinking coffee stimulates the upper parts of the body as well. Thus, it is consistent with our macrobiotic understanding that recent studies show a connection between coffee, smoking, and fibrocystic disease of the breast.

Helpful Suggestions

OBJECTIVE	REMEDY
To remove excess	Apply an ALBI PLASTER over the lump as often as your schedule allows, changing it every 4 hours, until the lump disappears. A plaster may be applied before you go to sleep and may be left on throughout the night. This is helpful in removing the lumps (excess).

Dietary Recommendations

It is most helpful to change to a macrobiotic dietary approach (see page 11) that is lower in the percentage of calories derived from protein.

☐ Avoid especially: animal products, alcohol, coffee, cigarettes, all sugary foods and drinks. Note that we are not suggesting a no-protein diet; the body needs a certain amount for repair and normal growth of cells.

See also BREAST CANCER.

FINGER INFECTION

A finger infection involves pus or an abscess resulting in pain and swelling of the finger. According to our macrobiotic understanding, the underlying cause of this type of infection is the overconsumption of protein (usually animal protein) and of simple carbohydrates such as sugar, honey, and fruit. Too much animal protein leads to the infecton, and too much sweet food contributes to the infection's growth and directs the energy of the infection to the extremities, in this case, the fingers.

Helpful Suggestions:

OBJECTIVE	REMEDY
To relieve severe pain	Remove the bones from a small catfish, roach (a European freshwater fish), or eel. Place the fish, skin side down, directly on the infection. Secure with a bandage and leave on until it is half-dried out or about 1 hour. Continue with new applications until the severe pain is gone. The skin of the fish will help absorb the poison of the infection.
To reduce pain and swelling	Immerse your hand in a warm CEDAR LEAVES BATH for 30 minutes and the pain and swelling should stop.
To alleviate persistent pain, swelling	Try applying an ALBI PLASTER on the affected area, changing it every 4 hours.
	or
	Lightly rub *UME EXTRACT* on the infected finger for 5 to 10 minutes followed by a GREEN LEAVES APPLICATION, secured with a bandage. Change the leaves every 1 to 2 hours.

Dietary Recommendations

The following dietary suggestions may be used until the infection is over or for one month. Then, widen your food choices using a macrobiotic dietary approach (see page 11).

☐ Main foods: Brown Rice Balls.
☐ Side dishes (less than one-third of main foods): Tekka Miso, Shio Kombu, Hijiki Nitsuke, Burdock Carrot Nitsuke, Carp Soup, Takuan Pickles, Miso Pickles.
☐ Miso soup ingredients: wakame, tororo kombu, daikon, scallions, burdock, Homemade Agé.
☐ Beverages: Brown Rice Tea, Brown Rice Bancha Tea, Bancha Tea. Drink a maximum of 2 cups of beverages per day.
☐ Avoid especially: all animal protein, fish, shellfish, dairy foods, eggs, meat-based soups, sweet foods and drinks, vinegar, hot spices, tomatoes, potatoes, eggplant, mushrooms, alcohol.

FLU

The flu (influenza) is a common and very contagious respiratory infection. According to modern medicine, the cause of the flu is any of several varieties of viruses that are spread by personal contact. After an incubation period of twenty-four to forty-eight hours, the flu comes on abruptly with chills, fever, severe headaches, and aches in the back, muscles, and joints. There may also be nausea and vomiting. In addition, there are cold symptoms such as runny nose, sneezing, sore throat, cough (usually with little or no sputum), and flushed face. Usually it takes one to fourteen days to recover from the flu. Because one is in a weakened condition, the flu may lead to bacterial infections such as bronchitis, pneumonia, or middle-ear infections.

According to our macrobiotic understanding, one who suffers from the flu is someone who has eaten too much yang food such as animal food or too much yin food such as sugary food, fruit, butter, and alcohol. Also, one who has a lowered resistance for any reason such as too much stress, overworking, poor diet, fatigue, recent or chronic illness, or a low amount of sodium in bodily fluids will more easily contract the flu.

Helpful Suggestions

OBJECTIVE	REMEDY
To relieve sore throat	Try gargling with warm-to-hot *BANCHA TEA WITH SALT* every 4 hours and using an ALBI PLASTER on the outside of the throat, changing it every 4 hours.
To reduce high fever in strong adults	Try drinking 1 cup of *DAIKON GINGER TEA* 3 times per day.
To reduce high fever in children, older adults, or weak people	Drink ½ to 1 cup (depending on age; younger or more frail persons use the lesser amount) of *BROWN RICE TEA WITH DRIED PERSIMMON AND TANGERINE SKIN* 3 times per day.
	Use the 3 preceding teas for 3 days only, then, if still needed, use only Brown Rice Tea with Dried Persimmon and Tangerine Skin for up to 1 week.
To relieve headache	MASSAGE the scalp and temples with GINGER SESAME OIL.
	or
	Use an APPLE or DAIKON PLASTER applied to the forehead. Change every 2 hours or as needed to help relieve headache pain.
To quiet a cough	Try drinking ½ cup of *LOTUS ROOT TEA* 3 times per day.

Dietary Recommendations

The following dietary suggestions may be used until you are recovered or for one month. Then, widen your food choices using a macrobiotic dietary approach (see page 11).

☐ Main foods: warm-to-hot Brown Rice Gruel with Miso and Scallions, Brown Rice Gruel with Grated Daikon served with Homemade Agé and miso, Brown Rice Gruel with Miso and Mochi. If the person is strong, use Brown Rice Gruel with Shiitake Mushrooms adding miso and mochi.

☐ Side dishes (less than one-fourth of main foods): Tekka Miso, Shio Kombu, Scallion Miso, Hijiki Lotus Root Nitsuke, Burdock Carrot Nitsuke, Tororo Kombu Soup, Oysters Cooked with Miso, boiled vegetables, Vegetable Tempura, Umeboshi, Miso Pickles.

☐ Miso soup ingredients: wakame, scallions, daikon, Homemade Agé, Brown Rice Mochi.

☐ Beverages: Brown Rice Tea, Brown Rice Bancha Tea, Sho-Ban Tea, Bancha Tea, Mu Tea, Grain Coffee, Grain Milk, Kombu Tea, Amasake Drink. Drink a maximum of 2 cups of beverages per day.

☐ Avoid especially: all meat, fish, shellfish, dairy (including ice cream), fruit, sweet foods, salads, melons, vinegar, sweet drinks, hot spices, tomatoes, potatoes, eggplant, alcohol, coffee, cocoa.

FOOD POISONING

When any of many harmful bacteria are ingested, food poisoning may result. The symptoms are so similar to stomach or intestinal disorders such as dysentery that it is often hard to tell whether or not food poisoning is involved. Nausea, vomiting, abdominal cramps, and diarrhea are the symptoms most often associated with food poisoning.

Here we discuss poisoning from only some specific foods and food combinations. If you have a severe case or suspect food poisoning that was contracted at a commercial eating establishment, contact medical help and/or call your local health department so that others may be warned.

Helpful Suggestions

OBJECTIVE	REMEDY
To alleviate food poisoning from any source	A BEACH SAND BATH for 6 to 8 hours will have the greatest healing power for any food poisoning.
To alleviate food poisoning from meat	Adults drink ⅓ cup and children drink 1 to 2 tablespoons of BURDOCK JUICE every 3 hours for 1 day to help neutralize the poison with the potassium from the Burdock Juice.
To alleviate food poisoning from fish	Try drinking ½ cup BLACK SOYBEAN TEA every 3 hours for 1 day to help break up excess phosphorus. *or* Chop and grind fresh beefsteak leaves in a suribachi or blender and squeeze out the juice. Drink ½ cup every 3 hours for 1 day.
To alleviate food poisoning from tuna or bonita fish	Drink 2 cups of SHIITAKE TEA, SOYBEAN POWDER TEA, or CHERRY TREE BARK TEA every 3 hours for 2 days to help balance excess protein and fat. If you are poisoned by bonita, do not drink ice water since this will congeal the fish oil.
To alleviate food poisoning from crab	Drink ½ to 1 cup SCALLION or LEEK JUICE every 3 hours for 1 day to help melt hardened fat.
To alleviate food poisoning from eggs	Drink 3 tablespoons natural vinegar or eat ¼ to ½ teaspoon sea salt every 3 hours for 2 days to help break up excess phosphorus.
To alleviate food poisoning from buckwheat	Eat 1 to 2 tablespoons fresh GRATED DAIKON every 3 hours for 2 days to help in the digestion of buckwheat protein.
To alleviate food poisoning from udon or somen	Drink 1 cup DAIKON JUICE every 3 hours for 2 days to help digest starchy food.
To alleviate food poisoning from tempura	Drink ½ cup DAIKON SOY SAUCE TEA or 2 cups of ORANGE PEEL TEA every 3 hours for 2 days to help in the digestion of excess oil (fat).
To alleviate food poisoning from watermelon	Drink 1 cup of SALT WATER DRINK once only to help induce vomiting.
To alleviate food poisoning from vinegar	Eat 1 teaspoon of GOMASHIO or TEKKA MISO every 3 hours for 2 days to help protect the heart.
To alleviate food poisoning from water	Drink ½ cup of UMEBOSHI JUICE TEA or UME EXTRACT TEA every 3 hours for 2 days to help weaken the bacteria.

FROSTBITE

Frostbite refers to tissue damage resulting from exposure to sub-freezing temperatures. During the exposure, there is gradual numbness, hardness, and paleness in the affected area, most commonly the fingers, toes, nose, and ears. Rewarming causes pain; a tingling or burning sensation, sometimes severe; and a change in color from white to red to purple in the affected area. This may be accompanied by shivering, slurred speech, and memory loss.

Blisters form in severe cases and amputation may be required. In mild cases, full recovery is possible with treatment.

According to our macrobiotic understanding, a contributing factor to frostbite is eating too much yin food such as sugary food, soft drinks, fruit, butter, alcohol, and vinegar. Smoking, windy weather, and certain diseases such as diabetes also increase a person's susceptibility to frostbite.

Helpful Suggestions

The suggestions for severe cases are for emergency care until medical help is available or if help is unavailable.

OBJECTIVE	REMEDY
To relieve mild cases	Soak the affected area in a warm GINGER BATH for 30 minutes per day.
To relieve more severe cases	Extreme care must be taken. Once the frost bite victim is inside (out of the extreme cold), remove any clothing from the affected area. It is important *never* to massage damaged tissue directly as this may destroy the tissue completely.
	then
	Use a *warm* (not hot) GINGER BATH (approximately 100°F) for 20 to 30 minutes. Higher temperatures or using a hot ginger compress before gently warming the area may cause further damage.
	then
	Try applying a GINGER COMPRESS to the area for 20 minutes followed by an ALBI PLASTER for up to 4 hours. Repeat both the compress and plaster as needed.
	and
	Don't smoke or use the affected limbs until your condition improves or medical attention is received.
To relieve very severe cases	Follow the preceding suggestions up to the point of applying an Albi Plaster. To help improve circulation to the area, follow the Ginger Compress with a RICE BRAN MASSAGE around *but not on* the frostbitten area.
	then
	Try putting good-quality sesame oil on the frostbitten area; *do not rub it in*. Follow with an ALBI PLASTER as above. This helps remove dead tissues. If albi is unavailable, you may use an APPLICATION of 2 or 3 GREEN LEAVES over the area, covered by soft cloth bandages to hold the leaves secure. Change the leaves every 2 hours.

Dietary Recommendations

Follow a macrobiotic dietary approach (see page 11), cutting down on all beverages until your condition improves.

☐ Avoid especially: sweet fruits, vinegar, alcohol, all yin foods.

GALLSTONES

A gallstone is a noncancerous solid mass, usually of cholesterol, formed in the gallbladder or bile duct. Sometimes there is pain in the upper right abdomen or between the shoulder blades, loss of appetite, nausea, vomiting, headache, fever, jaundice, and an intolerance for fatty foods leading to indigestion, bloating, and belching. However, there are no symptoms in over 40 percent of cases. Gallstones are more common among women, and 10 percent of the people in America are affected. This increases to 20 percent for those over the age of 40. The cause of gallstones is generally considered to be unknown, but there are many theories ranging from the gallbladder's failure to function properly to infections in the bile ducts.

According to our macrobiotic understanding, gallstones and kidney stones have the same underlying cause. They are caused by too much oxalic acid in the blood, too little salt in the body, and overconsumption of animal protein, especially beef or pork, as well as too much green-skinned fish and red-colored shellfish (lobster, shrimp). These conditions lead to excess acidity in the gallbladder or kidney fluids. To maintain a balanced pH, alkaline substances such as calcium are changed into soluble form and transported to the area. When the substances reharden or crystalize, a gallstone or kidney stone results. Although it is not scientific proof, the fact that older Americans are more often affected—especially those who eat a high-fat and cholesterol diet—leads one to the conclusion that gallstones are directly connected to one's diet and are not a natural result of the aging process.

Helpful Suggestions

Avoid hot baths and refrain from sex until the pain is gone and your condition is improved. Showers are okay.

OBJECTIVE	REMEDY
To relieve mild pain	Try drinking 1 cup of *UMESHO BANCHA TEA WITH GRATED DAIKON* every 3 hours.

| To relieve more severe pain | Apply a GINGER COMPRESS on top of the gallbladder (see Figure 3.8 on page 176) for 20 minutes. When the pain lessens, use an ALBI PLASTER for up to 4 hours. Repeat, using a Ginger Compress followed by an Albi Plaster as often as needed until the pain subsides.

then

Drink 1 cup of UMESHO BANCHA TEA WITH GRATED DAIKON every 3 hours. To relieve sharp pain, add 1 more tablespoon of grated daikon to the tea. |

Dietary Recommendations

The following dietary suggestions may be used until your condition improves or for about one month. In order to prevent the future development of gallstones and any other disorders, widen your food choices using a macrobiotic dietary approach (see page 11).

☐ Main foods: Brown Rice, Azuki Rice, Brown Rice Mochi, Grain Milk; serve grains with Gomashio made with 70 percent sesame seeds (black sesame seeds if available) and 30 percent salt. Chew each mouthful of rice 100 times.

☐ Side dishes (one-third of main foods): Tekka Miso, Oily Miso, Hijiki Lotus Root Nitsuke, Shio Kombu, Vegetable Stew, Vegetable Stew with Fish, Carp Soup, Burdock Carrot Nitsuke, Deep-Fried Kombu, Nori Roasted with Oil, Vegetable Tempura served with Grated Daikon, Natural Caviar.

☐ Miso soup ingredients: wakame, tororo kombu, onions, scallions, Homemade Agé, Brown Rice Mochi.

☐ Beverages: Bancha Tea, Brown Rice Bancha Tea, Sho-Ban Tea, Kombu Tea, Grain Milk, Amasake Drink. Drink less than 2 cups of liquid per day.

☐ Avoid especially: all animal foods, fish (except carp and fish in stew) and shellfish, dairy foods (including ice cream), soy milk, sweet drinks and foods, alcohol, black tea, green tea, cocoa, coffee, vinegar, tomatoes, eggplant, potatoes, mushrooms, peanuts, Rice Bran Pickles, chemicalized foods, melons, spicy foods.

GASTRIC JUICE, LACK OF

Gastric juice, which is produced and secreted by the glands in the mucous membrane lining of the stomach with the help of salt (NaCl), is also referred to as stomach juice or hydrochloric acid (HCl). Hydrochloric acid is needed for the proper digestion of protein because it helps the protein-based enzyme pepsin to digest protein.

Therefore, without salt in the diet, one may not be able to produce enough hydrochloric acid, leading to the improper digestion of protein. The improper digestion of protein may result in a shortage of some tissue cells, organ cells, red blood cells, white blood cells, and especially enzymes, because all of these are made of proteins.

One cannot digest protein, even if stomach enzymes are sufficient, unless there is acid in the stomach juice. With an insufficient amount of acid the body will, therefore, reject proteins that come from food or from the environment as in the case of pollen. This is an allergic reaction. Lack of gastric juice or hydrochloric acid is, then, one of the causes of an allergic reaction. When foods high in protein such as red meat, chicken, eggs, or cheese are eaten, the undigested protein may cause putrefaction in the stomach, intestines, and appendix leading to gastritis, gastroenteritis, or appendicitis. Also, insufficient hydrochloric acid usually leads to a lack of intrinsic factor, an enzyme made in the stomach that is essential for the absorption of vitamin B_{12}. Therefore, lack of hydrochloric acid in the stomach may result in pernicious anemia. See also the appropriate sections if you have any of these disorders.

Helpful Suggestions

OBJECTIVE	REMEDY
To increase hydrochloric acid	Drinking ½ cup UMESHO BANCHA TEA before breakfast and supper for 2 to 3 weeks is helpful because it will promote production of hydrochloric acid in the stomach.

Dietary Recommendations

Dietary changes will be the most helpful. Eat a more balanced diet, eat less protein, and use a little sea salt when cooking vegetables or sea vegetables. Use the following dietary suggestions for a week or two, then widen your food choices using a macrobiotic dietary approach (see page 11).

☐ Main foods: Brown Rice Balls with Gomashio; chew each mouthful 200 times.

☐ Side dishes (one-fourth of main foods): Tekka Miso, Burdock Carrot Nitsuke, Hijiki Lotus Root Nitsuke, Shio Kombu, Vegetable Tempura, Takuan Pickles.

☐ Miso soup ingredients: wakame, onion, scallion, Homemade Agé.

☐ Beverages: Brown Rice Tea, Brown Rice Bancha Tea, Sho-Ban Tea, Bancha Tea, Grain Coffee, Morning Tea.

☐ Avoid especially: all meat, including fish and shellfish, dairy foods (including ice cream), all fruit, sweet foods and drinks, mushrooms, melons, all alcohol, black tea, hot spices, tomatoes, vinegar.

GASTRITIS

Gastritis is a general term referring to any inflammation, irritation, or infection of the mucous membrane of the stomach. In general, gastritis symptoms include severe burning pain and pressure in the stomach, nausea, vomiting, diarrhea, loss of appetite, fever, weakness, coated tongue, and belching or passing gas. There are three forms of acute gastritis and a chronic type as well.

Acute simple gastritis is characterized by severe burning pain or pressure in the stomach, loss of appetite, nausea, coated tongue, and vomiting. These symptoms usually disappear in a couple of days. Acute erosive gastritis is distinguished by severe stomach pain, very fast pulse, cyanosis (a bluish discoloration), and excessive thirst. Acute infectious gastritis is indicated by lack of appetite, vomiting, and a full feeling in the stomach. Chronic gastritis has symptoms of mild nausea, a loss of appetite, constipation, acid taste in the mouth, bad breath, and stomach pain. It may last for months or even years and may lead to stomach cancer, so care should be taken if you have chronic gastritis.

The underlying causes of gastritis vary with the form of the condition but are similar in nature. Acute simple gastritis is caused by drinking too much alcohol because alcohol is absorbed in the stomach instead of the intestines. It may also be caused by the excessive use of certain drugs such as aspirin, coal-tar products such as MSG, and ammonium chloride, bromides, and quinine. Acute erosive gastritis results from the excess consumption of strong alkaline foods such as umeboshi or from drinking too much coffee (also alkaline-forming). Acute infectious gastritis is caused by diseases such as the flu, diphtheria, pneumonia, or any intestinal fever. According to our macrobiotic understanding, the underlying cause of these infections is the overgrowth of microbes brought about by a diet too high in simple carbohydrates such as sugary foods and drinks, ice cream, alcohol, and fruit juice along with an excess of protein foods, especially animal proteins. Simple carbohydrates break down into glucose in the stomach and increase the level of glucose in the intercellular fluid of the stomach. If there is also a low level of salt solution (normal is 0.85 percent), there is a greater chance for the overgrowth of microbes, leading to infections and thus to gastritis.

Chronic gastritis occurs as a result of the continuous overconsumption of alcohol, drugs, or coffee, or as a result of a general weakening of the system due to repeated cases of the acute forms of gastritis. If your constitution and physical condition are more weak or tired, you will tend to experience the acute forms of gastritis.

This is a warning that a change in dietary habits is needed; if you don't change, the chronic form develops. However, if you are strong in constitution and physical condition, you may go for years with no apparent problem only to be struck by the chronic form of gastritis more suddenly. Such a condition is usually severe and dangerous, so be careful when thinking that your excesses don't or won't affect you.

Helpful Suggestions

Do not take hot baths until the pain subsides.

OBJECTIVE	REMEDY
	WITH ACUTE GASTRIC PAIN
To relieve sharp pain	Induce vomiting by drinking ½ cup of strong SALT WATER DRINK, ½ cup of BANCHA TEA WITH SALT, or ½ to 1 cup (children and frail persons use the lesser amount) of strong SHO-BAN TEA once only. This will also help clean out the poisons and can cause diarrhea.
	then
	Eat 1 tablespoon of good-quality sesame oil; follow with 1 to 2 days, FASTING to help clean out the intestines. If you are weak, eat ⅓ cup of thick BROWN RICE CREAM (SPECIAL) 2 or 3 times per day instead of fasting. Chew well.
To relieve more severe pain	Use a ROASTED SALT PACK or GINGER COMPRESS on the stomach for 20 minutes every 4 hours.
To relieve diminished or generalized pain	Use an ALBI PLASTER on the stomach, changing it every 4 hours, or use a TOFU PLASTER on the stomach, changing it every hour.
	and
	Try drinking ½ cup of UMESHO BANCHA TEA 4 to 6 times per day when pain starts.
	and
	Applying a GINGER COMPRESS on the stomach for 20 minutes 1 to 3 times per day is very helpful.
	WITH CHRONIC GASTRIC PAIN
To improve the system	Make sure to eat a balanced diet since this condition shows a weakened system overall. For side dishes use only 1 teaspoon of TEKKA MISO and 2 or 3 slices of RICE BRAN PICKLES with every meal for a couple of weeks. This should improve your condition. Then, use the dietary recommendations for the yin type.

To ease heartburn	Try drinking ½ to 1 cup of thick *SHO-BAN TEA* 2 times per day or ½ cup of *DAIKON SOY SAUCE TEA* once a day until the heartburn stops.
To alleviate dizziness	Drink 1 cup of *SHO-BAN TEA* or ½ to 1 cup of *BANCHA TEA WITH SALT* 2 to 3 times per day.
To relieve constipation	Eat ¼ to ⅓ cup *AZUKI BEANS WITH KOMBU* once a day, adding a little salt to taste when cooking. *and* Eat 1 cup of *GREEN LEAFY VEGETABLES WITH HOMEMADE AGÉ* once a day.

Dietary Recommendations

The general cause of gastritis is overeating, so FASTING one to two days at first is recommended if your condition allows it. If you are weak, eat only one-third cup of thick Brown Rice Cream two to three times per day instead of fasting. Use the following suggestions for up to one month, then widen your food choices using a macrobiotic dietary approach (see page 11). Remember to chew each mouthful 200 times, and to eat less—two meals per day maximum. This will rest the stomach. If you are uncertain as to which type of gastritis you have, use the suggestions for the yin type first.

FOR THE YANG TYPE

☐ Main foods: Brown Rice Balls with a little Gomashio, and Azuki Rice Balls. To regain lost appetite, eat thick Brown Rice Cream (Special). Chew each mouthful 200 times.

☐ Side dishes (one-fourth of main foods): Tekka Miso, Burdock Carrot Nitsuke, Grated Daikon with Soy Sauce, Rice Bran Pickles.

☐ Miso soup ingredients: daikon, tofu, eggplant.

☐ Beverages: Brown Rice Bancha Tea, Bancha Tea, Grain Coffee, Grain Milk.

☐ Avoid especially: all animal foods (including fish, and shellfish), dairy foods, beer, wine, soy milk, all beans (except azuki), vinegar, hot spices, tomatoes, potatoes, melons, fruit, sweet foods.

FOR THE YIN TYPE

☐ Main foods: Brown Rice Balls or Azuki Rice Balls with Gomashio, Brown Rice Gruel with Mochi, Baked Mochi with Soy Sauce (once a day).

☐ Side dishes (one-fourth of main foods): Tekka Miso, Oily Miso, Shio Kombu, Burdock Carrot Nitsuke, Takuan Pickles, Miso Pickles.

☐ Miso soup ingredients: wakame, tororo kombu, scallions, onions.

☐ Beverages: Umesho Bancha Tea, Sho-Ban Tea, Bancha Tea, Brown Rice Bancha Tea. Drink only when thirsty.

☐ Avoid especially: all animal foods, fish, dairy foods, alcohol, soy milk, all beans (except azuki), vinegar, hot spices, tomatoes, potatoes, melons, fruit, sweet foods and drinks.

GINGIVITIS

See PERIODONTAL DISEASE.

GLAUCOMA

Glaucoma is a condition in which fluid pressure inside the eye increases. If not controlled, the pressure may cause permanent damage to the optic nerve. There are two types of glaucoma, chronic and acute. In chronic glaucoma, there are no symptoms in the early stages to warn the patient; by the time visual loss is noticed, it may be considerable. Later, one sees halos or rainbows around electric lights, has blind spots, and sees poorly at night. In the case of acute glaucoma, the loss of sight is rapid and is accompanied by severe throbbing pain in the eyeball, severe headaches, and vomiting. The cause of increased fluid pressure inside the eye is an abnormal accumulation of fluid in the eye due to an obstruction such as fatty material, mucus, or dead microbes. The obstruction doesn't allow the normal draining of fluid into and out of the eye. Dietary causes may be excess consumption of fruit or sugary food such as cakes or candy; excess drinking of sweet drinks, coffee with sugar, or milk; or overeating of fatty food such as ice cream.

Helpful Suggestions

A more balanced approach to diet is the best preventative. Avoid cigarette smoke, emotional stress, overworking, and prolonged eye stress such as watching television.

OBJECTIVE	REMEDY
To alleviate bacterial infection	Use a warm to hot SALT BANCHA EYE BATH 4 to 5 times per day until glaucoma improves.
To lower eye temperature	Use an UMEBOSHI EYE PLASTER or SESAME OIL EYE TREATMENT every night for 1 month or for as long as the condition persists.

or

Apply an ALBI PLASTER on each temple (see Figure 3.8 on page 176) before going to sleep and leave it on all night. This will help speed up the recovery.

Dietary Recommendations

Use the following dietary suggestions as long as glaucoma symptoms are present or for about one month. Then, widen your food choices using a macrobiotic dietary approach (see page 11).

☐ Main foods: Brown Rice, Azuki Rice, Brown Rice Balls, Brown Rice Mochi, all served with Gomashio.

☐ Side dishes (one-third of main foods): Tekka Miso, Hijiki Nitsuke, Burdock Carrot Nitsuke, Azuki Beans with Kombu and Winter Squash, Oily Miso; use sesame oil in your cooking and have sea vegetables every day.

☐ Miso soup ingredients: wakame, onions, carrots, scallions.

☐ Beverages: Bancha Tea, Brown Rice Tea, Grain Coffee. Drink a maximum of about 1 cup of beverages per day.

☐ Avoid especially: all meat, fish, shellfish, shrimp, crab, fruit, tomatoes, potatoes, eggplant, refined sugar, sweet foods, vinegar, dairy foods including cheese and butter, coffee, alcohol, fruit drinks.

GOITER

Goiter refers to an enlargement of the thyroid gland, causing swelling in the front part of the neck. There are many varieties of goiter with different kinds of swelling occurring in different parts of the thyroid gland, from a smooth, balloon-like swelling of the whole gland to a bumpy, grapelike enlargement affecting the sides of the gland.

Goiter is thought to be caused by enlargement of the thyroid due to iodine deficiency. According to our macrobiotic understanding, goiter affects those who eat overly yin foods and those who are in a yin condition. An overly yin diet creates a salt (sodium) deficiency in the body, causing an increased growth of microbes. Thus, children raised on cow's milk instead of mother's milk, or anyone who eats too many fruits, potatoes, yams, and other yin foods, can develop this disease.

Helpful Suggestions

OBJECTIVE	REMEDY
To reduce swelling	Try applying a GINGER COMPRESS on the throat for 20 minutes followed by an ALBI PLASTER for up to 4 hours. Repeat both the compress and the plaster as often as needed. This will promote healing by improving the circulation around the throat.

Dietary Recommendations

A change in dietary habits to rid yourself of the overly yin condition is best. Use the following dietary suggestions until the symptoms disappear or for one month. Then, widen your food choices using a macrobiotic dietary approach (see page 11).

☐ Main foods: Brown Rice Balls with Gomashio, Azuki Rice, Brown Rice Gruel with Mochi, Baked Mochi with Soy Sauce. Chew each mouthful 200 times.

☐ Side dishes (one-fourth of main foods): Tekka Miso, Oily Miso, Sesame Miso, Shio Kombu, Hijiki Burdock Nitsuke, Burdock Carrot Nitsuke, Carp Soup, Oysters Cooked with Miso, Oyster Tempura, Small Fish Tempura served with Grated Daikon, Miso Pickles, Umeboshi.

☐ Miso soup ingredients: wakame, onions, scallions, tororo kombu, Homemade Agé, Brown Rice Mochi.

☐ Beverages: Brown Rice Tea, Brown Rice Bancha Tea, Sho-Ban Tea, Bancha Tea, Grain Coffee, Bancha Tea with Gomashio.

☐ Avoid especially: all meat (except oysters and small fish), dairy foods (including ice cream), soy milk, all fruit, all sweet foods and drinks, potatoes, tomatoes, eggplant, vinegar, melons, coffee, alcohol.

GONORRHEA

Gonorrhea is a sexually transmitted infectious disease of the reproductive organs. It can affect both sexes and all ages, even infants, though it is most common among those aged twenty to thirty. Males usually experience more pronounced symptoms, and females often have few or no symptoms. Symptoms may include burning urination that is often slow and difficult and a thick green-yellow discharge from the penis or vagina. Sometimes there is also a mild sore throat, rectal itching and discharge, or tenderness or pain during sexual intercourse.

The cause of gonorrhea is an infection from gonococcus bacteria *(Neisseria gonorrhoeae)*. These bacteria flourish on soft, delicate, moist tissue. Although the bacteria are usually transmitted sexually, the origin in some cases is unknown. According to our macrobiotic understanding, since the symptoms of this disease are all yin, your chances of contracting gonorrhea greatly increase when you consume too much yin food such as fruit, sugary foods and drinks, and alcohol.

Helpful Suggestions

Home remedies are ineffective and antibiotics, especially penicillin, are the usual treatment. However, a macrobiotically balanced diet improves your resistance to the bacteria. A balanced diet is also helpful in neutralizing the effects of the antibiotics.

Dietary Recommendations

Gonorrhea is a very yin condition, so a more yang diet and more yang preparations are recommended. Use the following dietary suggestions while the symptoms persist or for one month. Then, widen your food choices using a macrobiotic dietary approach (see page 11).

☐ Main foods: Brown Rice, Azuki Rice, Gomashio with each meal.
☐ Side dishes (one-third of main foods): Carp Soup (2 cups per day), all sea vegetables, Shio Kombu, Burdock Carrot Nitsuke, Tekka Miso, scallions (the best vegetable for gonorrhea). Cook side dishes with sesame oil and soy sauce, and cook dishes a long time.
☐ Miso soup ingredients: scallions, Brown Rice Mochi, Homemade Agé.
☐ Beverages: Grain Coffee, Brown Rice Tea, Brown Rice Bancha Tea, Bancha Tea, Sho-Ban Tea, Azuki Kombu Drink. Drink as much as possible for 3 days only.
☐ Avoid especially: all animal foods (except carp), alcohol, coffee, black tea, fruit, sweet foods and drinks. Caffeine and alcohol irritate the urethra.

See also TESTICULAR INFLAMMATION.

HAIR, GREY

Long-term overconsumption of yang food may result in premature (before the age of fifty) greying of the hair. In this case, the hair root becomes contracted, limiting the supply of nutrition to the hair shaft. People who have eaten too much meat and fish during their childhood and then change to a macrobiotic dietary approach may have a tendency to eat too much salt. This may cause their hair roots to contract, resulting in silver hair. The

proper amount and use of salt is very important in maintaining a healthy condition.

Helpful Suggestions

OBJECTIVE	REMEDY
To open hair roots	Try applying a GINGER COMPRESS on the head for 20 minutes once a day.
	then
	Use a GINGER SESAME OIL MASSAGE on the scalp once a day.
	or
	You may try rubbing the scalp with *EGG OIL* for 5 minutes at a time.

Dietary Recommendations

Follow a macrobiotic dietary approach (see page 11) with plenty of kombu, hijiki, arame, wakame, and nori sea vegetables. These are good because sea vegetables contain nutrients that nourish the hair.

HAIR LOSS (BALDNESS)

Western medicine considers pattern baldness a hereditary condition and the result of aging, while general thinning may follow an acute illness like influenza, anemia, tuberculosis, or diabetes. General hair loss (thinning) ceases as one recovers from the acute illness. Since hair loss may affect men as young as twenty and since women are rarely affected before the age of fifty, hormonal factors are thought to contribute to pattern baldness. The presence of the male hormone testosterone seems to contribute to pattern baldness while the female hormone estrogen is theorized to protect women from hair loss.

According to our macrobiotic theory, excessive consumption of alcoholic beverages or yin foods such as potatoes, tomatoes, or eggplant contributes to general hair loss. We know that people who have high fevers sometimes lose their hair. Since the underlying cause of fever is usually the overeating of yang foods, there is a relationship between general hair loss and an excessively yang diet. The reasons for hair loss can be seen easily by looking at the condition of the intestines, since the condition of the intestines and the condition of the hair are considered to be related according to Eastern medicine.

Pattern baldness that develops at the back of the head, the most yang part of the head, is caused by the intake of too much yang food such as meat. Baldness that develops at the top of the head is caused by eating too much sugary food. Baldness in the front of the head is

---

CORNELLIA'S NATURAL HEALING AT WORK

Old-fashioned Japanese women had very long black hair. They washed their hair only once a month. Every day, they combed their hair with a very fine bamboo comb to take out the dirt and stimulate the skin, scalp, and hair roots. I remember that I used a bamboo comb after a car accident when my hair was cut very short, and it grew back very quickly. However, do not use a fine comb if you lose hair suddenly for no apparent reason or during times of hair loss due to an acute illness. Normally, you lose fifty to one hundred hairs a day, so you need not be concerned unless you begin to lose more. Medicated shampoos and ointments are useless and should be avoided. Use only natural products on the hair and change these often, especially if an allergic reaction is suspected.   ■

HAIR LOSS

---

due to the overconsumption of fruit. Eating too much of all these foods will cause total baldness.

Although there are primarily two causes (yin or yang) of any kind of hair loss as mentioned above, the mechanism that results in baldness seems the same to me. In either case, the mechanism is the loosening up or expansion of the tissue that holds the roots of the hair. In the case of yin baldness, expansion comes from sugar, fruit, vinegar, and alcohol. In the case of yang baldness, the expansion is caused by the fat in animal (yang) foods. Therefore, by not eating extreme yin foods or yang foods one can prevent baldness.

Helpful Suggestions

Eating sea vegetables helps hair growth. Cold weather also stimulates hair growth.

OBJECTIVE	REMEDY
To promote hair growth	Try using a PINE NEEDLE SCALP MASSAGE once a day to stimulate the scalp. This helps promote hair growth.
	and
	Vigorously rub the hair once a day with vegetable oil, but not mineral oil. Sesame oil, camellia oil, or EGG OIL are best.
	or
	Use a GINGER COMPRESS once or twice a day. Leave the towels on the scalp or massage the head with the ginger-compress-water until the scalp turns red. Follow each treatment by MASSAGING the head with GINGER SESEAME OIL, pressing it into the scalp.
	or

You may finely grate about ¼ cup of lotus root and squeeze out the juice. Mix the juice with a pinch of salt and then vigorously rub the head with this or with CHARCOALED MULBERRY BARK once a day.

Dietary Recommendations

To minimize pattern baldness, avoid the overconsumption of both extreme yin and yang foods. Use the following dietary suggestions until your condition improves or for about one month. Then, widen your food choices using a macrobiotic dietary approach (see page 11).

FOR THE YANG TYPE

☐ Main foods: Brown Rice with Barley (boiled) in 3 to 1 ratio, Azuki Rice served with a small amount of Gomashio.

☐ Side dishes (half of main foods): Ginger Miso, Hijiki Nitsuke, Green Salad served with Lemon Dressing or Rice Vinegar Dressing.

☐ Miso soup ingredients: wakame, tofu, sweet potatoes, and other yin vegetables.

☐ Beverages: Brown Rice Tea, Kombu Tea, Grain Coffee.

☐ Avoid especially: all animal foods, butter, eggs, and alcohol.

FOR YIN TYPES

☐ Main foods: Brown Rice, Azuki Rice served with a little Gomashio.

☐ Side dishes (one-third of main foods): Tekka Miso, Oily Miso, Hijiki Carrot Nitsuke, Hijiki Lotus Root Nitsuke, Hijiki Burdock Nitsuke, Azuki Beans with Kombu, root vegetable dishes, Burdock Carrot Nitsuke, Nori Roasted with Oil, Miso Pickles, and Rice Bran Pickles. Use more miso and soy sauce.

☐ Miso soup ingredients: scallions, onions, wakame, dried daikon, dried seitan, Brown Rice Mochi, and seasonal vegetables.

☐ Beverages: Brown Rice Tea, Sho-Ban Tea, Kombu Tea, Bancha Tea.

☐ Avoid especially: all meat, fish, shellfish, all dairy foods (including ice cream), eggs, sugar, sugary drinks, fruit, vinegar, hot spices, tomatoes, eggplant, potatoes, and melons.

HALITOSIS

See BAD BREATH.

HEADACHE

Headaches are one of the most common sicknesses of man. Symptoms range widely from mild to piercing pain. Headaches can be general or regional such as in the frontal lobe, temporal lobe (one side or both), or occipital lobe area. They can be intermittent, or constantly hitting, hammering, pressuring, etc. There are acute headaches and chronic headaches.

According to *Symptoms, The Complete Home Medical Encyclopedia*, there are over 150 chemicals that can cause headaches. A few examples are fumes of any kind, alcohol, ammonia, barbiturates, benzene, ephedrine, gasoline, kerosene, morphine, nitrous oxide, opium, privine, the sulfa drugs, high doses of vitamin A or D, tetracycline, chloromazine (used in tranquilizers), oral contraceptives, and excessive dosage of steroids. There are many other contributing factors such as tension, exhausting work, anxiety, depression, lack of sleep, excessive eating or drinking, eye strain, low blood sugar, hormonal changes, and allergic reactions, just to name a few.

There is little doubt that the agents and contributing factors listed above may result in headaches; however, there is no explanation as to why these agents and factors may cause headaches. In keeping with my experi-

ence, I believe that these agents cause a shortage of oxygen in the nerve cells in the body and in the brain. Thus, any factor that results in less oxygen available to the brain's nerve cells ultimately results in a headache. A diet too high in fatty, animal foods may cause constricted blood vessels, or a diet too high in sugar and other yin foods may cause dilated blood vessels that can result in headaches, especially when the agents or factors listed above also are present. This shortage of oxygen in the nerve cells is the cause of pain sensations.

Helpful Suggestions

OBJECTIVE	REMEDY
To relieve headache pain	Try MASSAGING your head every 3 hours with GINGER SESAME OIL, APPLE JUICE, or DAIKON JUICE.
	or
	Use an APPLICATION of GREEN LEAVES over the painful area; change the leaves every 2 hours.
To reduce fever	Apply a TOFU PLASTER to the forehead; change it every hour.
To relieve tension headache	Try applying an UMEBOSHI PLASTER on the temples.
	also
	Place 2 to 3 drops of DAIKON JUICE in each nostril and then sleep.
	and
	Every 4 hours, sip 1 tablespoon DAIKON JUICE WITH RICE SYRUP or drink 1 cup of *SHIITAKE DAIKON LOTUS ROOT TEA.*

Dietary Recommendations

The following dietary suggestions may be used any time you have a headache. Then use a macrobiotic dietary approach (see page 11) in order to help insure a good and unrestricted flow of oxygen throughout the body and brain.

☐ Main foods: Brown Rice with Barley (3 parts to 1 part), Azuki Rice served with a little Gomashio.
☐ Side dishes (half of main foods): Ginger Miso, Hijiki Nitsuke, vegetable nitsuke, Green Salad served with Lemon Dressing or Rice Vinegar Dressing.
☐ Miso soup ingredients: wakame, tofu, fresh vegetables other than sea vegetables.
☐ Beverages: Bancha Tea, Brown Rice Tea, Brown Rice Bancha Tea, Grain Coffee.
☐ Avoid especially: all fatty foods and extremely yin or yang foods.

See also HEADACHE, MIGRAINE.

HERMAN'S NATURAL HEALING AT WORK

When I was ten years old, I was living in my parents' home, which had a bathtub. This was not common for a Japanese family because family members usually went to public bathhouses in the evening instead of taking baths at home. According to Japanese custom, I had been taking a bath every day before dinner.

One night, I took my bath as usual. A few minutes later, I started to get a headache. I then started to hit my head against the bathroom wall, probably from instinct. Strangely enough, my headache lessened and I repeated hitting the wall. But soon I lost consciousness and fell on the bathroom floor. My parents, who had heard the loud banging, rushed to the bathroom and found me lying on the floor. By attracting my parents' attention, hitting the wall had saved my life.

My parents found that gas was leaking into the bathroom. I was a victim of carbon monoxide poisoning. But why would it cause a headache? I concluded, years later, that carbon monoxide causes a shortage of oxygen in the nerve cells. Then the nerve cells crave oxygen. The sensation associated with that craving is pain. Therefore, my reasoning for the cause of any pain, including headache, is that there is a shortage of oxygen in the nerve cells. ■

HEADACHE

HEADACHE, MIGRAINE

A migraine headache is an intense, often incapacitating headache that is accompanied by other symptoms and is often experienced in periodic attacks. These attacks vary in all characteristics from person to person and from time to time in the same person. However, the classic migraine follows a definite pattern of vision disturbances. These include an inability to see clearly, flashes, distortions, or bright spots that disappear once the headache begins with dull pain in the temple area spreading to an entire side of the head and resulting in intense, throbbing pain. Nausea and vomiting may follow. Sometimes a person becomes pale, experiences dizziness or ringing in the ears, or has bloodshot eyes or a runny nose. When a migraine headache occurs, it usually continues for six to twelve hours. Migraine headaches often afflict only one side of the head, usually the left side.

The left hemisphere of the brain controls the right side of the body because the nerves are crossed at the neck. Right-handed people use the right side of the body more. Therefore, a right-handed person will tend to experience a shortage of oxygen in the left side of the brain. Since most people are right-handed, there are more migraine headaches in the left side of the brain. By the same token, left-handed people will have more migraine headaches on the right side.

Migraine headaches occur when the blood vessels that go to the scalp and brain become constricted (narrow) followed by a dilation (widening) and inflammation. But what causes the blood vessels to act in this way? According to Western medicine, attacks may be started by tension or emotional upset, although the attack often occurs after stress is reduced; abnormal menstruation; fatigue; the overconsumption of alcohol; allergies to certain foods; and the use of oral contraceptives. Interestingly, migraines are more common in females. Anger, constipation, heredity, smoking, the use of many drugs, and lack of exercise greatly increase your risk of getting migraine headaches.

According to our macrobiotic understanding, however, these conditions may be contributing factors, but they are not the fundamental cause of migraines. In my opinion, the primary cause of a migraine headache is a shortage of oxygen supply to part of the brain. There are yin and yang causes of oxygen shortage that result in yin and yang types of migraine headaches. With a yang migraine, the body temperature goes up, the cheeks become red, and the pupils become smaller. A yin migraine causes the temperature to go down, the face to become pale, and the pupils to dilate.

The yin cause of oxygen shortage is eating too many yin foods and drinks such as sugary foods, fruits, other simple carbohydrates, alcoholic drinks, and butter. These foods are quickly oxidized, consuming a great deal of oxygen and causing a shortage of oxygen in the brain's nerve cells; butter is not a simple carbohydrate, but it is easily oxidized and turned to heat. In this process, butter consumes twice as much oxygen as simple carbohydrates consume. Therefore, a high consumption of butter also causes yin migraine headaches. In addition, the red blood cells made from overly yin foods are weaker and not able to carry as much oxygen as the red blood cells made from a more balanced diet. This rapid depletion of oxygen causes pain in the head and results in a yin migraine headache. Furthermore, these foods stimulate the sympathetic nervous system, causing the pupils to dilate, skin color to pale on the affected side of the brain, and brain cells to expand.

The yang cause of oxygen shortage occurs when excessive amounts of fatty, animal foods are consumed. Fat clogs the capillaries of the brain and blocks blood circulation in the brain. This causes an oxygen shortage and, ultimately, migraine headaches. Unlike yin food, animal food, containing much sodium, is yang and will stimulate the parasympathetic nerves, causing the pupils to contract, skin color to redden on the affected side of the brain, and the temperature to go up. This is the mechanism of a yang migraine headache.

Another cause of yin migraine headaches is too much water in the body. The metabolism of simple carbohydrates produces water, which is added to the fluid one consumes. As a result, the fluid in the brain increases too much and makes the brain cells expand, causing the nerves to press against the skull and produce pain.

Helpful Suggestions

OBJECTIVE	REMEDY
To relieve headache without fever	Try applying a GINGER COMPRESS on the top of the head for 20 minutes any time for pain. *and* Use a GINGER SESAME OIL MASSAGE on the scalp after the compress.
To relieve headache with a low fever	Wash the head with warm water and use an APPLE PLASTER on the forehead for 20 minutes up to 3 times per day.
To relieve headache with fever over 100°F	Apply a TOFU PLASTER to the forehead; change it every hour *and* Place an APPLICATION OF GREEN LEAVES on a pillow and lie down with the pillow under the back of your neck. Change leaves every 2 hours.

Dietary Recommendations

There is no long-term remedy as effective as changing dietary habits to a macrobiotic approach. Follow this approach (see page 11), avoiding both extreme yang and yin foods. The following suggestions may be helpful at the time of each attack.

☐ Main foods: Brown Rice with Barley in a 3 to 1 ratio, Azuki Rice served with a little Gomashio.
☐ Side dishes (half of main foods): Ginger Miso, Hijiki Nitsuke, vegetable nitsuke, Green Salad served with Lemon Dressing or Rice Vinegar Dressing.
☐ Miso soup ingredients: wakame, tofu, vegetables other than sea vegetables.
☐ Beverages: Bancha Tea, Brown Rice Tea, Brown Rice Bancha Tea, Grain Coffee.
☐ Avoid especially: all fatty foods and extremely yin or yang foods.

HEART ATTACK

A heart attack (myocardial infarction) refers to the death of heart-muscle cells that results from an interruption of the blood supply to the area. Many times, there are no previous symptoms, and the first perceived indication of illness may be a life-threatening disorder that results in irreparable damage to the heart. Warning signs are most often present, but may be mistaken for stomach pain or some other disorder.

Symptoms that occur just prior to a heart attack may include mild or severe chest pain or heavy pressure (angina pectoris), sweating, shortness of breath, nausea, and vomiting. The pain usually radiates from the chest to the jaw, neck, and left arm. The area between the shoulder blades or the upper abdomen may also experience pain. These symptoms and thus a heart attack are often brought on by a heavy meal, an emotional crisis, or heavy exercise, especially in the heat or cold and wind.

The cause of a heart attack is a partial or complete blockage of coronary arteries resulting in a reduced or obstructed blood flow, thus cutting the supply of oxygen to the heart. The lack of oxygen results in pain, as was discussed in the headache section. There are many high risk factors including a diet that is high in fat and sugar along with too much salt, high blood-cholesterol levels, smoking, stress, obesity, sedentary life-style, fatigue or overwork, and diabetes. These factors indicate the need for dietary and life-style changes for most Americans.

Unfortunately, since heart attacks are more common among men over the age of forty, many people have begun to think of heart attacks as a normal part of the aging process. However, the causes and risk factors as well as the incidence of heart attacks in women and younger men indicate otherwise. According to our macrobiotic understanding, a balanced diet that is low in fat, protein, and simple carbohydrates and high in complex carbohydrates is the best preventative for heart attacks. The United States Senate Select Committee on Nutrition and Human Needs and the American Medical Association agree with our macrobiotic understanding in this regard.

Helpful Suggestions

By the time you have a heart attack, you may require hospitalization and even surgery. Statistics show that most persons recover from a first heart attack, especially if the person receives immediate emergency care. Unfortunately, many do not change their diet or life-style and succeeding and more deadly heart attacks follow.

OBJECTIVE	REMEDY
To relieve chest pain	Apply an ALBI PLASTER on the painful area, changing it every 4 hours.
To quiet a too strong pulse	Every 4 hours, try drinking SOUR APPLE JUICE made from 1 small apple. A large person may use 2 to 3 apples. The grated apple juice goes to the intestines to help take away the heat, and the lemon juice goes to the kidneys to activate urination.
	and
	A DAIKON PLASTER over the heart area is helpful. If you are really in pain, change the plaster every 5 minutes. The daikon will become hot even in such a short time. If you have no daikon, use an APPLE PLASTER. Use the plaster for only 1 hour because grated daikon or apple reduces the heart's heat and can make the heart too cold (yin). The Daikon (or Apple) Plaster is used only to relieve the symptoms.
To alleviate palpitations	Try drinking ½ to 1 cup of *SHO-BAN TEA* 2 to 3 times per day.
	and
	Use a DAIKON or APPLE PLASTER on the heart (see Figure 3.8 on page 176) for no more than an hour, changing it every 20 minutes. If this treatment is not effective, try a TOFU PLASTER applied to the heart area for 1 hour.
To eliminate (melt away) fats and crystalized salt	Take a FAR-INFRARED SAUNA several times per week.
To maintain alkaline condition	Avoid hot baths. Short, warm showers are okay.

Dietary Recommendations

The following dietary suggestions may be used until your heart condition improves or for about one month. Then, widen your food choices based on a macrobiotic dietary approach (see page 11).

☐ Main foods: Brown Rice (or any whole grains) served with Gomashio, Brown Rice Mochi.
☐ Side dishes (one-third of the main foods): Tekka Miso, Hijiki Nitsuke, Nori Nitsuke, Shio Kombu, Vegetable Tempura, Azuki Beans with Kombu and Winter Squash, Burdock Carrot Nitsuke. Use less salt than usual in the cooking of side dishes.
☐ Miso soup ingredients: wakame, tororo kombu, daikon, burdock.
☐ Beverages: Brown Rice Tea, Bancha Tea, Grain Coffee.
☐ Avoid especially: all animal foods including fish and shellfish, all sweet foods and drinks, ice cream, all fruit, all alcohol.

See also ARTERIOSCLEROSIS.

HEARTBEAT, RAPID (TACHYCARDIA)

When the heartbeat is much more rapid than usual and is not caused by overexertion, it is referred to as "tachycardia." Normally, the heart beats from 70 to 90 times per minute in adults and from 80 to 110 times per minute in children. During exercise or other periods of exertion, a person's heartbeat rate may rise to 160 or more. This is normal and various goals are set for elevating the heart rate during what is called pulse-related exercise. Tachycardia refers to a heart rate above 100 beats per minute in adults who are not exercising.

Someone with tachycardia will have a pounding heart, rapid pulse at the wrist or neck, faintness, loss of breath, increased urination, coughing, and chest pain. The cause of this condition is unknown although it is known that heart muscle and the electrical system of the heart are involved. Stress, smoking, caffeine or other drugs, overworking or fatigue, and heart disease increase your chances of experiencing tachycardia. Uninterrupted episodes may lead to life-threatening heart disorders and so your health-care advisor should be consulted.

According to our macrobiotic understanding, too much yin food, especially food rich in potassium (fruits such as bananas and vegetables such as potatoes), along with too little sodium (salt) is the underlying cause.

Potassium increases the excitability of the sympathetic nervous system while sodium decreases it. The sympathetic nervous system stimulates the heart to beat faster. Thus, a proper balance between potassium and sodium is the best preventative and the best remedy for repeated attacks of tachycardia.

Helpful Suggestions

Physical fitness is known to help prevent tachycardia and regular exercise is recommended. However, this exercise does not need to be strenuous; check with your health-care advisor before embarking on an exercise program if you have heart problems.

OBJECTIVE	REMEDY
To strengthen a weak pulse	Drink the RANSHO DRINK prepared from 1 egg, once a day for 3 days before bedtime. If once a day is not enough, eat a second 1-egg preparation of ransho per day until the heart becomes stronger (shows a stronger pulse).
	and/or
	Eat 1 teaspoon of TEKKA MISO once a day at any meal for 1 week.
To improve circulation	Apply a MUSTARD PLASTER to the heart until the skin begins to turn a red color (about 10 minutes), then apply an ALBI PLASTER for up to 4 hours. Apply these plasters for 1 week.
	and
	Eat ½ teaspoon of EGG OIL 3 times per day for 1 week to help make the heart stronger.
To relieve chest pain	Apply an ALBI PLASTER on the painful area, changing it every 4 hours as needed.
To relieve cough	Drink ½ to 1 cup of LOTUS ROOT TEA 2 or 3 times per day.
To eliminate (melt away) fat and crystalized salt	Take a FAR-INFRARED SAUNA several times per week.

Dietary Recommendations

The following dietary suggestions may be used until your heart condition improves or for about one month. Then, widen your food choices based on a macrobiotic dietary approach (see page 11).

☐ Main foods: Brown Rice, Azuki Rice served with Gomashio, Fried Rice, Brown Rice Mochi. Chew each mouthful more than 100 times.
☐ Side dishes (one-fourth of main foods): Tekka Miso, Oily Miso, Hijiki Lotus Root Nitsuke, Burdock Carrot Nitsuke, Carp Soup, Vegetable Tempura, Nori Roasted with Oil, Miso Pickles. Slowly increase the amount of

salt, measured by taste, in side dishes.

☐ Miso soup ingredients: wakame, scallions, onions, Brown Rice Mochi, tororo kombu.

☐ Beverages: Brown Rice Bancha Tea, Sho-Ban Tea, Kombu Tea, Mu Tea. Drink less than usual.

☐ Avoid especially: all animal foods including fish, shellfish, dairy foods (especially ice cream), and eggs; all fruit; sweet foods; all forms of caffeine such as coffee, cola drinks, and chocolate; all alcohol since alcohol depresses the heartbeat; vinegar; mushrooms; melons; all beans except azuki beans.

HEART BLOCK

Heart block refers to an interference with the normal conduction of electrical impulses that control heart muscle activity. Thus, the regulatory mechanism that speeds heartbeat during stress or exertion and slows it down at other times does not function normally. Sometimes, there are no apparent symptoms, especially in less severe forms, and at other times symptoms range from a slow irregular heartbeat to a sudden loss of consciousness or convulsions. Heart block can result from clotting in the coronary arteries, atherosclerosis (hardening of the arteries), a congenital heart defect, or the ingestion of too many drugs such as digitalis.

Helpful Suggestions

Severe cases are sometimes controlled with the surgical implantation of a pacemaker. However, the macrobiotic approach is to try a change in diet and life-style first, and thus possibly avoid the need for an operation.

OBJECTIVE	REMEDY
To strengthen a weak pulse	Drink the RANSHO DRINK prepared from 1 egg, once a day for 3 days before bedtime. If once a day is not enough, eat a second 1-egg preparation of ransho per day until the heart becomes stronger (shows a stronger pulse). *and/or* Eat 1 teaspoon of TEKKA MISO once a day at any meal for 1 week.
To improve circulation	Apply a MUSTARD PLASTER to the heart just until the skin turns a red color (about 7 minutes), then apply an ALBI PLASTER for up to 4 hours. Apply these plasters for 1 week. *and* Eat ½ teaspoon of EGG OIL 3 times per day for 1 week to help make the heart stronger.

To relieve chest pain	Apply an ALBI PLASTER on the painful area, changing it every 4 hours as needed.
To eliminate (melt away) fat and crystalized salt	Take a FAR-INFRARED SAUNA several times per week.

Dietary Recommendations

The following dietary suggestions may be used until your heart condition improves or for about one month. Then, widen your food choices based on a macrobiotic dietary approach (see page 11).

☐ Main foods: Brown Rice, Azuki Rice served with Gomashio, Fried Rice, Brown Rice Mochi. Chew each mouthful more than 100 times.

☐ Side dishes (one-fourth of main foods): Tekka Miso, Oily Miso, Hijiki Lotus Root Nitsuke, Burdock Carrot Nitsuke, Carp Soup, Vegetable Tempura, Nori Roasted with Oil, Miso Pickles. Slowly increase the amount of salt, measured by taste, in side dishes.

☐ Miso soup ingredients: wakame, scallions, onions, Brown Rice Mochi, tororo kombu.

☐ Beverages: Brown Rice Bancha Tea, Sho-Ban Tea, Kombu Tea, Mu Tea. Drink less than usual.

☐ Avoid especially: all animal foods including fish, shellfish, dairy foods (especially ice cream), and eggs; all fruit; sweet foods; all forms of caffeine such as coffee, cola drinks, and chocolate; all alcohol since alcohol depresses the heartbeat; vinegar; mushrooms; melons; all beans except azuki beans.

HEARTBURN

Heartburn is a symptom and not a disease and has nothing to do with the heart. It refers to any discomfort in the upper digestive tract and may signal a hiatal hernia, ulcers of the esophagus, or a condition in which stomach acid rises into the esophagus. Some of the common signs of heartburn are an uncomfortable, burning sensation in the esophagus and the upper part of the stomach, difficulty in swallowing, and on rare occasions severe abdominal pain and vomiting. According to our macrobiotic understanding, an unbalanced diet, especially one that creates an overacidic condition, is the root of heartburn. Animal foods such as red meats and sugary foods including alcohol are all acid-forming in the body. Spicy dishes, coffee, and acid fruits, while they may be alkaline-forming in overall effect, stimulate heavy stomach-acid secretion as does an overconsumption of protein-rich foods.

Helpful Suggestions

Reducing or avoiding stress, obesity, smoking, alcohol consumption, and the use of drugs including aspirin will help lower your risk of heartburn.

OBJECTIVE	REMEDY
To relieve pain	Try drinking 1 cup of *SHO-BAN TEA, SHO-BAN TEA WITH GRATED DAIKON*, or *BANCHA TEA WITH GOMASHIO* 2 or 3 times per day. or Eat a 1-inch square of *ROASTED KOMBU*, 1 teaspoon of *GOMASHIO*, or 1 umeboshi as needed.

Dietary Recommendations

Many people take nonprescription liquid antacids for mild discomfort and these may be helpful. However, recurrence of heartburn is common especially if the underlying cause is not controlled. The best way to remedy heartburn is to change your diet to a more balanced one by following a macrobiotic dietary approach (see page 11). Otherwise, you may develop an ulcer, or stomach or esophageal cancer. In other words, heartburn, like other symptoms, is a signal that dietary and life-style changes are needed. If these changes are made and you continue to have episodes of heartburn after one month, then try eating two to three pieces of rice bran pickles (preferably homemade using daikon) or takuan pickles per meal to aid in proper digestion.

HEART FAILURE, CONGESTIVE

Congestive heart failure occurs when the heart loses its full pumping capacity; it is most likely caused by an overworking of the heart muscle. If some of the muscles of the heart are damaged as is the case in a heart attack, even normal activity may cause the heart to overwork. Arteriosclerosis leads to a similar condition. Actually, any heart disease or an infection complicating the heart disease may lead to congestive heart failure, so it is important to deal also with the underlying heart disorders. An overworked heart may damage more heart muscle, in which case, the heart cannot work to full capacity. In this case, blood backs up into other organs such as the lungs and liver. Symptoms associated with congestive heart failure are shortness of breath; fatigue; weakness or faintness; coughing; abnormal sodium and water retention, resulting in swelling of the abdomen, legs, and ankles; irregular heartbeat; low blood pressure; enlarged liver; and enlarged pupils.

Helpful Suggestions

OBJECTIVE	REMEDY
To strengthen a weak pulse	Drink the *RANSHO DRINK* prepared from 1 egg, once a day for 3 days before bedtime. If once a day is not enough, eat a second 1-egg preparation of ransho per day until the heart becomes stronger (shows a stronger pulse). and/or Eat 1 teaspoon of *TEKKA MISO* once a day at any meal for 1 week.
To improve circulation	Apply a *MUSTARD PLASTER* to the heart just until the skin turns a red color (about 7 minutes), then apply an *ALBI PLASTER* for up to 4 hours. Apply these plasters for 1 week. and Eat ½ teaspoon of *EGG OIL* 3 times per day for 1 week to help make the heart stronger.
To relieve chest pain	Apply an *ALBI PLASTER* on the painful area, changing it every 4 hours as needed.
To eliminate (melt away) fat and crystalized salt	Take a *FAR-INFRARED SAUNA* several times per week.
To maintain a strong condition	Avoid hot baths. Short, warm showers are okay. and Drinking 1 cup of *ENMEI TEA* 2 or 3 times per day for 1 week is effective for congestive heart failure.

Dietary Recommendations

The following dietary suggestions may be used until your heart condition improves or for about one month. Then, widen your food choices based on a macrobiotic dietary approach (see page 11).

☐ Main foods: Brown Rice, Azuki Rice served with Gomashio, Fried Rice, Brown Rice Mochi. Chew each mouthful more than 100 times.

☐ Side dishes (one-fourth of main foods): Tekka Miso, Oily Miso, Hijiki Lotus Root Nitsuke, Burdock Carrot Nitsuke, Carp Soup, Vegetable Tempura, Nori Roasted with Oil, Miso Pickles. Slowly increase the amount of salt, measured by taste, in side dishes.

☐ Miso soup ingredients: wakame, scallions, onions, Brown Rice Mochi, tororo kombu.

☐ Beverages: Brown Rice Bancha Tea, Sho-Ban Tea, Kombu Tea, Mu Tea. Drink less than usual.

☐ Avoid especially: all animal foods including fish, shellfish, dairy foods (especially ice cream), and eggs; all fruit; sweet foods; alcoholic drinks; vinegar; mushrooms; melons; all beans except azuki beans.

HEART-RHYTHM IRREGULARITY

Heart-rhythm irregularity (arrhythmia) refers to abnormalities in the rhythm of the heartbeat. These abnormalities may be occasional or constant and are most likely to occur in persons over age sixty-five, especially if they have had a history of other heart diseases or endocrine disorders, or have used any of a number of drugs such as digitalis, stimulants, diuretics, and antidepressants. Symptoms of irregular heart rhythm may be occasional or constant and include skipped heartbeats, shortness of breath, or sudden weakness or fainting. Frequently, there are no symptoms.

Irregular heart rhythm may also be due to an electrolyte imbalance, especially from too much or too little potassium, that, in turn, may be caused by kidney weakness. Kidney weakness may result from the side effects of certain drugs, especially digitalis, diuretics, and/or other stimulants, or from a long-term diet too high in both fatty animal foods and yin foods such as sugar and alcohol. (See Kidney Failure for a more detailed discussion.) Whatever the cause of irregular heart rhythm, the underlying problem of improper diet must be dealt with and changed.

Helpful Suggestions

OBJECTIVE	REMEDY
To strengthen a weak pulse	Drink the RANSHO DRINK prepared from 1 egg, once a day for 3 days before bedtime. If once a day is not enough, eat a second 1-egg preparation of ransho per day until the heart becomes stronger (shows a stronger pulse).
	and/or
	Eat 1 teaspoon of TEKKA MISO once a day at any meal for 1 week.
To improve circulation	Apply a MUSTARD PLASTER to the heart just until the skin turns a red color (about 7 minutes), then apply an ALBI PLASTER for up to 4 hours. Apply these plasters for 1 week.
	and
	Eat ½ teaspoon of EGG OIL 3 times per day for 1 week to help make the heart stronger.
To eliminate (melt away) fat and crystalized salt	Take a FAR-INFRARED SAUNA several times per week.
To maintain a strong condition	Avoid hot baths. Short, warm showers are okay.

Dietary Recommendations

The following dietary suggestions may be used until your heart condition improves or for about one month. Then, widen your food choices based on a macrobiotic dietary approach (see page 11).

☐ Main foods: Brown Rice, Azuki Rice served with Gomashio, Fried Rice, Brown Rice Mochi. Chew each mouthful more than 100 times.

☐ Side dishes (one-fourth of main foods): Tekka Miso, Oily Miso, Hijiki Lotus Root Nitsuke, Burdock Carrot Nitsuke, Carp Soup, Vegetable Tempura, Nori Roasted with Oil, Miso Pickles. Slowly increase the amount of salt, measured by taste, in side dishes.

☐ Miso soup ingredients: wakame, scallions, onions, Brown Rice Mochi, tororo kombu.

☐ Beverages: Brown Rice Bancha Tea, Sho-Ban Tea, Kombu Tea, Mu Tea. Drink less than usual.

☐ Avoid especially: all animal foods including fish, shellfish, dairy foods (especially ice cream), and eggs; all fruit; sweet foods; alcoholic drinks; vinegar; mushrooms; melons; all beans except azuki beans.

HEART-VALVE PROBLEMS

The four valves of the heart are the mitral or bicuspid, tricuspid, pulmonary, and aortic valves. If the heart chambers are expanded (yin) so that the valves cannot be closed completely, blood will flow backward when the heart is in a constriction cycle, causing an insufficient supply of blood to the body. Signs of heart-valve problems are fatigue and weakness, dizziness, fainting, chest pain, shortness of breath, lung congestion, irregular heart rhythm, and heart murmurs.

Although a heart-valve problem can arise as a side effect of a chest or heart operation, this disorder is generally thought to be inherited or caused by other disorders such as high blood pressure, endocarditis (inflammation of the membrane lining the heart), atherosclerosis, rheumatic fever, and syphilis. According to our macrobiotic understanding, the underlying cause of these diseases or of the inherited condition is a diet that is too high in yin foods and drinks such as sugary foods, cow's milk, and alcohol, resulting in a heart-valve problem. In this case, the heart is overly expanded, the blood is very thin, the person is generally anemic, and the pulse is very weak.

Helpful Suggestions

Don't take hot baths if you have any heart disease. Short, warm showers are okay. However, the use of a FAR-INFRARED SAUNA is recommended because the sauna will eliminate (melt away) fats and crystalized salt. Perspiring and eliminating fat are especially good for atherosclerosis and high blood pressure. When fat inside of the capillaries and arteries melts and is eliminated through blood circulation, the blood pressure goes down. This can also be achieved by sweating. However, in order to sweat enough to eliminate fat from the arteries and capillaries, a person must run about two to three miles. This is almost impossible for someone who has heart and circulatory troubles. And a normal sauna is too hot for people with heart trouble. Therefore, a far-infrared sauna, which is much safer for persons with heart problems, is preferable.

OBJECTIVE	REMEDY
To strengthen a weak pulse	Drink the RANSHO DRINK prepared from 1 egg, once a day for 3 days before bedtime. If once a day is not enough, eat a second 1-egg preparation of ransho per day until the heart becomes stronger (shows a stronger pulse).
	and/or
	Eat 1 teaspoon of TEKKA MISO once a day at any meal for 1 week.
To improve circulation	Apply a MUSTARD PLASTER to the heart just until the skin turns a red color (about 7 minutes), then apply an ALBI PLASTER for up to 4 hours. Apply these plasters for 1 week.
	and
	Eat ½ teaspoon of EGG OIL 3 times per day for 1 week to help make the heart stronger.
To alleviate palpitations	Try drinking ½ to 1 cup of SHO-BAN TEA 2 to 3 times per day.
	and
	Use a DAIKON or APPLE PLASTER on the heart for no more than an hour, changing it every 20 minutes. If this treatment is not effective, try a TOFU PLASTER applied to the heart area for 1 hour.
To relieve chest pain	Apply an ALBI PLASTER on the painful area; change it every 4 hours as needed.
To alleviate constipation	Eat ½ cup of AZUKI BEANS WITH KOMBU once a day for 1 week, and use less salt than usual.

Dietary Recommendations

The following dietary suggestions may be used until your heart condition improves or for about one month. Then, widen your food choices based on a macrobiotic dietary approach (see page 11).

☐ Main foods: Brown Rice, Azuki Rice served with Gomashio, Fried Rice, Brown Rice Mochi. Chew each mouthful more than 100 times.

☐ Side dishes (one-fourth of main foods): Tekka Miso, Oily Miso, Hijiki Lotus Root Nitsuke, Burdock Carrot Nitsuke, Carp Soup, Vegetable Tempura, Nori Roasted with Oil, Miso Pickles. Slowly increase the amount of salt, measured by taste, in side dishes.

☐ Miso soup ingredients: wakame, scallions, onions, Brown Rice Mochi, tororo kombu.

☐ Beverages: Brown Rice Bancha Tea, Sho-Ban Tea, Kombu Tea, Mu Tea. Drink less than usual.

☐ Avoid especially: all animal foods including fish, shellfish, dairy foods (especially ice cream), and eggs; all fruit; sweet foods; alcoholic drinks; vinegar; mushrooms; melons; all beans except azuki beans.

HEAT RASH

See PRICKLY HEAT.

HEATSTROKE

See SUNSTROKE.

HEAVY METAL POISONING

Heavy metal poisoning can result from exposure to heavy metal contaminants such as mercury, lead, cadmium, arsenic, antimony, and thallium. Even a brief exposure can cause acute symptoms while a chronic condition arises after a long-term exposure to low to moderate levels. Heavy metal poisoning is due to the absorption, or inhalation, of any of the heavy metals, and the incidence is increasing as industrial wastes are deposited into the environment. Symptoms vary greatly depending on the heavy metal and on whether the poisoning is acute or chronic. For example, acute mercury poisoning symptoms include vomiting, stomachache, bloody diarrhea, urination problems, and ulcers in the digestive organs; chronic mercury poisoning symptoms include tremors, lack of coordination, bleeding gums, a loosening of the teeth, excessive saliva, and stomachaches; cadmium poisoning symptoms range from joint soreness, hair loss, anemia, a dulled sense of smell, appetite loss, and dry, scaly skin to high blood pressure, emphysema, cancer, and a shortened lifespan. Symptoms of lead poisoning include headaches, loss of appetite and of weight, dizziness, constipation, anemia, irritability, and moderate hypertension.

It has been claimed that a far-infrared sauna can melt deep body fat (4 inches into the body) and heavy metals such as mercury and cadmium are eliminated with sweat. According to experiments with the far-infrared sauna, aluminum (although not a heavy metal) was reduced by 15 percent, cadmium almost disappeared, and arsenic was reduced by more than 50 percent. Mercury and lead levels were initially reduced and later increased, although not to their original levels.

Helpful Suggestions

Removing sources of heavy metals (paints, air pollutants) from your environment as much as possible will help to prevent heavy metal poisoning. For symptoms of heavy metal poisoning, such as insomnia, anemia, constipation, abdominal pain, diarrhea, headaches, etc., see those sections for specific remedies.

OBJECTIVE	REMEDY
To relieve symptoms of acute or chronic poisoning	Try using saunas or salt baths. Take a SAUNA once a day at 120° to 150°F until you sweat, then shower with warm water to wash off the sweat. Take saunas until symptoms disappear.
	also
	Take a warm (not hot) 1 percent SALT BATH for 30 minutes to 1 hour each day.
	or
	Take a BEACH SAND BATH for 6 to 8 hours.
	and
	If you become weak, drink ½ to 1 cup of *SHO-BAN TEA* after the saunas or baths.

Dietary Recommendations

Follow a macrobiotic dietary approach (see page 11) using ceramic cooking utensils that have been tested to be lead free. (Note that regulations in foreign countries may not be as strictly enforced as in the United States.) Some macrobiotic thinkers believe that miso helps rid the body of heavy metals, and while there is no scientific evidence to confirm this claim, it can't hurt to eat miso soup every day. Removing the heavy metals from your environment as much as possible is also recommended. It is especially important to test your water and buy an adequate filter if necessary.

HEMORRHOIDS

Hemorrhoids (piles) are dilated veins of the rectum or anus. External hemorrhoids generally cause itching and constipation. Internal hemorrhoids are quite painful with clotting, rectal bleeding, itching or mucous discharge after bowel movements, and the continuing urge to evacuate the bowels even though excretion is completed. Internal hemorrhoids can result from a serious illness such as syphilis or tuberculosis.

According to our macrobiotic understanding, hemorrhoids are most commonly caused by the overconsumption of yang foods, especially those lacking in dietary fiber. Straining during bowel movements aggravates the hemorrhoids and the pain but is not the underlying cause. If the following suggestions and a change to a diet high in dietary fiber does not help or if there is extreme pain or excessive rectal bleeding, consult with your healthcare advisor.

Helpful Suggestions

If hemorrhoids are the result of another illness, see the helpful suggestions for that condition. If you do not change the condition of your whole body through dietary changes, then you are not eliminating the primary cause of the hemorrhoids and they will return. Good physical conditioning has a positive effect on bowel functioning; therefore, exercising is important.

OBJECTIVE	REMEDY
To relieve pain	Try taking a DAIKON or ARAME HIP BATH for 20 minutes followed by an ALBI PLASTER placed directly on hemorrhoids, changing the plaster every 4 hours and continuing as long as needed.
To reduce hemorrhaging piles	Use the same remedies as for pain and MASSAGE the area with SESAME OIL 2 to 3 times per day.

Dietary Recommendations

The following dietary suggestions may be used as long as the hemorroids persist or for about one month. Then, widen your food choices using a macrobiotic dietary approach (see page 11).

☐ Main foods: Brown Rice, Azuki Rice, Brown Rice Mochi served with Gomashio.
☐ Side dishes (one-third to one-half of main foods): Tekka Miso, Scallion Miso, Burdock Nitsuke, Hijiki Nitsuke, Shio Kombu, Vegetable Tempura (especially

using burdock), Carp Soup, hijiki, Homemade Agé, Takuan Pickles.

☐ Miso soup ingredients: wakame, scallions, onions, Homemade Agé, Brown Rice Mochi.

☐ Beverages: Brown Rice Tea, Brown Rice Bancha Tea, Kombu Tea. Drink a maximum of 2 cups of beverages per day.

☐ Avoid especially: all meats and red-meat fish, shell-fish, dairy foods (including ice cream), meat-based soups, fruit, sweet foods and drinks, alcohol, mushrooms, sweet potatoes, peanuts, tomatoes, eggplant.

HEPATITIS

Hepatitis is an inflammation of the liver. In the beginning stages of hepatitis, there may be an enlargement of the liver, fever, fatigue, nausea, vomiting, diarrhea, and loss of appetite. Later, a yellow color that is caused by too much bile in the blood appears in the skin and eyes, and the urine becomes darker because of the overflow of bile into the urine.

Acute viral hepatitis is caused by an infection of any of three different but related viruses known as type A, type B, and type non-A, non-B. The type A virus usually moves through contaminated water or food while type B virus usually is spread by blood transfusions, non-sterile needles or syringes, and oral-anal sexual practices. Type non-A, non-B is most commonly spread through contaminated blood transfusions. The most common forms of hepatitis are hepatitis A (infectious hepatitis) and hepatitis B (serum hepatitis). All forms are contagious.

Your risk of getting hepatitis increases with exposure to areas with poor sanitation or to persons with hepatitis, the need for blood transfusions or injections, and contact with anything that lowers the body's resistance to viral infections such as an illness, poor nutrition, or alcoholism. Beyond taking care of the symptoms, the macrobiotic approach is to make the body as resistant to infections as possible through a balanced diet and a positive life-style.

Helpful Suggestions

To test for an enlarged liver, lay down on your back and bend your knees. Push in under the center of your right ribs with your third and fourth fingers. You should be able to push the fingers in to the second finger joint (two full finger sections from the tip). If your liver is enlarged, you will not be able to do this. If your liver is in a healthy condition, you will not experience any pain or tenderness.

OBJECTIVE	REMEDY
To reduce an enlarged liver	Try applying a GINGER COMPRESS over the liver area (see Figure 3.8 on page 176) for 20 minutes, followed by an ALBI PLASTER for up to 4 hours. Continue these remedies each day for 2 to 3 weeks until the liver is no longer enlarged.
To relieve pain	Put a ROASTED SALT PACK on the stomach (see Figure 3.8 on page 176) to keep abdomen warm and to increase circulation.
To reduce a bloated stomach	Try applying a GINGER COMPRESS to the stomach for 20 minutes, then apply a BUCK-WHEAT PLASTER once a day for 4 hours. Place a ROASTED SALT PACK on top of the BUCKWHEAT PLASTER to keep it warm. Do this for up to 10 days.
To reduce fever	Place a TOFU PLASTER on the forehead; change it every hour.
To relieve nausea	Eat 1 or 2 BROWN RICE BALLS WITH GOMASHIO, chewing very well.
In all cases	The best remedy is FASTING for 3 days to 1 week if your condition allows it. Complete fasting with water only is used for extreme cases only and is not generally recommended.

Dietary Recommendations

Use a macrobiotic dietary approach (see page 11) with less oil and eat less for about a week. Drink Brown Rice Tea, Brown Rice Bancha Tea, Bancha Tea, and Grain Coffee.

☐ Avoid especially: all animal foods and overly yin foods, especially alcohol.

HERNIA

A hernia is an abnormal protrusion of an organ or part of an organ through the structures that usually contain it. There are several kinds of hernias depending on where the breakthrough occurs. A hiatus hernia is a protrusion of the stomach at the juncture of the esophagus and the stomach. In hiatus hernias, the onset of pain occurs immediately after meals. Pain may occur during sleep as well. Bleeding may occur, which can cause severe anemia. An inguinal hernia is a protrusion of the tissues or muscles at the lower end of the abdominal cavity. A lump under the pubic hair is an indication of an inguinal hernia. Sometimes there is no pain, but in the case of an acute hernia, there is severe pain in the area of the hernia.

According to our macrobiotic understanding, a hernia is the result of a yin condition of the muscles. Eating too much yin food causes some muscles to expand and lose their flexibility, resulting in a hernia. Therefore, the cause of a hernia is the long-time consumption of yin food or a mother's excess consumption of yin foods—fruit, candy, dairy foods, tomatoes, eggplant, and potatoes—during pregnancy. If the mother drinks cow's milk while breastfeeding, this may cause a hernia as well. Hernias can be an acquired condition, too, but the same remedies and dietary suggestions apply.

Helpful Suggestions

Avoid hot baths until your condition improves. Heavy lifting and straining should be avoided as well. Hernias take a long time to remedy so you will need to continue applying plasters each day as time permits. A hernia belt is all right to use if surgery can be avoided by its use. Be aware that the long-term use of a tight hernia belt (truss) may injure or weaken tissues, making surgery difficult if not impossible.

OBJECTIVE	REMEDY
To relieve symptoms of a hernia	Try using an ALBI PLASTER over the hernia, with a ROASTED SALT PACK on top; change both the plaster and the compress every 2 hours. *and* The affected area may be lightly rubbed with good-quality sesame oil and gently pushed inward.

Dietary Recommendations

The following dietary suggestions may be used for about one month. Then, widen your food choices using a macrobiotic dietary approach (see page 11).

☐ Main foods: Brown Rice, Azuki Rice, Fried Rice served with Gomashio. Chew well.
☐ Side dishes (one-third of main foods): Tekka Miso, Oily Miso, Hijiki Nitsuke, Shio Kombu, Burdock Carrot Nitsuke, Vegetable Stew, Carp Soup, Vegetable Tempura, Nori Roasted with Oil, natural caviar, Takuan Pickles, Miso Pickles.
☐ Miso soup ingredients: wakame, tororo kombu, Homemade Agé, seitan, Brown Rice Mochi.
☐ Beverages: Brown Rice Tea, Brown Rice Bancha Tea, Bancha Tea, Sho-Ban Tea, Kombu Tea, Grain Coffee.
☐ Avoid especially: all meats, red-meat fish, shellfish, eggs, dairy foods, milk, cheese, butter, ice cream, soy milk, all mushrooms, peanuts, hot spices, rice bran pickles.

Hiccups

Hiccups are repeated, sudden, violent, involuntary contractions of the diaphragm indicated by a characteristic sound made by the sudden closure of the vocal cords. Hiccups result from the failure of synchronization between the movement of the lid that shuts off the airways during swallowing and the diaphragm. The phrenic nerve that connects the diaphragm to the brain is also involved. Hiccups are a symptom and not a disease, and short episodes usually don't indicate the presence of disease. However, hiccups that last longer than eight hours may signal a serious disease and your health-care advisor should be consulted.

The cause of short episodes is usually considered to be unknown while longer episodes may result from many causes including emotional disturbances, the use of certain drugs (both prescription and nonprescription), alcoholism, swallowing irritating substances. Hiccups are also associated with any number of disorders involving the stomach, esophagus, large intestine, bladder, pancreas, lung, or liver. According to our macrobiotic understanding, the underlying cause of short hiccup episodes is eating too much yin food such as hot peppery foods, overeating any foods, and/or faulty swallowing due to eating or drinking in a hurry. These factors also contribute to longer episodes.

Helpful Suggestions

There are many common remedies for short hiccup episodes, ranging from breathing into a paper (not plastic) bag and rebreathing the air in the bag to drinking a glass of water rapidly while upside down. Any of your favorites may be tried.

OBJECTIVE	REMEDY
To control hiccups	It is important to breath deeply. *or* Holding a pinch of salt in the mouth or eating 2 teaspoons of GOMASHIO may be helpful. Chew well. *or* Biting on a small piece of fresh ginger is also beneficial, although very potent.

Dietary Recommendations

Those who practice macrobiotics experience a great reduction in the number of hiccuping episodes, if not a total cessation, and episodes that do occur are less intense.

Following a macrobiotic dietary approach (see page 11) while paying particular attention to chewing each mouthful very well is most helpful for preventing hiccups and for dealing with the underlying factors that can result in longer episodes.

☐ Avoid especially: hot spicy foods, overeating, and eating or drinking in a hurry.

HUNCHBACK (KYPHOSIS)

Hunchback or kyphosis refers to an abnormally increased convexity in the curvature of the thoracic spine as viewed from the side. Other conditions associated with hunchback include swollen knees, severe diarrhea, and dry heaves. According to Western medicine, a hunchback spine is caused by birth injury or by nerve or bone diseases.

According to our macrobiotic understanding, the cause is the mother's diet during pregnancy and/or while she is nursing. If during these times the mother eats too much yin food such as potatoes, fruit, sweet foods, milk, and vinegar, the child may develop a hunchback.

Helpful Suggestions

If the baby has a hunchback, the mother should change her diet and therefore her milk supply. Small children recover easily from a hunchback spine, but it is much harder to remedy in children over the age of ten.

OBJECTIVE	REMEDY
To reduce swollen knees	Try applying an ALBI PLASTER on the knees, changing it every 4 hours.
To control severe diarrhea	Give a DAIKON or ARAME HIP BATH WITH GRATED GINGER for 20 minutes once a day. *and*
	Give children beyond the age of breastfeeding ½ cup of UMESHO KUZU TEA 2 times per day.
To alleviate dry heaves	If a baby or child is trying to vomit and needs help, give ⅓ to ½ cup (the lesser amount to younger babies or children) of UMESHO BANCHA TEA once to help induce vomiting.

Dietary Recommendations

Children or nursing mothers may use the following dietary suggestions for about one month. Then, widen the food choices using a macrobiotic dietary approach (see page 11).

☐ Main foods: Brown Rice Balls with Gomashio, Azuki Rice, Azuki Millet Rice, Brown Rice Gruel with Mochi and Miso.

☐ Side dishes (one-fourth to one-third of main foods): Tekka Miso, Hijiki Carrot Nitsuke, Carp Soup, Winter Squash and Onions, Burdock Carrot Nitsuke, Vegetable Tempura, Deep-Fried Kombu, Azuki Beans with Kombu.

☐ Miso soup ingredients: wakame, tororo kombu, scallions, onions, Brown Rice Mochi, dried seitan.

☐ Beverages: Brown Rice Tea, Brown Rice Bancha Tea, Sho-Ban Tea, Grain Milk, Kombu Tea.

☐ Avoid especially: all yin foods including sweet foods and fruit, especially vitamin D milk with fruit.

HYPERACTIVITY

Hyperactivity is a disorder of the central nervous system that results in abnormally increased activity such as lack of concentration, temper tantrums, impatience, quick frustration, clumsiness, sleep disturbances, head-knocking, and an inability to sit still. Those suffering from the disorder often exhibit failure at school. Many factors have been associated with hyperactivity, ranging from oxygen deprivation at birth and the mother's smoking during pregnancy to environmental pollutants, artificial additives in food, and refined sugar.

However, according to our macrobiotic understanding, the primary cause of hyperactivity is a diet with too much sugary food, including fruit and fruit juices, combined with the overconsumption of animal protein such as meat, chicken, fish, and eggs. Overeating, even of grains, is a contributing factor. Children may exhibit symptoms of hyperactivity after eating large amounts of sugar; however, some do not. The difference seems to be the amount of animal food in the diet because animal foods contain phosphorus, which is used in the production of ATP (brain energy). Vegetarian children, for example, often become lethargic after eating sugar. Thus, it is the combination of too much animal food with too much sugar that leads to hyperactivity.

Dietary Recommendations

Most important is to chew each mouthful 100 times and to eat only when hungry. Follow a macrobiotic dietary approach (see page 11).

☐ Avoid especially: all meat and animal foods, sugary foods, fruit, fruit juices, and foods with artificial additives and preservatives.

HYPERTHYROIDISM

The thyroid gland is the part of the endocrine system that regulates metabolism. The endocrine system includes the pituitary gland, parathyroid glands, pancreas, adrenal glands, and ovaries or testicles; a problem in one part of the system may signal a disorder in other or all parts of the system.

When the thyroid gland is overactive, the condition is called hyperthyroidism. Symptoms include hyperactivity, sweating, rapid heartbeat, itchy skin, a constant warm or hot feeling, weight loss even with overeating, anxiety, hand tremors, sleeplessness, fatigue, and weakness. Sometimes there is also diarrhea, goiter, hair loss, protruding eyes, and/or double vision. Because hyperthyroidism develops gradually, symptoms are often difficult to recognize and the condition may be well-developed by the time it is noticed. The specific causes of hyperthyroidism are generally thought to be thyroid nodules or tumors, ovarian disorders, or pituitary problems.

According to our macrobiotic understanding, hyperthyroidism is a very yin illness caused by eating too many yin foods such as fruits and sugary foods including cakes, candy, and soft drinks, and/or by eating too little salt or salty foods over a long period of time. Unless there is a medical emergency, you should try a change in diet first before taking drugs or having surgery, especially because drugs or surgery for hyperthyroidism may lead to hypothyroidism, the underproduction of thyroid hormone. Drugs may also produce side effects. A balanced diet is the best way to ensure proper thyroid functioning.

Helpful Suggestions

OBJECTIVE	REMEDY
To alleviate rapid heartbeat and/or dizziness	Try drinking 1 cup of SHO-BAN TEA 1 or 2 times per day. Start with weak Sho-ban Tea and gradually make it stronger by adding more soy sauce as your condition improves.
To relieve heart pain	Apply an ALBI PLASTER directly over the heart, changing it every 4 hours.
To reduce sweating	Try eating 1 cup of MOCHI SOUP once a day.
To relieve headache	Use an APPLE JUICE or GINGER SESAME OIL MASSAGE on the head.

Dietary Recommendations

Follow a macrobiotic dietary approach (see page 11) with one cup of Miso Soup served with five to six pieces of small dried fish and rice-bran pickles every day. Use condiments such as tekka, umeboshi, and gomashio. Occasionally—once a week—freshwater or white-meat fish may be eaten.

☐ Avoid especially: sugary foods and drinks, fruits, dairy products, stimulants, tomatoes, potatoes, eggplant, and mushrooms.

HYPOGLYCEMIA

Hypoglycemia, commonly known as low blood sugar, refers to an abnormally diminished amount of glucose (sugar) in the blood. Functional hypoglycemia is low blood sugar caused by the abnormal function of the pancreas. In this case, excess insulin is produced by the pancreas in response to a high consumption of refined sugar and other simple carbohydrates, heavy exercise, pregnancy, or other causes that are unknown. Nervousness, sweating, trembling hands, drowsiness, fatigue, dizziness, headache, irritability, and excessive hunger may indicate a functional hypoglycemic condition.

Another form of low blood sugar occurs in patients taking medication for diabetes; symptoms vary depending on the severity of the reaction. Mild reaction symptoms include weakness, emotional instability and difficulty concentrating, nervousness, excessive hunger, headache, and sweating. A moderate reaction is indicated by increased weakness, memory loss, staring expression and unawareness of one's surroundings, pounding heartbeat, difficulty walking, double vision, numbness around the mouth or fingers, and excessive sweating leading to cold, clammy skin. Symptoms of a severe hypoglycemic reaction include lack of urinary control, muscle twitching, convulsions, and unconsciousness. Fatigue, stress, smoking, the use of certain drugs, improper diet, illness with fever, and liver or pancreas disorders increase the risk of hypoglycemia.

According to our macrobiotic understanding, there are two underlying causes of hypoglycemia. If the blood has too much glucose, the pancreas produces insulin, which changes glucose to glycogen (form of carbohydrate used as storage material) in order to keep a nearly constant amount of glucose in the blood stream. When too much simple carbohydrate such as refined sugar is eaten, it quickly becomes glucose in the intestines. This stimulates the pancreas to produce insulin in an excessive amount. The result is that too much glucose is changed to glycogen. Thus, eating too much refined sugar and other simple carboydrates is one primary cause of hypoglycemia.

The other underlying cause of hypoglycemia is a malfunctioning of the adrenal glands. These glands normally produce glucocorticoids in the case of low blood sugar. The glucocorticoids change liver glycogen to blood sugar. When the adrenal glands are weak, then too few glucocorticoids are produced and the body is unable to adequately raise the amount of blood sugar. The result is hypoglycemia. The primary cause of weak adrenal glands is weak kidneys from drinking too much liquid (water, tea, coffee, alcohol, etc.), eating a low- or high-salt diet, or eating too much acid-forming food such as meat, eggs, cheese, fish, chicken, oily foods, fatty foods, high-protein foods, and all sugary foods. Smoking excessively may also weaken the adrenal glands.

Helpful Suggestions

Avoid stress and cigarette smoke as much as possible. See Kidney Failure for ideas on making the kidneys and thus the adrenal glands stronger.

Dietary Recommendations

Following a macrobiotic dietary approach (see page 11) with plenty of whole grains is the best way to remedy this condition. Chew very well. Eating five or six small meals a day is helpful. If you crave sweets, eat Winter Squash and Onion, or Baked Yams or Sweet Potatoes.

☐ Avoid especially: alcohol, refined sugar, and other simple carbohydrates.

HYPOTHYROIDISM

Hypothyroidism refers to an underactive thyroid gland and is more common than hyperthyroidism, an overactive thyroid gland. The thyroid gland, located in the neck just below the Adam's apple, is part of the endocrine system and a disorder in it may signal problems in other parts of the system such as the pituitary or adrenal glands, pancreas, or ovaries or testicles. Signs of hypothyroidism include decreased tolerance for cold; decreased tolerance for medication; reduced appetite, sex drive, and sweating; irregular heartbeat; weight gain or extreme thinness; fatigue or anemia; fluid retention, especially around the eyes; chest pain; constipation; irregular sleep patterns; mental and menstrual disorders; muscle weakness; and coarse skin. It is highly unlikely that one person will have all these symptoms, but most will have several.

The cause of hypothyroidism is sometimes unknown. In cases where the cause is known, several factors may be involved. These include autoimmune disease, the use of certain drugs, iodine deficiency, surgery for hyperthyroidism, and decreased activity of the pituitary gland.

According to our macrobiotic understanding, hypothyroidism is a very yang illness caused by eating too many yang foods such as animal foods and not enough vegetables, sea vegetables, and occasional fruit. While thyroid-replacement hormones are available and often prescribed, taking them does nothing to remedy the underlying cause. A balanced diet over a long period of time is the best remedy and the only way to ensure proper thyroid functioning.

Helpful Suggestions

For the symptoms of hypothyroidism such as constipation, fatigue, anemia, menstrual disorders, etc., see the appropriate sections. In general, dietary change is the only way to begin to remedy this condition. Avoid radiation treatments as these can lead to the destruction of the thyroid gland and the need for thyroid replacement therapy for the rest of your life. Hypothyroidism is very difficult to identify in infants. Therefore, it is very important to prevent the condition by not giving babies animal foods such as eggs, meat, chicken, pork, fish, cheese, and cow's milk.

Dietary Recommendations

Follow a macrobiotic dietary approach (see page 11) with one cup of miso soup and several Rice Bran Pickles every day. Occasionally (once a week) freshwater or white-meat fish can be eaten by adults.

☐ Avoid especially: all animal foods (except fish), sugary foods and drinks, fruits, dairy products, stimulants, tomatoes, potatoes, eggplant, and mushrooms. Until your condition improves, avoid small dried fish, tekka, umeboshi, and gomashio.

HYSTERIA

Hysteria is a psychoneurosis characterized by lack of control and emotional overreactions, anxiety, overexaggeration of sensory impressions, and morbid self-consciousness. Symptoms may include pain and tenderness in the ovaries, spine, and head; an abnormally increased sensitivity or the loss of feeling and other sensory disturbances; dimness of vision; retention of urine; fever; and vasomotor disturbances. More severe cases may result in paralysis, convulsions, hallucinations, and catalepsy.

According to our macrobiotic understanding, hysteria is the result of an unbalanced condition caused by eating an excess of both extreme yin and yang foods. Thus, the only true remedy is to change the whole body's condition by changing your diet.

Helpful Suggestions

In severe cases or if these suggestions are not helpful, consult with your health-care advisor.

OBJECTIVE	REMEDY
To relieve headache	Try applying a GINGER COMPRESS on the head for 10 to 20 minutes *or* MASSAGE the entire head with GINGER SESAME OIL.
To relieve severe headache	Apply a TOFU PLASTER on the forehead and place a GREEN LEAVES APPLICATION under a headband at the back of the neck, changing each every 2 hours.
To alleviate numbness or pain	Place a GINGER COMPRESS on the affected area for 20 minutes. *and* Take a DAIKON or ARAME HIP BATH every day for 20 minutes. *and* Drinking 1 cup of *MU TEA* 2 or 3 times per day for 1 week may be helpful.

Dietary Recommendations

The following dietary suggestions may be used until your condition improves or for about one month. Then, widen your food choices based on a macrobiotic dietary approach (see page 11).

☐ Main foods: Brown Rice, Azuki Rice, Millet Rice, Brown Rice Gruel with Mochi, Fried Rice, and Gomashio served with each meal. Chew each mouthful 200 times.

☐ Side dishes (one-fourth of main foods): Tekka Miso, Scallion Miso, Hijiki Nitsuke, Azuki Beans with Kombu, Shio Kombu, Nori Roasted with Oil, Burdock Carrot Lotus Root Nitsuke, Vegetable Tempura served with Grated Daikon, Takuan Pickles, Miso Pickles.

☐ Miso soup ingredients: wakame, tororo kombu, onions, scallions, Brown Rice Mochi.

☐ Beverages: Brown Rice Tea, Brown Rice Bancha Tea, Bancha Tea, Sho-Ban Tea, Kombu Tea, Grain Coffee, Mu Tea.

☐ Avoid especially: all animal foods, fish, shellfish, dairy foods (including ice cream), eggs, meat-based soups, fruit, sweet foods and drinks, tomatoes, potatoes, eggplant, vinegar, mushrooms, melons, black tea, peanuts.

IMPOTENCE

Impotence refers to a lack of power or virility in the male and is characterized by the inability to have or maintain an erection of the penis. Often there is no erection or it may be too weak, brief, or painful for satisfactory sexual intercourse. Occurences of impotence are most common in men over the age of forty-five, but men of any age can be affected.

Impotence may be due to disorders of the central nervous system, particularly spinal-cord injury, stroke, or multiple sclerosis; endocrine system disorders involving the pituitary, thyroid, adrenal, or sexual glands; other illnesses including diabetes, syphilis, or atherosclerosis or hardening of the arteries. Alcoholism and abuse of both prescription drugs such as some antihypertensive medications and illicit drugs such as marijuana, cocaine, tranquilizers, sedatives, and hallucinogenics may be the cause. There are many other physiological causes, and impotence may be due to something as simple as temporary fatigue or stress.

However, about 80 percent of impotence cases have psychological causes such as guilt feelings; depression; anxiety; a loss of contact with reality; a lack of sexual information, especially regarding female anatomy and physiology; and a lack of sexual attraction or feelings of aggressiveness towards one's partner. Brief counseling or improved communication with one's partner often leads to quick recovery. If physical origins are the cause, then improvement of the underlying disorder is needed.

According to our macrobiotic understanding, the underlying causes of impotence are the overconsumption of yin acid-forming foods such as sugary foods; weak kidneys that cannot keep the body fluids alkaline enough; the dietary lack of alkaline-forming elements, especially calcium and sodium, leading to an overly acidic condition; and eating too much yin food such as sugary foods and drinks, alcohol, cow's milk, and fruit; or taking too many yin drugs, such as those previously mentioned, over a long period of time without enough yang foods, such as salty foods, for balance. This kind of diet weakens the system in general and makes one more susceptible to many illnesses. And since dietary causes are often behind disorders of the central nervous, endocrine, and cardiovascular systems, a good, balanced diet is very important as a preventative and for dealing with periods of impotence.

Helpful Suggestions

Strenuous exercise, saunas, and hot tubs may reduce sperm counts and should be avoided during periods of impotence. However, regular, mild exercise is important for keeping the body in good physical condition and for maintaining one's self-esteem. Avoiding stress, cigarette smoke, and drugs is also recommended.

OBJECTIVE	REMEDY
To improve circulation	A GINGER COMPRESS applied on the sexual organs for 20 minutes once a day may be helpful.

Dietary Recommendations

The following dietary suggestions may be used during periods of impotence or for about one month. Then, widen your food choices using a macrobiotic dietary approach (see page 11).

☐ Main foods: Brown Rice, Azuki Rice, Mochi Soup, Baked Mochi with Soy Sauce and nori, and Gomashio served with each meal.
☐ Side dishes (one-third of main foods): Tekka Miso, Sesame Miso, Scallion Miso, Shio Kombu, Burdock Carrot Nitsuke, Deep-Fried Chuba Iriko (5 pieces every day).
☐ Miso soup ingredients: wakame, tororo kombu, scallions, onions, Homemade Agé.
☐ Beverages: Even if you are thirsty, drink less and chew your food more. You can drink Brown Rice Tea, Brown Rice Bancha Tea, and Sho-Ban Tea.
☐ Avoid especially: eggs, all dairy foods (including ice cream), meat-based soups, red meat, alcohol, soy milk, sweet drinks and foods, all fruit, vinegar, hot spices, tomatoes, mushrooms.

INFERTILITY

Infertility occurs in 10 percent of all couples and is characterized by the inability of a woman to conceive or by the inability of a male to impregnate a fertile woman. Feelings of guilt or inadequacy may contribute to the problem and are often more troublesome than the fertility problems, which may be minor and reversible. There are many possible causes of infertility from anatomical abnormalities and infections to emotional stress and the use of drugs and some medications, including oral contraceptives. Use of birth control pills or devices may impede fertility even after use has been discontinued.

According to our macrobiotic understanding, fertility problems of a nonanatomical nature in females or males are caused by eating too much yin food such as sweet foods, coffee, or fruit over a long period of time.

In this case, a yin type of infertility is the result. However, occasionally too much yang food, especially fatty animal foods, is the cause and a yang type of infertility results. In my opinion, if a woman eats too much fruit, it will be difficult for her to become pregnant as the uterus becomes cool and the sexual appetite is diminished. There are so many reasons for infertility that medical help or counseling may be needed. However, positive results have been achieved by many with the use of simple suggestions so there is reason for optimism.

Helpful Suggestions

If you are uncertain which type of infertility you have, try the suggestions for the yin type first.

OBJECTIVE	REMEDY
	FOR THE YANG TYPE
To balance hormones	Once a day before sleeping (or 2 hours after supper), take a DAIKON or ARAME HIP BATH WITH GRATED GINGER for 20 minutes.
To relieve ovarian or testicular pain	Apply an ALBI PLASTER to the painful area, changing it every 4 hours.
	FOR THE YIN TYPE
To balance hormones	Once a day before sleeping (or 2 hours after supper) take a DAIKON or ARAME HIP BATH with a handful of salt added. Stay in the bath for 20 minutes. Before or after the hip bath, drink 1 cup of SHO-BAN TEA.
To relieve ovarian or testicular pain	Use an ALBI PLASTER on the painful area, changing it every 4 hours. Avoid long hot baths; short baths or showers are okay. Refrain from sex until your condition improves.
	FOR YANG OR YIN TYPES
To increase the likelihood of fertilization	Both partners should avoid overexercising prior to intercourse. Men should avoid tight underwear or athletic supporters and also avoid ejaculation for at least 3 days prior to making love to the ovulating woman. During love-making, use only saliva as a lubricant since other lubricants may interfere with sperm mobility. A quick withdrawal after ejaculation is suggested so as not to reduce the number of sperm that can swim toward the egg. Placing pillows under the woman's bottocks immediately after intercourse may ease the sperm's swim.

Dietary Recommendations

It is most important to change dietary habits in order to change the body's condition, especially if a hormonal imbalance is present. Try the following dietary suggestions for about one month. Use the suggestions for the yin type if you have been overeating both yin and yang foods. Then, widen your food choices based on a macrobiotic dietary approach (see page 11).

FOR THE YANG TYPE

☐ Main foods: Brown Rice, Azuki Rice served with Gomashio.

☐ Side dishes (less than one-fourth of main foods): Sesame Miso, Ginger Miso, Carp Soup, Vegetable Stew, Okara Nitsuke, Grated Daikon with Soy Sauce, Daikon Nitsuke with Homemade Agé, Boiled Daikon (1-inch thick) served with Lemon Miso, Azuki Beans with Kombu, Burdock Carrot Daikon Nitsuke, Vegetable Tempura, Eggplant Nitsuke with Miso, Green Leafy Vegetables, Sour Cabbage.

☐ Miso soup ingredients: daikon, daikon greens, tofu, eggplant, carrots, sweet potatoes, yams, Chinese cabbage, green leafy vegetables, Brown Rice Mochi.

☐ Beverages: Brown Rice Tea, Brown Rice Bancha Tea, Vegetable Broth, Grain Coffee.

☐ Avoid especially: all animal foods including fish, shellfish, eggs, dairy foods (including ice cream), sweet foods and drinks, meat-based soups, hot spices.

FOR THE YIN TYPE

☐ Main foods: Brown Rice, Azuki Rice, Millet Rice, all served with Gomashio.

☐ Side dishes (one-third or less of main foods): Tekka Miso, Scallion Miso, Hijiki Lotus Root Nitsuke, Carp Soup, Vegetable Stew, Vegetable Stew with Fish, Oysters Cooked with Miso, Shio Kombu, Burdock Carrot Nitsuke, Vegetable Tempura served with Grated Daikon, Nori Roasted with Oil, Kombu Rolls with Chuba Iriko, Takuan Pickles, Miso Pickles.

☐ Miso soup ingredients: wakame, tororo kombu, scallions, onions, Homemade Agé, Brown Rice Mochi.

☐ Beverages: Brown Rice Tea, Brown Rice Bancha Tea, Bancha Tea, Kombu Tea, Grain Milk, Mu Tea.

☐ Avoid especially: all meat and fish (except oysters and carp), eggs, dairy foods (including ice cream), all fruit, sweet foods and drinks, alcohol, tomatoes, vinegar, potatoes, peanuts, hot spices, black teas, melons.

INFLUENZA

See FLU.

INSOMNIA

Insomnia refers to a habitual inability to sleep or an abnormal wakefulness that is characterized by difficulty either falling asleep or remaining asleep. Underlying causes are many and include anxiety resulting from stress, sexual problems, erratic work hours, or a new or noisy environment; disorders such as depression, an overactive thyroid gland, allergies, heart or lung conditions that disturb breathing, any illness involving pain, and urinary or gastrointestinal problems; the use of some medications; alcoholism; drug abuse or withdrawal from addictive substances; consumption of stimulants such as coffee; and lack of physical exercise.

According to our macrobiotic understanding, one cause of insomnia is overeating. In addition, people who overeat yang food such as animal foods will experience the shallow sleep of carnivorous animals. Consumption of too much yin food such as fruit, sugar, alcohol, and sweet foods also results in shallow sleep even though the sleep may be long. Some people at these extremes become so sensitive and nervous that they cannot sleep at all. Another cause of insomnia is insufficient sodium in the bodily fluids. This occurs when one eats a very low- or no-salt diet. A lack of salt (yang) inhibits the function of yang organs such as the heart, liver, and kidneys. As a result, blood circulation is slow, metabolism is low, and acid accumulation is high. Overeating fatty, animal foods results in the same condition. On the other hand, when you eat an adequate amount of salt, the circulation is good, metabolism is improved, and acids are cleaned up. Therefore, you can sleep well.

Another cause of insomnia is weak kidneys, which cannot maintain the proper amount of sodium in the bodily fluids. Then, the nerves become too active because the potassium to sodium ratio increases too much (potassium stimulates the nerves). In order to remedy this condition, one has to increase the amount of sodium in the blood. However, if the kidneys are weak, it is not wise to increase salt intake as this can further damage the kidneys. This creates a very difficult situation. In this case, you need to increase the amount of sodium in the blood in a nondietary way. See the section on Kidney Failure for ideas to help improve the condition of the kidneys.

Helpful Suggestions

If you have a weak condition, avoid hot baths and refrain from sex until your condition improves. Regular exercise and a change in diet are most helpful in establishing a life-style that promotes good sleep patterns.

OBJECTIVE	REMEDY
To aid in relaxation	Before going to sleep, wash your head with warm water or use a WARM TOWEL COMPRESS every night for 20 minutes. and The BREATHING EXERCISE for 10 minutes or a WATER FOOT BATH for 20 minutes before going to sleep is also effective.
To increase the proportion of sodium in the blood in a nondietary way	Try taking a SALT BATH that contains 2 pounds of salt in 24 gallons of warm water. Continue this until you can sleep easily.
To help you go to sleep	If you have been eating too much yang food, try placing scallions or onions near your pillow at night. The smell of the onions may make you sleepy. and Eating 1 tablespoon of SCALLIONS SEASONED WITH MISO or SCALLION MISO is helpful for insomnia.
To remove old medications from your system	Drink 1 cup of MU TEA WITH BLACK SOYBEANS 2 to 3 times per day for 2 to 3 weeks to help remove old medications from your body.

Dietary Recommendations

Use the following dietary suggestions during periods of insomnia or for about one month. Then, widen your food choices using a macrobiotic dietary approach (see page 11). If you have overeaten both yin and yang foods in the past, try the suggestions for the yin type first.

FOR THE YANG TYPE

☐ Main foods: Brown Rice Balls served with a little Gomashio, Azuki Rice. Chew each mouthful 200 times.

☐ Side dishes (one-fourth of main foods cooked to a less salty taste than usual): Sesame Miso, Wakame or Hijiki Lotus Root Nitsuke, Tororo Kombu Soup, Natto with Soy Sauce and Scallions served with Grated Daikon, Azuki Beans with Kombu, Carp Soup, Vegetable Tempura served with Grated Daikon, Steamed Vegetables, Eggplant Nitsuke with Miso and Lemon, Cucumber Pressed Salad, pressed salad, Umeboshi.

☐ Miso soup ingredients: daikon, tofu, green peas, string beans, sweet potatoes or yams.

☐ Beverages: Brown Rice Tea, Brown Rice Bancha Tea, Bancha Tea, Grain Coffee. Drink a maximum of 2 cups of beverages per day.

☐ Avoid especially: all animal protein, shellfish, fish (except carp), meat-based soups, eggs, all dairy foods, sweet foods and drinks, coffee.

FOR THE YIN TYPE

☐ Main foods: Brown Rice served with Gomashio. Chew each mouthful 200 times.

☐ Side dishes (one-third of main foods): Tekka Miso, Hijiki Nitsuke, Burdock Carrot Nitsuke, Vegetable Tempura served with Grated Daikon, Homemade Agé, Azuki Beans with Kombu, Takuan Pickles, Miso Pickles, Carp Soup, Vegetable Stew with Fish.

☐ Miso soup ingredients: wakame, scallions, onions, Homemade Agé, Brown Rice Mochi.

☐ Beverages: Brown Rice Tea, Brown Rice Bancha Tea, Bancha Tea, Kombu Tea, Grain Coffee. Before going to sleep, drink Sho-Ban Tea or 1 teaspoon of Gomashio swallowed with some water.

☐ Avoid especially: all animal protein, fish (except carp and fish in stew), shellfish, eggs, meat-based soups, all tomatoes, mushrooms, coffee, cocoa, ice cream, all alcohol, sugar and sugary foods, vinegar, hot spices, and pressed salad.

JAUNDICE

Jaundice is a condition caused by any of various liver or bile duct diseases that result in bile pigment buildup in the blood. Because of this buildup, bile pigment is deposited in the skin and mucous membranes, giving a yellow appearance to the skin and whites of the eyes. Thus, jaundice is a symptom of liver and blood disorders. It may also be a signal of an obstruction in the normal flow of bile from the liver to the intestinal tract through what is called the biliary tract. As a result, the bile backs up into the blood stream. When jaundice is caused by a biliary obstruction, there will be dark urine and light stools. Mild jaundice (yellowing) is common in newborn babies, especially those born early, and usually clears up in a couple of days with exposure to sunlight. If it lasts longer or appears to be more severe, consult with your health-care advisor.

According to our macrobiotic understanding, overworking the liver is usually caused by the overconsumption of yang foods, especially fatty, animal foods. This results in yang jaundice. Sometimes the liver is overworked by eating and drinking too much yin food, especially sweet and/or oily foods, and this results in yin (chronic) jaundice. Too much fat or oil in the diet may also precede a tumor, gallstones, or inflammation resulting in a biliary tract obstruction.

Helpful Suggestions

If jaundice is accompanied by dark urine, light stool, fever and itching, consult your health-care advisor.

OBJECTIVE	REMEDY
To relieve itchy skin	Use hot GINGER BATH water as a sponge bath 2 to 3 times per day.
To cleanse the system of toxins	Drink ½ cup of salty SHO-BAN TEA 2 times for 1 day only. This may induce diarrhea or vomiting.
	and/or
	FASTING or partial fasting with 1 to 3 cups of MUGWORT TEA per day for 1 week is helpful if your condition allows it. If you fast, follow the recommendations for breaking a fast in the FASTING remedy. In cases where fasting is not possible, eat ½ cup of RAW BROWN RICE for breakfast for 1 week.

Dietary Recommendations

Use the following dietary suggestions for meals other than breakfast during the week of raw brown rice (see Fasting remedy above) and until the jaundice clears up or for one month. Then, widen your food choices using a macrobiotic dietary approach (see page 11). If you have eaten a lot of animal foods in the past, use the suggestions for the yang type.

FOR THE YANG TYPE

☐ Main foods: Brown Rice Balls, Azuki Rice, both served with a little Gomashio.

☐ Side dishes (one-fourth of main foods using less salt than usual): Sesame Miso, Hijiki Nitsuke, Boiled Daikon served with Oily Miso, Daikon Nitsuke with Homemade Agé, Okara Nitsuke, Vegetable Tempura served with Grated Daikon, Burdock Carrot Nitsuke, Eggplant Nitsuke with Miso, Pressed Salad, Sour Cabbage, Umeboshi.

☐ Miso soup ingredients: daikon greens, green leafy vegetables.

☐ Beverages: Bancha Tea, Brown Rice Bancha Tea, Vegetable Broth, Grain Coffee.

☐ Avoid especially: all animal food including fish and shellfish, all dairy foods (including ice cream), all sweet foods, sweet drinks, alcohol, black tea, and coffee.

FOR THE YIN TYPE

☐ Main foods: Brown Rice Balls, Azuki Rice, Brown Rice Mochi served with Gomashio.

☐ Side dishes (one-half of main foods): Tekka Miso, Oily Miso, Hijiki Nitsuke, Oysters Cooked with Miso, Vegetable Tempura served with Grated Daikon, Burdock Carrot Nitsuke, Azuki Beans with Kombu, Deep-Fried Kombu, Takuan Pickles, Miso Pickles.

☐ Miso soup ingredients: wakame, tororo kombu, onions, scallions, dried daikon, Homemade Agé, dried seitan, Brown Rice Mochi.

☐ Beverages: Brown Rice Tea, Brown Rice Bancha Tea, Sho-Ban Tea, Bancha Tea, Kombu Tea, Grain Milk. Drink a maximum of 2 cups of beverages per day.

☐ Avoid especially: all overly yin foods and overly yang foods especially mushrooms, tomatoes, eggplant, hot spices.

KIDNEY FAILURE

There are two types of kidney failure, acute and chronic. In the early stages of acute kidney failure, there is little or no urination and swelling occurs in the face, especially under the eyelids. In the later stages, symptoms include severe itching, high or low blood pressure, unexplained bruising, mental changes such as irritability or drowsiness, nausea, appetite loss, vomiting, diarrhea, vertigo, convulsions, and coma. Acute kidney failure is characterized by the sudden failure of the kidneys to function and usually has a short course that is relatively severe.

The cause of acute kidney failure usually involves underlying conditions, including blood poisoning; congestive heart failure; blood transfusion reaction; extensive muscle injury; problems in blood vessels supplying blood to the kidneys; kidney stones that obstruct the passage of urine; an overly anemic condition; overdose of many poisons or drugs, especially mind-altering drugs; use of certain medications for a long time such as anesthesia or antibiotics; and fluid or electrolyte imbalances. Prompt treatment of the underlying condition will most likely lead to a complete recovery.

Chronic kidney failure is characterized by the inability of the kidneys to eliminate the body's nitrogen waste products. Symptoms do not appear until the kidneys lose over 60 percent of their filtration function. They include itching skin, anemia, fatigue, bad breath, shortness of breath, tingling and burning in the legs and feet, water retention, high blood pressure, mental confusion, mouth and gum disorders, abdominal pain, and decreased sex drive. A person with chronic kidney failure will exhibit one or more of these symptoms.

Causes of chronic kidney failure include an overdose of many drugs, chemicals, and preservatives; diabetes; blood circulation problems, especially in or around the arteries in the kidneys; chronic urinary tract infections and other infections; drinking too much water, coffee, tea, or juice; eating too many animal foods, chemical additives, or salty foods. Many life-threatening disorders

CORNELLIA'S NATURAL HEALING AT WORK

At the beginning and middle of each month, it is a Japanese tradition to eat azuki rice (brown rice and azuki beans cooked together). The reason for this custom is that azuki beans, even though they are acid-forming, are good for stimulating urination and bowel movements thus eliminating the body's toxins. Ancient Japanese wise men initiated the custom because of their belief in the benefits azuki beans have for the kidneys.

An American couple in Japan thought that since azuki beans were yang, they could have azuki rice every day. They gave this to their children, and one daughter developed a type of hunchback. Although azuki beans are good, eating them every day will make the blood too acidic. When calcium (an alkaline substance) is taken from the blood to balance the excess acid, the bones become weak. We do recommend that people with urination troubles eat azuki beans (cooked with kombu) every day, but this is only until they are better. If your urination is normal, it is not good to eat beans every day in North America. ∎

KIDNEY FAILURE

can result from this condition, and kidney failure usually worsens gradually and eventually ends in death. Kidney dialysis or transplant is the usual course of treatment.

According to our macrobiotic understanding, acute and chronic kidney failure can be further divided into yang and yin kidney failure. Whether acute or chronic, yang kidney failure is the result of eating too much yang food such as animal foods and salty foods and the result of ingesting too many yang chemicals and drugs. Eating too much salt over a long period of time can also lead to a condition called atrophic kidney, in which the kidney is diminished in size. This condition may lead to high blood pressure or kidney failure. Yin kidney failure results from the overconsumption of liquids and other yin foods such as sugary foods, alcohol and fruit, and from taking too many yin drugs and medications.

Helpful Suggestions

For the yang type, try taking hot baths two to three times per day for two to three weeks. The baths promote sweating. Stop eating salt for this period of time. With the yin type, slowly increase salt in the diet. Avoid yin foods. Avoid hot baths (showers are okay) and refrain from having sex until your condition improves. With either type, it is a good idea to improve the general condition of the kidneys over an extended period of time. Use one or more of the suggestions for either type per day.

OBJECTIVE	REMEDY
FOR THE YANG TYPE	
To relieve swollen limbs	Drink 1 cup of DAIKON TEA or BROWN RICE TEA up to 5 times per day until swelling goes down.
To induce urination	Drink 1 cup of WATERMELON RIND TEA 3 times per day for 1 week, or eat 1 raw persimmon 2 times per day for 1 week. These methods will produce urination, which will help cleanse the kidneys.
To improve atrophic kidney condition	For a period of 1 month, apply a GINGER COMPRESS on the kidney area (see Figure 3.8 on page 176) each day for 20 minutes followed by an ALBI PLASTER for up to 4 hours. The Ginger Compress helps relieve pain and improves circulation to kidneys, while the Albi Plaster helps remove excess toxins.
FOR THE YIN TYPE	
To reduce swelling	Drink 1 cup of PERSIMMON CAP TEA 3 times per day until swelling goes down.
To induce urination	You can also use the following for 1 week: 1 cup of BROWN RICE BROTH 2 times per day, ½ cup of AZUKI BEANS WITH KOMBU once a day, 1 cup of DAIKON TEA 2 times per day, or 1 to 2 pieces of BROWN RICE MOCHI WITH AZUKI BEANS once a day.
To relieve headache	Use an APPLE or DAIKON JUICE MASSAGE on the head.
FOR EITHER TYPE (YIN OR YANG)	
To strengthen kidneys	Apply a GINGER COMPRESS over the kidney area (see Figure 3.8 on page 176) for 20 minutes every day for a period of 1 month. If the kidneys are still weak, try another month of compresses.

and/or

Walking barefoot on the grass in the early morning for 5 to 20 minutes every day is very helpful. Both the compresses and the barefoot-walking help make blood circulation better and provide more oxygen to the kidneys, thus making them stronger.

and/or

Take a FAR-INFRARED SAUNA 2 or 3 times a week at about 140°F until you begin to sweat (about 20 minutes).

and/or

SALT BATHS in 1 percent salt solution are most helpful. Try to take 2 or 3 of these per week also.

and/or

If you live near a beach, you might want to try a BEACH SAND BATH. The saunas, salt baths, and beach sand baths help the kidneys by discharging excess acids through the skin, allowing the kidneys to rest.

Dietary Recommendations

The following dietary suggestions may be used until your condition improves or for about one month. Then, widen your food choices using a macrobiotic dietary approach (see page 11).

FOR THE YANG TYPE

☐ Main foods: Brown Rice Balls, Azuki Rice; chew each mouthful 200 times. In severe cases, use Brown Rice Cream (thick) with Grated Daikon.
☐ Side dishes (one-fourth of main foods): Sesame Miso, Hijiki Nitsuke, Burdock Nitsuke, Natto with Soy Sauce and Scallions, Okara Nitsuke served with Grated Daikon, Vegetable Tempura served with Grated Daikon, Azuki Beans with Kombu and Winter Squash (2/3–1 cup every day), Eggplant Nitsuke with Miso, Cucumber with Kuzu Sauce, Daikon Nitsuke with Homemade Agé, Chinese Cabbage Pickles, Mustard Green Pickles, Watermelon Syrup, Carp Soup.
☐ Miso soup ingredients: daikon, tofu, eggplant, Chinese cabbage, green leafy vegetables.
☐ Beverages: Brown Rice Tea, Brown Rice Bancha Tea, Bancha Tea, Grain Coffee, Azuki Kombu Drink.
☐ Avoid especially: all animal food including meat-based soups, eggs, dairy foods; sweet foods and drinks, and hot spices.

FOR ATROPHIC KIDNEY

☐ Main foods: Brown Rice, Azuki Rice, Brown Rice with Barley in a 3 to 1 ratio, whole-wheat spaghetti, Brown Rice Mochi.
☐ Side dishes (one-third to one-fourth of main foods): Natto with Soy Sauce and Scallions, Okara Nitsuke, Vegetable (eggplant) Tempura served with Grated Daikon, Azuki Beans with Kombu, Carp Soup, Tofu with Kuzu Sauce, Rice Bran Pickles, Sour Cabbage, and Pressed Salad. Use less salt than usual.
☐ Miso soup ingredients: wakame, daikon, tofu, eggplant, shiitake mushrooms, Chinese cabbage, bok choy.
☐ Beverages: Brown Rice Tea, Brown Rice Bancha Tea, Vegetable Broth, Brown Rice Cream (thin), Habucha Tea, Grain Coffee, Bancha Tea.
☐ Avoid especially: all animal food including dairy foods, fish, eggs, all alcohol, cocoa, coffee, hot spices, commercial sushi.

FOR THE YIN TYPE

☐ Main foods: Brown Rice Balls or Azuki Rice Balls served with Gomashio. In severe cases, use Brown Rice Cream (thick) with Grated Daikon. Eat 2 cups per day. Chew each mouthful 200 times.
☐ Side dishes (one-third of main foods): Tekka Miso, Oily Miso, Hijiki Nitsuke, Burdock Carrot Nitsuke, Shio Kombu, Vegetable Tempura, Carp Soup, Vegetable Stew, Azuki Beans with Kombu (every day eat 1/3 to 1/2 cup), Miso Pickles, Takuan Pickles.
☐ Miso soup ingredients: wakame, tororo kombu, onions, scallions, Homemade Agé, Brown Rice Mochi.
☐ Beverages: Brown Rice Tea, Brown Rice Bancha Tea, Sho-Ban Tea, Bancha Tea, Kombu Tea, Mu Tea.
☐ Avoid especially: all animal food, fish, shellfish, dairy foods (including ice cream), eggs, fruit, sweet foods and drinks, mushrooms, melons, all beans (except azuki), tomatoes, potatoes, eggplant, black tea, pressed salad.

KNOCK-KNEES

See LEG PROBLEMS, CHILDREN'S.

KYPHOSIS

See HUNCHBACK.

LARYNGITIS

The larynx is situated in the neck and is the entrance into the trachea and the lungs. Its main functions are speech, respiration, and protection of the airway during swallowing. The vocal cords of the larynx are two muscular bands that contract during swallowing to help prevent solids or liquids from entering the lungs. In humans, the vocal cords control the expulsion of air from the lungs into the mouth and throat. This release of air is formed into sounds or words by the tongue, lips, and cheek muscles. The larynx also allows inhaled air to enter the trachea and lungs.

Laryngitis refers to an inflammation of the larnyx accompanied by dryness and soreness of the throat, cough, hoarseness or loss of voice, and difficulty swallowing. A slight fever is sometimes present. Since the air passages of the throat are full of moisture, there are millions of microbes living around the larynx. An overgrowth of microbes will cause an infection in this area.

Thus, according to Western medicine, larynx inflammation is most often the result of an infection of microbes (viruses, bacteria) or of allergies. Excessive use of the voice may also result in laryngitis.

According to our macrobiotic understanding, this inflammation is the result of eating too much yin sugary food with an absence of salt (yang) in one's diet. This kind of diet promotes the growth of microbes. Your risk of getting laryngitis increases with smoking, which brings energy to the throat area, and with a host of yin factors such as excessive alcohol consumption, extremely cold weather, recent respiratory disorder, or exposure to irritants in the air.

Helpful Suggestions

Modern medical practitioners frequently administer antibiotics to kill microbes growing in the throat. However, according to our macrobiotic understanding, the habitual practice of using antibiotics creates a weaker immune system and invites more serious infectious diseases. Instead of antibiotics, try the following:

OBJECTIVE	REMEDY
To reduce swelling	Try GARGLING with 1 cup of BANCHA TEA WITH SALT 3 times per day. *and* Drink 1 cup of CHARCOALED UMEBOSHI TEA once a day until the swelling goes down. *or* Try drinking ½ to 1 cup of SALTY SHO-BAN TEA or 1 cup of strong KOMBU TEA 3 times per day until the swelling goes down.
To relieve pain	Apply a GINGER COMPRESS to the throat for 20 minutes, followed by an ALBI PLASTER for up to 4 hours. Repeat both the compress and the plaster as often as needed.
To alleviate hot feeling in the throat	Apply an ABLI TOFU PLASTER to the throat; change it every 4 hours.
To reduce fever	Drink ½ to 1 cup of DAIKON GINGER TEA, BROWN RICE TEA WITH SHIITAKE MUSHROOMS, or BROWN RICE TEA WITH DRIED PERSIMMON AND TANGERINE SKIN 3 times per day to reduce fever if needed.
To restore loss of voice	GARGLE with ½ cup of LOTUS ROOT TEA 3 times per day. Increasing the moisture in the air with a humidifier is also helpful.

Dietary Recommendations

The following dietary suggestions may be used until the laryngitis is over or for one week. Then, widen your food choices using a macrobiotic dietary approach (see page 11). Consume all food and drink when they are warm

until your normal appetite returns. If the symptoms of laryngitis last longer than two weeks, it may be a signal of cancer. Consult with your health-care advisor.

☐ Main foods: Brown Rice Gruel with scallions, Brown Rice Gruel with mochi and scallions (use miso and soy sauce to taste), Brown Rice Cream (thick).
☐ Side dishes (one-third of main foods): Tekka Miso, Oily Miso, Hijiki Carrot Nitsuke, Burdock Carrot Lotus Root Nitsuke or Burdock Carrot Nitsuke, Oysters Cooked with Miso, Boiled Daikon served with Oily Miso, Umeboshi with Soy Sauce.
☐ Miso soup ingredients: wakame, scallions, onions, daikon, Homemade Agé, tofu.
☐ Beverages: Brown Rice Tea, Brown Rice Bancha Tea, Bancha Tea, Kuzu Bancha Tea, Lotus Root Tea, Amasake Drink.
☐ Avoid especially: all meat, fish (except oysters), all sweet foods, all fruit, mushrooms, melons, tomatoes, eggplant, dairy, vinegar dishes, beer, wine.

LEAD POISONING

See HEAVY METAL POISONING.

LEG CRAMPS

Sporadic leg cramps that occur during or immediately after exercise, while relaxed or resting in bed, or while sitting in an unnatural or unusual position are common and do not signal an underlying disorder. Muscle cramps may also result from an adverse reaction to a drug such as a diuretic, or from heat exhaustion. Recurrent leg cramps with stiffness and weakness may signal a circulatory disorder or an inflammation of connective tissue.

According to our macrobiotic understanding, cramps are caused by too much yin food and by an overly acidic condition. When the muscles are too yin, they contract

---

HERMAN'S NATURAL HEALING AT WORK

When I was working in a peach orchard, I ate five freestone peaches every day. I had leg cramps every morning. This was caused by the peaches making the muscles too yin (cold or immobilized) along with overworking in the hot sun making my condition too acidic. Once I stopped eating the peaches and overworking, the cramps went away.   ∎

LEG CRAMPS

in order to counteract the expansive yin quality. Intracellular fluid that is too acidic causes the loss of calcium (an alkaline element) inside the cells. Such cells will then hold sodium—a yang, contracting, alkaline element—and when the neural signal for movement comes, cramping results. Fatigue, worry, too much work, and overeating and overdrinking are all acid-forming and also contribute to muscular cramping.

Helpful Suggestions

Try to identify any underlying disorder such as atherosclerosis and then see the suggestions in the appropriate section.

OBJECTIVE	REMEDY
To relieve sporadic leg cramps	MASSAGE the area just above the cramp. *and* Use ALTERNATING HOT TOWEL COMPRESSES.
To relieve recurrent cramps	Use massages and alternate compresses.

Dietary Recommendations

The only lasting remedy is a balanced diet. Follow a macrobiotic dietary approach (see page 11), avoiding fruit and yin acid-forming foods such as soy milk, beans, and tofu, until your condition improves.

LEG PROBLEMS, CHILDREN'S

Two common problems that can occur in children's legs are bowed legs (knees abnormally far apart) and knock-knees (knees abnormally close together). According to our macrobiotic understanding, there are two types of bowed legs, yin bowed legs in which the feet are turned outward and yang bowed legs in which the feet are turned inward. Yin bowed legs are caused by too much yin animal food such as dairy foods in the child's diet or in the diet of the pregnant or especially the nursing mother. Yang bowed legs are caused by eating too much salt.

Knock-knees are the result of a very yin diet, although at first glance it may appear to be more yang since the knees are closer (more yang) together. However, in this case the legs have turned inward at the knees because of weakness (more yin) and an inability to hold the upper body properly. Also, people with knock-knees are usually more pale in color and more skinny, both yin conditions.

CORNELLIA'S NATURAL HEALING AT WORK

My son Jiro was a heavy baby; when he started to walk at the age of 15 months, he developed bowed legs. I thought the reason was that my weak condition during pregnancy had prevented Jiro's getting enough calcium. At the time Jiro's condition became apparent, in the summer of 1960, we were in Southampton, New York. I was helping Lima Ohsawa in the kitchen of the first macrobiotic summer camp ever held in the United States. George Ohsawa saw Jiro and said, "You must cure him. This is a big piece of homework for you because Western medicine has no cure for bowed legs. Only our diet can cure this."

I was very ashamed to have a child with bowed legs. My husband Herman asked me, "Can you cure it?" I said, "Yes, I must do it."

I experimented by giving the children brown rice, miso soup, vegetable nitsuke, sea vegetables, and small fish bones. I gave deep-fried smelt bones to my children twice a week. The children ate the head and bones of the fish, and Herman ate the rest. One year later, Jiro's legs were straight. If you have no small fish, give dried chuba iriko after deep-frying. You can use only sea vegetables without fish, but it will take longer for the condition to improve; eating fish will speed up the process. ∎

LEG PROBLEMS, CHILDREN'S

Dietary Recommendations

Try using a macrobiotic dietary approach (see page 11) with the following added suggestions. For feet turned outward (yin bowed legs), eat Gomashio, Miso Soup, Burdock Carrot Nitsuke, and one small sour apple every day. The sour apple is to help digest excess protein. For feet turned inward (yang bowed legs), eat more Brown Rice with Barley (boiled), Fried Noodles, and vegetables, and less Pressure-Cooked Brown Rice. Eat two small sour apples every day. This condition takes longer to correct than yin bowed legs. A macrobiotic dietary approach will help correct knock-knees, but it also takes a long time.

LEPROSY

According to Western medicine, leprosy is a chronic, infectious disease caused by a specific microorganism, *Mycobacterium leprae*, which produces multiple areas of lesions in the skin, the mucous membranes, and the peripheral nervous system. Skin-type leprosy is an infection on the face, hips, arms and legs, causing red spots and numbness. The nodular type makes brown-colored nodules and also causes numbness. Nerve leprosy starts with oversensitivity and results in a loss of sensitivity to pain, cold, and heat; and the malfunctioning of one's metabolism.

According to our macrobiotic understanding, the underlying cause of leprosy is an inappropriate diet. It is not considered contagious to those eating a well-balanced diet. There are two types of leprosy, namely yin and yang. Yin leprosy is caused by eating too much yin food such as sugary foods, sweet foods, fruit, and potassium-rich food over a long time. Yin leprosy affects the nervous system. Yang leprosy is caused by the long-time overconsumption of yang food such as meat and other animal foods, which produce acidic toxins. Because of the excess of acidic toxins. Because of the excess of acidic toxins, yang leprosy affects the skin and/or nodules of the mucous membranes.

Helpful Suggestions

OBJECTIVE	REMEDY
	FOR THE YANG TYPE
To improve circulation	If a small area is affected, apply a GINGER, DAIKON GINGER, or ARAME COMPRESS on the affected area for 20 minutes.
	or
	If a larger area or the whole body is affected, use a GINGER, DAIKON, or ARAME BATH for 20 minutes.
To remove excess toxins	Follow either the compress or bath with an ALBI PLASTER on the most affected area for 4 hours to help remove excess toxins. Repeat both the compress (or bath) and plaster for a total of 2 to 3 times per day until recovered. Continue each day as often as possible and when practical. It is helpful to use the Albi Plaster for any length of time over an hour if you don't have 4 uninterrupted hours.
	also
	Steam baths or FAR-INFRARED SAUNAS once a day are very helpful.
	FOR THE YIN TYPE
To improve circulation	Take a DAIKON or ARAME BATH WITH SALT or a short DAIKON or ARAME BATH WITH MUSTARD POWDER for 10 to 15 minutes.
	or
	Using a GINGER SESAME OIL MASSAGE on the affected areas 2 or 3 times per day is very helpful.
To remove excess toxins	After the bath, apply an ALBI PLASTER on the most affected area. Repeat the bath and the plaster every 4 hours for a total of 2 to 3 times per day until recovered. Continue each day as often as is practical. If you don't have 4 hours of uninterrupted time, an albi plaster for longer than 1 hour is beneficial.

Dietary Recommendations

The following dietary suggestions may be used until your condition improves or for about one month. Then, widen your food choices using a macrobiotic dietary approach (see page 11).

FOR THE YANG TYPE

☐ Main foods: Brown Rice, Azuki Rice, whole-wheat spaghetti, Udon Noodles, Brown Rice Broth.
☐ Side dishes (one-third of main foods): Tekka Miso, Shio Kombu, Wakame Nitsuke, Arame Nitsuke or kombu dishes, Vegetable Stew, Okara Nitsuke, Natto with Soy Sauce and Scallions, Mochi Soup with Homemade Agé, Azuki Beans with Kombu, Vegetable Tempura served with Grated Daikon, Cucumber with Kuzu Sauce, Sour Cabbage, Rice Bran Pickles.
☐ Miso soup ingredients: wakame, daikon, sweet potatoes or yams, tofu, Chinese cabbage.
☐ Beverages: Brown Rice Tea, Bancha Tea, Grain Coffee.
☐ Avoid especially: all animal protein foods.

FOR THE YIN TYPE

☐ Main foods: Brown Rice served with lots of Gomashio, Millet Rice, Azuki Rice, Buckwheat Noodles, Buckwheat Groats, Brown Rice Mochi.
☐ Side dishes (one-third to one-half of main foods): Tekka Miso, Shio Kombu, Hijiki Nitsuke, Wakame Nitsuke, Nori Roasted with Oil, Vegetable Stew, Vegetable Stew with Fish, Carp Soup, Chuba Iriko Nitsuke, Vegetable Tempura, Takuan Pickles, Kombu Rolls with Chuba Iriko.
☐ Miso soup ingredients: wakame, onions, carrots.
☐ Beverages: Brown Rice Broth, Sho-Ban Tea.
☐ Avoid especially: all fruit, all sweet foods, potatoes, shiitake mushrooms, tofu, spices.

LEUKEMIA

Leukemia is a progressive, malignant disease of the blood-forming tissues. It is classified into various forms depending on the character and duration (acute or chronic), on the type of cell involved, and on whether or not there is an increase in the number of abnormal cells in the blood. Leukemia is a form of blood cancer that is often fatal.

Acute forms of leukemia are characterized by a malignant overgrowth of white blood cells in bone marrow or tissues of the lymphatic system (lymph glands, spleen, and liver). These excess cells accumulate and spill into the blood stream, eventually involving other tissues.

Symptoms of acute forms of leukemia include low fever, fatigue, anemia, headache, bruising and/or bleeding easily, increasing paleness, enlarged spleen, and abdominal pain. The cause of acute forms of leukemia is unknown but several underlying factors, especially viruses and radiation, are suspected. Your risk of getting leukemia increases with excessive exposure to x-rays, exposure to and use of certain drugs and chemicals, congenital disorders, and a family history of leukemia.

Chronic forms of leukemia develop more gradually and are characterized by increasing general weakness or fatigue. A common form occurring in over 30 percent of all persons with leukemia is chronic lymphocytic leukemia, a very slow-growing cancer of the blood-forming tissues (bone marrow, lymph glands, liver, and spleen) of older persons. Symptoms of chronic lymphocytic leukemia include general fatigue, mild anemia, enlarged lymph nodes, enlarged liver and spleen, unexplained weight loss, and increasing susceptibility to infections. In late stages, the preceding symptoms increase until incapacitating weakness and an inability to resist bacterial, viral, or fungal infections results. Again, the cause and specific preventive measures are unknown.

However, according to our macrobiotic understanding, the primary cause of leukemia is overeating yin foods, especially sugar and sugary foods. Stopping the consumption of overly yin foods along with following a macrobiotic dietary approach can be beneficial both to those who have leukemia already and to those seeking to prevent its development.

Helpful Suggestions

A good, balanced diet is best.

OBJECTIVE	REMEDY
To improve circulation and strengthen the system	Use a GINGER COMPRESS on the stomach (see Figure 3.8 on page 176) and back at the same time for 20 minutes. Especially apply the compress to the spine to help in the process of making new blood.
To strengthen the heart	Before bedtime for 3 days, drink the RANSHO DRINK made from 1 egg. Taking it then will not cause thirst.

Dietary Recommendations

Use the following dietary suggestions until your condition improves or for about one month. Then, widen your food choices using a macrobiotic dietary approach (see page 11).

☐ Main foods: Brown Rice Balls served with Gomashio.
☐ Side dishes (one-half of main foods): Tekka Miso,

Hijiki Nitsuke, natural caviar, Deep-Fried Chuba Iriko, Poached Fish, Organic (if possible) Pheasant, Burdock Carrot Nitsuke, Vegetable Tempura, Shio Kombu, Carp Soup, Vegetable Stew, Vegetable Stew with Fish, Miso Pickles.
☐ Miso soup ingredients: wakame, tororo kombu, onions, scallions, Brown Rice Mochi.
☐ Beverages: Brown Rice Tea, Brown Rice Bancha Tea, Bancha Tea with Gomashio, Sho-Ban Tea.
☐ Avoid especially: all animal protein (except those recommended above), red-meat fish, shellfish, all dairy foods (including ice cream), fruit, sweet foods and drinks, meat-based soups, eggplant, tomatoes, potatoes, melons, pressed salad, all alcohol.

LIVER CANCER

Liver cancer refers to the malignant growth of cells in the liver. Liver cancer may start in the liver itself or it may start in the bile duct or other places such as the rectum, colon, lungs, breasts, pancreas, esophagus, or skin (malignant melanoma). Some warning signs of liver cancer are loss of appetite, weight loss, tender mass in the right upper abdomen, pain in the upper abdomen, and sometimes yellow eyes, yellow skin, and fluid retention. According to modern medicine, the cause of liver cancer is unknown and there are no specific preventive measures.

However, according to our macrobiotic understanding, the underlying cause of liver cancer is the overconsumption of acid-forming foods in the form of simple carbohydrates such as sugar and alcohol, and fatty animal foods, especially cheese, butter, chicken, pork, and other meats. Cancer thrives in an overly acidic environment. Causing the bodily fluids to become more alkaline by eating more alkaline-forming foods and less acid-forming ones is the best preventative.

Helpful Suggestions

OBJECTIVE	REMEDY
To relieve pain	Try applying a GINGER COMPRESS over the liver (see Figure 3.8 on page 176) for 20 minutes followed by an ALBI PLASTER for up to 4 hours. Repeat both the compress and the plaster as often as needed and as time allows. The Albi Plaster may be left on overnight without being changed.

Dietary Recommendations

Liver cancer is one of the most difficult cancers to control. The best tactic is to follow a macrobiotic dietary approach (see page 11) over a long period of time, with an emphasis on alkaline-forming foods such as root vegetables and avoidance of overly acidic foods as mentioned above. This will at least slow (if not stop) the growth of the cancer cells and give the body a chance to heal itself.

LOW BLOOD SUGAR

See HYPOGLYCEMIA.

LUNG CANCER

Lung cancer is malignant cell growth in the lungs. Symptoms include intense cough, sputum that may contain blood, wheezing, chest pain, fatigue, and weight loss. More deaths are caused by lung cancer than any other form of cancer, and the incidence of lung cancer is increasing. Lung cancer may result from the spreading of cancerous cells from another part of the body, but 75 percent of the cases are linked to cigarette smoking. The risk of lung cancer also increases with exposure to certain chemicals and air pollutants.

According to our macrobiotic understanding, there are two kinds of lung cancer. The first is caused primarily by eating too much yang food such as eggs, beef, pork, and often fish, creating a toxic condition that can lead to the development of yang lung cancer. The yin type is caused primarily by eating too much yin food such as fruit, sugary foods, hot spices, and chemicalized foods. Moreover, the overconsumption of acid-forming foods such as meat and sugar and chemicals in foods is a major contributing factor to cancer development of either type. Cancer develops quickly for a meat-and-egg eater, but develops more slowly for a vegetarian. These dietary factors cause the development of many forms of cancer, but cigarette smoke and air pollutants bring the energy and excess toxins to the lung area and help ensure that lung cancer is the form of cancer that develops.

Helpful Suggestions

Avoid cigarette smoking, the cigarette smoke of others, and chemical and air pollutants as much as possible. Refrain from sex until your condition improves. For cancer from yin causes, avoid hot baths and hot springs.

OBJECTIVE	REMEDY
To relieve pain	Use a GINGER COMPRESS on the chest for 20 minutes followed by an ALBI PLASTER for up to 4 hours. Repeat both the compress and the plaster as often as needed and as time allows. The Albi Plaster may be left on overnight without being changed.

Dietary Recommendations

The best approach is to change your diet to a more balanced one. Use the following dietary suggestions for about one month. Then, widen your food choices using a macrobiotic dietary approach (see page 11). If you are uncertain which type of lung cancer you have, use the suggestions for the yin type first.

FOR THE YANG TYPE

☐ Main foods: Brown Rice, Brown Rice with Barley, and a little Gomashio as a condiment.
☐ Side dishes (one-fourth of main foods): Tekka Miso, Ginger Miso, Vegetable Tempura served with Grated Daikon, Eggplant Nitsuke with Miso, Okara Nitsuke, Burdock Nitsuke, Rice Bran Pickles, and Umeboshi. Make these dishes less salty.
☐ Miso soup ingredients: wakame, daikon, tofu, spinach, eggplant.
☐ Beverages: Barley Tea, Brown Rice Tea, Brown Rice Bancha Tea, Vegetable Broth, Grain Coffee. Drink a maximum of 2½ cups of beverages per day.
☐ Avoid especially: all meats (including fish, except carp, and shellfish), dairy (including ice cream), meat-based soups, sweet drinks, all alcohol, vinegar.

FOR THE YIN TYPE

☐ Main foods: Brown Rice Balls, Azuki Rice Balls with a little Gomashio, Brown Rice Gruel with Mochi, Baked Mochi with Soy Sauce. Chew each mouthful 200 times.
☐ Side dishes (one-third to one-half of main foods): Tekka Miso, Oily Miso, Hijiki Burdock Nitsuke, Shio Kombu, Burdock Carrot Nitsuke, Vegetable Tempura served with Grated Daikon, Carp Soup, Miso Pickles.
☐ Miso soup ingredients: wakame, tororo kombu, onions, scallions, and burdock.
☐ Beverages: Brown Rice Tea, Brown Rice Bancha Tea, Sho-Ban Tea, Bancha Tea with Gomashio. Drink a maximum of 2 cups of beverages per day.
☐ Avoid especially: all animal foods, dairy foods (including ice cream), fish, shellfish, all fruit, all sweet foods and drinks, salads, vinegar, tomatoes, eggplant, potatoes, pressed salads.

MALARIA

Malaria is an infection thought to be caused by a single-cell parasite that is transmitted by the bite of a mosquito. Blood cells and vessels, the liver, and central nervous system are affected. Symptoms include headache, fatigue, nausea, shaking, chills with fever for twelve to twenty-four hours, rapid breathing, and heavy sweating resulting in a lowering of temperature. Cases of malaria can range from quite mild to very serious, sometimes resulting in death. Recurrent episodes can continue for years every two to three days if left untreated and can be fatal without treatment or in persons who have low resistence to disease.

According to our macrobiotic understanding, the cause of this disease is not just parasites or mosquitoes. Malaria can also result from an inappropriate diet, an unsanitary environment, and bad weather and climatic conditions. Not eating the traditional balanced diet of a given region is the main underlying cause of this disease. As with any life-threatening disease, seek proper medical attention if you have a serious case that is not responding to the suggestions here.

Helpful Suggestions

OBJECTIVE	REMEDY
To relieve chills	Cover yourself with blankets. *and* Drink 2 to 3 cups of DAIKON GINGER TEA once only. *and* Eat 1 cup of thin BROWN RICE CREAM WITH GRATED DAIKON 3 times per day.
To reduce fever	Take a DAIKON or ARAME BATH WITH GRATED GINGER for 20 minutes once a day. The bath will promote sweating and help reduce fever.

Dietary Recommendations

Dietary changes are needed to help make the body strong. Use the following suggestions until your condition improves or for one month. Then, widen your food choices using a macrobiotic dietary approach (see page 11).

☐ Main foods: Brown Rice Cream, Brown Rice Gruel (make with Azuki Rice for variety).
☐ Side dishes (one-third of main foods): Umeboshi, Vegetable Tempura, Natto with Soy Sauce and Scallions, Cucumber with Kuzu Sauce, Grated Daikon, Shiitake Nitsuke, Vegetable Stew.
☐ Miso soup ingredients: wakame, daikon, Chinese cabbage.
☐ Beverages: Brown Rice Tea, Bancha Tea.
☐ Avoid especially: all medications, all animal foods, all sweet foods including fruit.

MEASLES

Measles is a contagious viral disease that affects the respiratory tract and skin. This is a common childhood disease although adults may be affected as well. Red measles is considered a serious disease; complications include pneumonia, encephalitis, and meningitis. Symptoms usually occur in the following order: temperature of 102°F or higher, fatigue, appetite loss, sneezing, runny nose, harsh cough, red eyes and sensitivity to light, tiny white spots in the mouth and throat, and a reddish rash that begins on the forehead and spreads to the whole body. The cause of red measles is thought to be a rubeola-virus infection with an incubation period of seven to fourteen days after exposure.

German measles (rubella) is also contagious but much more mild. However, serious birth defects can occur in babies if the mother develops this disease during the first three to four months of pregnancy. Symptoms of German measles include fever, fatigue, headache, muscle aches and stiffness, a reddish rash on head and body that lasts one to two days, and swollen lymph glands. German measles is caused by an RNA virus and is spread by person-to-person contact.

Immunization, administered to children after the age of one and combined with immunization against mumps, is required for children entering schools in many states. However, there are procedures for those who wish not to immunize. While many doctors recommend immunizations, there are many others who do not. In my opinion, immunizations are not natural and are harmful to the body's immune system. In other words, injecting an animal's antibody into human beings causes a degeneration contrary to the natural biological order. The macrobiotic approach always seeks to follow the natural order rather than to oppose it. On the other hand, if you are not committed to following the natural order and to ensuring that your children eat well, immunizations should be thoughtfully considered. Consult with your health-care advisor if you decide to take immunization and if you are pregnant or plan to become pregnant within three to four months of immunization.

According to our macrobiotic understanding, either

type of measles is a discharge of excess acid created by yang acid-forming food such as meat, chicken, eggs, cheese, and fish eaten by the mother during pregnancy. Thus, measles is often a natural discharge (cleansing) of acid, causing a rash during a child's growing years.

Most forms of measles may be allowed to run their course. However, if there are complications and a macrobiotic approach doesn't work or if you have a more severe case, it is best to consult your health-care advisor. A balanced macrobiotic dietary approach is a good preventative and helps reduce the severity of the disease if you do contract either type of measles. If you are pregnant, change your diet gradually since completely changing the sources of nutrition may cause discharges that are detrimental to your baby.

Helpful Suggestions

Do not give medications (like aspirin) or external treatments, especially to children. Just keep the room warm and moist and stay in bed. After the measles start, it is best to keep out of drafts and stay inside the house. If one gets chilled, the measles may start internally and can be very dangerous.

OBJECTIVE	REMEDY
To induce rash and aid in the discharge of the disease	A rash should appear within 3 to 7 days from the first symptoms of measles. (In German measles, no rash appears in 40 percent of cases, so don't worry if these suggestions do not bring about a rash.) Try drinking 1 tablespoon to ½ cup (increase the amount as age increases) of DAIKON MEASLES TEA 2 to 3 times per day. Use only until the rash appears. The quicker the rash appears the better. *and* If no rash appears after 1 day even with Daikon Measles Tea, try eating ⅓ to ½ cup of BROWN RICE GRUEL 3 times per day as your only food.
To relieve cough	Try eating ½ cup of BROWN RICE TEA WITH LOTUS ROOT AND TANGERINE SKINS every 3 hours. *or* Every 3 hours, try drinking 1 to 3 teaspoons of RICE SYRUP JUICE (older children use the larger amount).
To deal with a fever of 104°F or under	Do not use a tofu plaster or green leaves as you would in other fever cases, but let the measles run its course.
To deal with a fever over 104°F	Drink ½ cup of SOUR APPLE JUICE every hour until the fever lowers or consult your health-care advisor.

To alleviate persistent rash and fever	Follow the dietary suggestions for yang pneumonia (see page 126).
To relieve excessive itching	Rub the rash with daikon leaves from a DAIKON GINGER COMPRESS.
To cleanse the body	When the rash begins disappearing, use GINGER BATH water as a sponge bath to cleanse the body. *and* Use a GINGER SESAME OIL MASSAGE on the affected areas.

Dietary Recommendations

Use the following dietary suggestions until your condition improves or for one month. Then, widen your food choices using a macrobiotic dietary approach (see page 11).

☐ Main foods: Brown Rice Gruel with Grated Daikon.
☐ Side dishes (one-fourth of main foods): Boiled Daikon, Wakame Nitsuke, Scallion Miso, Tekka Miso, Burdock Carrot Nitsuke, Takuan Pickles, Boiled Daikon served with Scallion Miso, Vegetable Stew.
☐ Miso soup ingredients: daikon, green leafy vegetables, wakame.
☐ Beverages: Brown Rice Tea, Brown Rice Bancha Tea, Amasake Drink, Grain Milk.
☐ Avoid especially: cold drinks, cold foods, sweet foods, vinegar, potatoes, eggplant, tomatoes, candy, chocolate, all fruit, meat, fish, eggs, and dairy foods.

MENINGITIS

Meningitis refers to an inflammation of the meninges (membranes covering the brain and spinal cord) due to an infection from a bacteria, virus, or fungus usually emanating through the blood stream from other parts of the body. Spotted fever is thought to be caused by a meningococcal infection. A tubercle germ is thought to be the cause of tubercular meningitis. Pneumococcal, staphylococcal, and influenzal germs may each cause meningitis. Most cases occur in children aged six months to five years although all ages may be affected. The first symptoms of meningitis are usually vomiting followed by an intense headache and stiffness of the neck. Often there is an intolerance to light and sound. There can be twitching and convulsions. Additional developments include confusion, weakness, delirium, and often coma.

Tubercular meningitis lasts about a week to a month and there is loss of appetite, tiredness, and fever. Then, headaches, vomiting, fever, white tongue, and constipation follow. Many patients fully recover, but when the disease is fatal, the final disease stages include cramps and heart attack.

However, according to our macrobiotic understanding, germs are not the underlying cause because germs are the result of eating too much yin food, especially dairy foods, sugary foods, and fruit. These foods, eaten daily over a long period of time, create an environment inside the body favorable to the growth of microorganisms that can lead to diseases like meningitis. And any disease (or poor nutrition) that lowers your overall resistance increases your chances of getting meningitis. Thus, people who eat too much of both extreme yin and yang foods may contract meningitis also. In Japan, those who take commercial milk and dairy food as infants may be more susceptible to meningitis when they are sixteen to seventeen years old.

Helpful Suggestions

Meningitis is a serious disorder and usually requires prompt medical attention. The following suggestions are complementary.

OBJECTIVE	REMEDY
To reduce high fever	Try applying a 1-inch thick TOFU PLASTER to the whole head (shave off all hair for best results); change it every hour.
	also
	Drink 1 cup of DAIKON GINGER TEA slowly with a spoon 4 times per day. Resume normal activities as your strength allows.

Dietary Recommendations

If you do not want food, then don't eat anything; fast until hungry if your condition allows it. If you are hungry or need to eat, try eating one cup of thick Brown Rice Cream three to five times per day. When you are feeling better, eat only Brown Rice served with Gomashio or Tekka Miso. Once recovered and feeling better, you can add Miso Soup and side dishes to your diet. Follow this dietary approach of grains and vegetables until completely well, then widen your food choices using a macrobiotic dietary approach (see page 11).

MENSTRUAL IRREGULARITIES

When menstruation fails to occur at the expected age of puberty, a young woman is said to have primary amenorrhea. The cause of the absence of menstruation is usually unknown and treatment is often delayed unless the cause can be identified and treated safely. Possible underlying causes include emotional distress, eating disorders, tumors or infections of the endocrine system, and the use of certain drugs. Chromosome disorders or abnormalities of the reproductive system may result in primary amenorrhea that cannot be corrected.

If menstruation stops for reasons other than menopause for at least three months in a woman who has previously menstruated, this condition is known as secondary amenorrhea. Causes include pregnancy; breastfeeding; emotional stress; psychological disorders; various diseases such as disorders of the endocrine system, diabetes, or tuberculosis; obesity; strenuous exercise such as participating in competitive sports; surgical removal of the ovaries or uterus; and discontinued use of birth-control pills. The use of certain drugs and improper nutritional habits increase your likelihood of experiencing amenorrhea. Normal menstrual cycles resume after pregnancy or breastfeeding ceases, two months to two years after stopping the use of birth-control pills, and after strenuous exercise programs are reduced.

According to our macrobiotic understanding, the underlying cause of menstrual irregularities in premenopausal women who do not have congenital defects is imbalanced eating—too much yin and/or yang food. If there is no menstruation, the cause is overeating yin foods—assuming there are no abnormalities of the reproductive system or other fundamental causes such as a hysterectomy. If another disease is involved, it usually must be remedied before menstruation resumes. Amenorrhea is not considered a health risk; however, it may be a signal that greater disorders are present and that a change in dietary habits is needed.

Those who start a macrobiotic dietary approach sometimes stop menstruating for a time. I think menstruation stops because of the change from a diet of plenty of meat, fish, eggs, and milk to a macrobiotic approach. Generally speaking, one's physical condition does not change so fast, and when starting a macrobiotic diet there may not be enough yang food to compensate for what the body is used to. The result is that the body does not produce an excess of blood and menstruation stops.

Helpful Suggestions

OBJECTIVE	REMEDY
To increase circulation	Try taking a DAIKON or ARAME HIP BATH with ⅓ to ½ cup of salt added to either hip bath once a day until menstrual cycle becomes regular. Hip baths help increase circulation. Sit in the bath for 20 minutes and circulate the water into the vagina with your finger.
To increase circulation when there is pain	Apply a GINGER COMPRESS on the skin over the ovaries or a ROASTED SALT PACK over each ovary (see Figure 3.8 on page 176) every night for 20 minutes to help improve circulation and to help in cases of pain.
To relieve pain	If you change your diet and still have menstrual pain, eat 1 teaspoon of GOMASHIO with water.

and

Drinking ½ to 1 cup of SHO-BAN TEA 2 or 3 times a day may be tried. |

Dietary Recommendations

If menstruation stops for more than three months after your switch to a macrobiotic diet, try eating one bowl of Carp Soup every day for one week. This will help menstruation to begin again. If you can't find carp, use any freshwater fish in the soup. If you dislike fish, you can substitute Tekka Miso, Vegetables Cooked with Miso, or Brown Rice Gruel with Miso and Scallions. Also, Miso Soup with Mochi served with scallions may be eaten once a day.

Change your diet and your condition should improve. If you have eaten many yin, sugary foods in the past or if you are generally weak, use the following dietary suggestions until your condition improves or for about one month. Then, widen your food choices using a macrobiotic dietary approach (see page 11). If you are strong and haven't eaten too many sweet foods in the past, then use a macrobiotic dietary approach instead of the following suggestions. If your cycle continues to be irregular, it shows that you do not have enough salt in your diet. If you have a big body and no menstruation, it is because of the intake of yin foods such as fruit, potatoes, and yams.

☐ Main foods: Brown Rice Balls covered with Gomashio, Azuki Rice served with Gomashio, Brown Rice Mochi served with Grated Daikon, Fried Rice.

☐ Side dishes (one-fourth of main foods): Tekka Miso, Scallion Miso, Shio Kombu, Hijiki Burdock Nitsuke, Umeboshi, Takuan Pickles, Miso Pickles. Using miso in your cooking helps the body to yangize. Use sesame oil when you cook with miso. Miso is quite salty but sesame oil covers the miso (salty taste) so you do not get thirsty after eating it. Have Vegetables Cooked with Miso every day or every other day.

☐ Miso soup ingredients: wakame (have Wakame Miso Soup every morning), tororo kombu, onions, scallions, Homemade Agé, Brown Rice Mochi.

☐ Beverages: Brown Rice Tea, Brown Rice Bancha Tea, Sho-Ban Tea, Bancha Tea, Kombu Tea, Mu Tea. Drink a maximum of 2 cups of beverages per day.

☐ Avoid especially: meat, fish (except carp and freshwater fish for soups), pressed salads, dairy foods, eggs, sweet foods, fruit, and yin foods.

MISCARRIAGE AND PREMATURE BIRTH

A miscarriage is a premature termination of pregnancy before the fetus can survive outside the womb. When a child is born before thirty-seven weeks of pregnancy, it is considered a premature birth. Miscarriage may be preceded by uterine cramps and vaginal bleeding, although cramps and bleeding do not necessarily mean that a miscarriage is in progress. In this case, a miscarriage is only threatened. During the first three months of pregnancy, a miscarriage, often referred to as a spontaneous abortion, may result from abnormalities in the fetus or in the uterus. During the second three months, an abnormal uterine condition that causes the detachment of the fetus from the placenta may result in a miscarriage. The same effect may be produced by infections such as influenza or German measles and/or by the use of certain drugs. Factors such as stress, poor nutrition, smoking, alcohol, endocrine disorders, and anything that lowers one's resistance such as a recent infection increase the risk of miscarriage or premature birth.

According to our macrobiotic understanding, the underlying cause of miscarriage or premature birth is eating or drinking too many extreme yin foods such as wine and sugar or too much extreme yang food such as meat. Meat is yang but it produces an acidic condition with a similar effect as wine or sugar during pregnancy. Either causes abnormalities in the fetus or uterus that result in the detachment of the fetus and the placenta. The use of drugs that may destroy the fetus and/or make the fetus detach from the uterus and that may result in uterine infections can also cause a miscarriage or premature birth.

Dietary changes present special problems for pregnant women. The body makes adjustments to whatever diet one eats. According to our macrobiotic understanding, illnesses are part of the body's adjustment to an unbalanced or improper diet. A change in dietary habits will result in changes in your life on the physical, emotional, mental, and spirtual levels. Oftentimes, there is a temporary worsening of a condition while the body adjusts to making or obtaining the nutrients it needs from food sources that are new and thus foreign to it. While these changes and adjustments are generally not a problem, pregnant women need to monitor their reactions to dietary changes very closely. Consult with your midwife or obstetrician. Physical changes can be monitored easily through blood and urine analysis. However, often only you are aware of emotional or spiritual changes. If you have doubts or experience too many changes, slow down the dietary changes by eating some foods that you might otherwise avoid. Buy the best quality of these foods with the fewest added chemicals so that you may enjoy this very special time of pregnancy and childbirth.

Helpful Suggestions

When a miscarriage threatens, refrain from sexual intercourse until the symptoms disappear and you are sure a miscarriage is no longer a possibility. Bed rest is important for either a threatened miscarriage or an actual miscarriage. Resume normal activities after a couple of days.

OBJECTIVE	REMEDY
To deal with overconsumption of meat	Each night for 1 month, take a DAIKON or ARAME HIP BATH for 20 minutes before going to sleep.
To deal with overconsumption of yin food or drugs	Add 1/3 to 1/2 cup of salt to the DAIKON or ARAME HIP BATH.
To improve circulation	Drink 1/2 cup of MU TEA 2 to 3 times per day for 1 to 2 months.
To provide calcium for a developing fetus	Eat 1 to 2 tablespoons of sea vegetable dishes and 2 to 3 small dried fish every day.
To contract the uterus	GOMASHIO is good in the case of a miscarriage. Eat 1 teaspoon daily or put it in a capsule and swallow it.

Dietary Recommendations

During pregnancy or during times of threatened miscarriage, maintaining a macrobiotic dietary approach (see page 11) will be beneficial. The following special dietary suggestions may be used during periods of threatened miscarriage or for a few weeks after a miscarriage. Otherwise, follow a macrobiotic approach with a wide and healthy variety of foods. If you have eaten large quantities of meat and sugar, use the suggestions for the yin type first.

FOR THE YANG TYPE

☐ Main foods: Brown Rice, Brown Rice Mochi, a little Gomashio.

☐ Side dishes (one-third of main foods cooked with less salt than usual): Roasted Wakame, Azuki Beans with Kombu, Vegetable Tempura served with Grated Daikon, steamed vegetables, Takuan Pickles.

☐ Miso soup ingredients: wakame, daikon, tororo kombu, spinach, tofu, Homemade Agé, Brown Rice Mochi.

☐ Beverages: Brown Rice Tea, Brown Rice Bancha Tea, Bancha Tea, Grain Coffee, Kombu Tea.

☐ Avoid especially: all animal food, fish and shellfish (except carp), dairy foods, sweet foods, fruit, vinegar, eggplant, tomatoes, potatoes, alcohol.

FOR THE YIN TYPE

☐ Main foods: Brown Rice served with Gomashio, Brown Rice Mochi.

☐ Side dishes (one-third to one-half of main foods): Tekka Miso, Scallion Miso, Shio Kombu, Hijiki Burdock Nitsuke, Vegetable Stew, Carp Soup, Oysters Cooked with Miso, Azuki Beans with Kombu, Burdock Carrot Nitsuke, Vegetable Tempura, Kombu Rolls with Chuba Iriko.

☐ Miso soup ingredients: wakame, tororo kombu, onions, scallions, dried daikon, Brown Rice Mochi.

☐ Beverages: Brown Rice Tea, Brown Rice Bancha Tea, Bancha Tea, Kombu Tea, Grain Milk.

☐ Avoid especially: all animal food, fish and shellfish (except carp and oysters), dairy foods, sweet foods, fruit and foods rich in vitamin C, vinegar, eggplant, tomatoes, potatoes, alcohol.

MORNING SICKNESS

Morning sickness is a type of nausea, sometimes with vomiting, that may accompany pregnancy. It usually occurs in the morning—hence the name—although it may occur at any time of day during the first three months of pregnancy. During pregnancy, the body produces more progesterone and other hormones. These hormones cause certain involuntary muscles to relax, probably slowing the movement of food through the stomach and intestines, resulting in a nauseous feeling. In addition, low blood sugar may contribute to this problem.

However, according to our macrobiotic understanding, eating too much extreme acid-forming foods, both yin and yang, is the underlying cause. During pregnancy, a woman produces more acid because of the fetus. Eating too many acid-forming foods at this time disturbs the nervous system and metabolism, especially the functioning of the kidneys. The result is morning sickness. Very yang foods such as miso or umeboshi or very yin foods such as potatoes and coffee do not cause morning sickness because they are easily balanced with fresh vegetables and salty condiments. However, pregnant women who are following a macrobiotic dietary approach may have morning sickness if their kidneys are weak. In this case, even a mild acid-forming food such as brown rice can cause morning sickness. See Kidney Failure for general ideas for improving the kidneys.

Helpful Suggestions

The following small snacks are helpful any time you have morning sickness. Avoid large meals, especially those with high amounts of fat.

OBJECTIVE	REMEDY
To relieve nausea	Try eating ¼ cup of GRATED DAIKON WITH SOY SAUCE once only, 1 UMEBOSHI WITH SOY SAUCE to help make the body more alkaline, or 2 to 3 BROWN RICE BALLS WITH GOMASHIO. *and* If you are still nauseated after eating Brown Rice Balls with Gomashio, try eating a 1-inch-square piece of ROASTED KOMBU as needed.
To quench thirst	Drink ½ to 1 cup of BROWN RICE TEA or up to 2 cups of SHO-BAN TEA per day.

Dietary Recommendations

The following dietary suggestions may be used during periods of morning sickness. Otherwise, eat a wide and healthy variety of foods according to a macrobiotic dietary approach (see page 11).

☐ Main foods: Brown Rice Balls with Gomashio, Azuki Rice served with Gomashio, Brown Rice Mochi served with Grated Daikon, Fried Rice.

☐ Side dishes (one-fourth of main foods): Tekka Miso, Scallion Miso, Shio Kombu, Hijiki Burdock Nitsuke, Umeboshi, Takuan Pickles, Miso Pickles.

☐ Miso soup ingredients: wakame, tororo kombu, onions, scallions, Homemade Agé, Brown Rice Mochi.

☐ Beverages: Brown Rice Tea, Brown Rice Bancha Tea, Sho-Ban Tea, Bancha Tea, Kombu Tea, Mu Tea. Drink a maximum of 2 cups of beverages per day.

☐ Avoid especially: all animal protein, fish, eggs, shellfish, dairy foods (including ice cream), all fruit and sweet foods, vinegar, coffee, alcohol, tomatoes, eggplants, potatoes, mushrooms, melons, peanuts, pressed salads.

MOTION SICKNESS

Motion sickness occurs when a person riding in an airplane, boat, car, or other vehicle is subjected to movement that results in dizziness, nausea, vomiting, appetite loss, weakness, unsteadiness, and headaches. It is commonly thought that the brain's vomiting center misinterprets signals that are transmitted by fluid changes in the inner ear. Recent studies indicate that motion sickness occurs most often when the body senses movement that conflicts with what other senses indicate.

But why are some people affected and others not? According to our macrobiotic understanding, the underlying cause of motion sickness is weak intestines. Therefore, the best prevention is to make the intestines and stomach strong by eating a balanced diet.

Helpful Suggestions

OBJECTIVE	REMEDY
To relieve nausea	Try eating 1 to 3 teaspoons of rice vinegar 1 hour before traveling. *and* Drinking 1 cup of UMEBOSHI JUICE TEA, omitting the ginger, 1 hour before traveling may be helpful.
To prevent nausea	The common macrobiotic preventative is to tape an umeboshi pit to your navel 1 hour before traveling, leaving it in place until you arrive at your destination. If you have recurring motion sickness, this may be worth a try. Other preventatives include avoiding large meals just before traveling, staying in well-ventilated areas and away from cigarette smoke if possible, breathing slowly and deeply, and sitting or standing where you can see the motion coming, such as on the deck of a ship.

Dietary Recommendations

Following a macrobiotic dietary approach (see page 11) with Miso Soup and Rice Bran Pickles every day helps make the intestines, stomach, and liver strong and is the best recommendation. Bread, noodles, and condiments can also be eaten. Chew well, especially grains. This is most important for the prevention of motion sickness.

☐ Avoid especially: fatty foods; animal foods including fish, cheese, butter; all sweetened foods including sugar, candy, alcohol, beer, wine.

MUMPS

Mumps is an acute communicable viral infection that causes painful swelling of the salivary (parotid) glands. However, it frequently affects other oral glands, the pancreas, or the sexual organs. Symptoms of mumps are inflammation, pain in the parotid glands that increases with chewing or swallowing, fever, headache, and sore throat. Pain in the testicles, abdominal pain near the ovaries and/or pancreas, and/or a severe headache in addition to the symptoms listed above indicate a case of mumps with complications. This is a very dangerous virus because it can kill a woman's eggs and may cause sterility in adult males.

According to our macrobiotic understanding, the underlying cause of mumps is eating too much extreme yang and extreme yin food at the same time. Too many animal foods and sugary cakes and candy weaken the immune system and make one more susceptible to infections.

Helpful Suggestions

OBJECTIVE	REMEDY
To reduce high fever	Apply a TOFU PLASTER on the forehead and on the mumps (parotid glands) (see Figure 3.8 on page 176), changing the plaster every hour. *and* Use a GREEN LEAVES APPLICATION on the back of the neck; change the leaves every 2 hours. *and* Drink ½ to 1 cup of DAIKON GINGER TEA, BROWN RICE TEA WITH SHIITAKE MUSHROOM, BROWN RICE TEA WITH DRIED PERSIMMON AND TANGERINE SKIN, or BROWN RICE TEA WITH GINGER 3 times per day.
To protect against sterility	Use an ALBI PLASTER on the sex organs, changing it every 4 hours, to lower body temperature around sexual organs and to help in protecting against sterility. A high fever can damage or destroy sperm and egg cells.
To relieve pain	Try applying a DAIKON PLASTER to the painful area, changing it every hour.
To relieve ear pain in adults	Finely grate a daikon and squeeze out the juice. Put 2 to 3 drops of this juice on a small cotton ball and insert it in the ear for 10 to 20 minutes. Then, fold the ear forward and apply a TOFU PLASTER to the back of the ear for 1 hour. Secure with a cotton bandage. Repeat both the juice drops and the plaster up to 4 times per day.
To relieve ear pain in children	Do not use the Daikon Juice ear drops for children. You may try the plasters, but it's best to consult a health-care advisor. Usually the plasters will relieve the pain.
To relieve persistent pain	Apply an ALBI PLASTER to the swollen area; change the plaster every 4 hours.
To reduce infection	Try using an ALBI PLASTER to help draw out all the infection; change the plaster every 4 hours.
To relieve headache	Use a GINGER SESAME OIL or APPLE JUICE MASSAGE on the entire head up to 4 times per day.

Dietary Recommendations

The following dietary suggestions may be used until you recover, usually about ten days to two weeks. Then, widen your food choices using a macrobiotic dietary approach (see page 11). When your appetite returns to normal, be sure to chew grains very well.

☐ Main foods: Brown Rice Cream, Brown Rice Gruel with mochi and scallions seasoned with miso.
☐ Side dishes (one-fourth of main foods): especially Tekka Miso, Hijiki Nitsuke, Burdock Nitsuke, Burdock Carrot Nitsuke, Carp Soup, Miso Pickles.
☐ Miso soup ingredients: wakame, daikon, onions, scallions, Homemade Agé.
☐ Beverages: Sho-Ban Tea, Bancha Tea, Brown Rice Bancha Tea, Grain Milk, Amasake Drink.
☐ Avoid especially: all animal foods including dairy foods and eggs, all sweet foods and drinks including ice cream and candy, all fruit, all beans including fresh soybeans, tomatoes, eggplant, potatoes, pressed salads, vinegar, and vinegar pickles.

MUSCLE CRAMPS

According to our macrobiotic understanding, muscle cramps in parts of the body other than the stomach are often caused by eating too much yin food such as fruit or iced foods. If you eat a lot of fruit or cold, iced foods or drinks, the muscles become cool. Then, around 2 A.M. to 3 A.M. the next morning when air temperature is lowest, muscles, especially in the feet, become very yin (cold). As a result, the cold (yin) muscles attract yang (sodium) from the intercellular fluid. Then, the muscle cells may become too yang and constrict or cramp.

Helpful Suggestions

OBJECTIVE	REMEDY
To relieve muscle cramps	Lay down and relax. Apply a HOT TOWEL COMPRESS on the affected area for 20 minutes followed by a MUSTARD PLASTER until the skin turns red.
	or
	Apply a GINGER COMPRESS for 20 minutes followed by an ALBI PLASTER with a ROASTED SALT PACK on top of the plaster to keep it a little warm. Leave the Albi Plaster on for up to 4 hours and repeat both the compress (either) and its corresponding plaster as needed for relief of cramps.

Dietary Recommendations

Following a macrobiotic dietary approach (see page 11) is very helpful.

☐ Avoid especially: fruit and cold, iced foods or drinks.

MYELITIS

See SPINAL CORD INFLAMMATION.

NASAL POLYPS

Nasal polyps are nonmalignant growths in the nasal mucous membranes. They may be indicated by a loss of the sense of smell, headache, excessive nasal discharge, and nasal obstruction resulting in a chronic "stuffy nose" feeling. Usually both sides of the nose are equally affected. Nasal polyps affect all ages but are much more common in adults. The cause of nasal polyps is thought to be a chronic infection or allergy in the nose. In this case, the nasal mucous membranes swell and excess fluid is produced. However, there is no proven cause for the underlying allergy or chronic infection.

According to our macrobiotic understanding, the underlying cause of nasal polyps is weak kidneys, resulting primarily from taking too much medication or from eating too much fatty food. Even though the symptoms can be alleviated with surgery, if nothing is done to remedy the uderlying cause, the polyps will return. Thus, recurrence is common even after surgery because the true cause is misunderstood. A change in dietary habits that removes the underlying allergy or chronic infection is best.

Helpful Suggestions

OBJECTIVE	REMEDY
To alleviate stuffy nose or excessive nasal discharge	Try using a SALT BANCHA NASAL BATH 3 to 4 times per day until your condition improves. *and* Use a GINGER SESAME OIL MASSAGE on the outside of the nose.
To remove excess mucus	Apply an ALBI PLASTER to the nose overnight. Do this until the nose is clear of excess mucus.

Dietary Recommendations

Following a macrobiotic dietary approach (see page 11) that is low in fatty foods and high in dietary fiber is most helpful. Eat plenty of root vegetables, sea vegetables, and Deep-Fried Chuba Iriko for calcium.

☐ Avoid especially: all overly yin foods such as ice cream, cookies, cakes, fruit, refined sugar, and fatty foods.

NERVE PAIN

See PAIN, FACIAL AND NERVE.

NERVOUS SYSTEM MALFUNCTION

A general nervous system malfunction may be indicated by slow reactions and the inability to feel pain. The nervous system, along with the endocrine system, correlates one's adjustments and reactions to internal and environmental conditions. The central nervous system consists of the brain and spinal cord and any malfunction may signal the beginning of a greater disorder such as leprosy. According to our macrobiotic understanding, a nervous system malfunction is caused by overeating animal foods, sugary foods, dairy foods, refined foods, chemicalized food, and other acid-forming foods.

Helpful Suggestions

Avoiding hot baths and refraining from sex is helpful until your condition improves.

OBJECTIVE	REMEDY
To cleanse the body	If your condition allows, it is a good idea to FAST for 1 to 7 days to help clean up the body. Drink up to 2 to 3 cups per day of water, *KUZU TEA*, or *BROWN RICE TEA* during the fast.
	or
	Try a special BROWN RICE BALL FAST with 2 to 3 RICE BALLS twice a day. Chew very well. This will aid in a quick recovery.

Dietary Recommendations

Use the following dietary suggestions until your condition improves or for about one month. Then, widen your food choices using a macrobiotic dietary approach (see page 11).

☐ Main foods: Brown Rice, Azuki Rice, Millet Rice, Fried Rice, all eaten with Gomashio.

☐ Side dishes (one-fourth of main foods): Tekka Miso, Sesame Miso, Shio Kombu, Hijiki Nitsuke, Roasted Wakame, Azuki Beans with Kombu and Winter Squash, Takuan Pickles, Miso Pickles.

☐ Miso soup ingredients: wakame, kombu, onions, scallions, Homemade Agé, Brown Rice Mochi.

☐ Beverages: Brown Rice Tea, Brown Rice Bancha Tea, Bancha Tea, Kombu Tea, Mu Tea, Grain Coffee. Drink only when thirsty, except while fasting.

☐ Avoid especially: all meats and animal foods, fish, shellfish, eggs, dairy foods (including ice cream), vinegar, tomatoes, potatoes, eggplant, sweet foods, fruit, sweet drinks, peanuts.

NIGHT BLINDNESS

Night blindness refers to a failure or loss of vision at night or in dim light. Normally, the eye receives light and it is focused on the retina. The retina changes light energy to nerve energy and sends a nerve impulse to the brain through the nervous system. The condition of night blindness results when someone cannot create enough nerve energy for a nerve impulse to reach the brain from the retina. On bright days or in bright light, there is more energy and vision is better if not normal.

According to our macrobiotic understanding, the underlying cause of night blindness is an overly yin diet and also a lack of good quality vegetable oil in the diet. Eye problems often signal greater disorders in the body. In this case, a general overall weakness leading to a greater susceptibility to disease is indicated and thus the need for a change in dietary habits.

Helpful Suggestions

OBJECTIVE	REMEDY
To improve circulation in and around the eye	Try using a SALT BANCHA EYE BATH 3 times per day and just before sleeping until your eyesight improves.
	also
	Before going to sleep, use a SESAME OIL EYE TREATMENT to nourish the eyes.

Dietary Recommendations

Following a macrobiotic dietary approach (see page 11) is recommended; eat especially whole grains with root vegetables, Tekka Miso and Burdock Carrot Nitsuke as main foods; seasonal vegetables sautéed with good quality sesame oil as side dishes; and wakame, tororo kombu, burdock, Brown Rice Mochi, and Homemade Agé as miso soup ingredients.

NOCTURNAL EMISSION

Nocturnal emission is the involuntary loss of semen during sleep. While these emissions are completely normal in pubescent boys, adult males may want to stop them. According to our macrobiotic understanding, the underlying cause of this condition is eating too much animal food, and the only real remedy is to stop eating animal foods.

Dietary Recommendations

Eating dinner early is helpful. Use the following dietary suggestions until the noctural emissions stop or for about one month. Then, widen your diet using a macrobiotic dietary approach (see page 11).

☐ Main foods: Brown Rice, Brown Rice with Barley, whole-wheat spaghetti, Udon Noodles.

☐ Side dishes (one-third of main foods): Okara Nitsuke, Natto with Soy Sauce and Scallions served with Grated Daikon, Eggplant Nishime, vinegar salad dressing, Shiitake Nitsuke, Tofu with Kuzu Sauce.

☐ Miso soup ingredients: daikon, tofu, sweet potatoes, eggplant, green leafy vegetables.

☐ Beverages: Green Tea, Bancha Tea, hot water, Grain Coffee. Drink a maximum of 2 cups of beverages per day.

☐ Avoid especially: all animal foods, fish, shellfish, meat-based soups, sweet foods and drinks, dairy foods (including ice cream), alcohol.

NOSE, OBSTRUCTED

An obstructed nose accompanies such sicknesses as a common cold, chronic rhinitis, deviated septum, nasal polyps, adenoiditis, and cancer of the pharynx. Western medicine considers that these sicknesses are the cause of an obstructed nose. However, according to our macrobiotic understanding, these sicknesses are themselves only symptoms of dietary habits with excessive amounts of yin foods such as sugary foods, potatoes, tomatoes, coffee, fruit, and alcohol. Fatty animal foods contribute as well.

Helpful Suggestions

OBJECTIVE	REMEDY
To clear nasal passages	Using a SALT BANCHA NASAL BATH 3 to 4 times per day until nasal passages clear is most helpful.
	also
	You may try using a LOTUS ROOT JUICE APPLICATION; leave the cotton ball in each nostril for 30 minutes.
	or
	Place a HOT TOWEL COMPRESS over the nose for 15 minutes 5 to 6 times per day; change when compress cools.
To remove excess mucus in adults	Apply an ALBI PLASTER on the nose and leave on overnight.
To remove excess mucus in children	Use a LOTUS ROOT JUICE APPLICATION for 30 minutes in each nostril 1 time only.
	or
	Place the white part of a raw scallion in each nostril for 15 to 20 minutes 3 or 4 times per day.

Dietary Recommendations

A change in dietary habits is most helpful. Use the following dietary suggestions until the nose clears or for one month. Then, widen your food choices using a macrobiotic dietary approach (see page 11).

☐ Main foods: Brown Rice, Azuki Rice, Fried Rice with a little Gomashio.

☐ Side dishes (less than one-third of main foods): Tekka Miso, Scallion Miso, Hijiki Lotus Root Nitsuke, Burdock Carrot Lotus Root Nitsuke, Shio Kombu, Burdock Carrot Nitsuke, Vegetable Tempura, Carp Soup, Deep-Fried Chuba Iriko, Miso Pickles.

☐ Miso soup ingredients: wakame, tororo kombu, bur-dock, scallions, onions, Homemade Agé, dried seitan, Brown Rice Mochi.

☐ Beverages: Sho-Ban Tea, Brown Rice Tea, Bancha Tea, Kombu Tea, Grain Milk. Less drinking is better, a maximum of 2 cups total per day.

☐ Avoid especially: all animal protein, all dairy food including ice cream, all fruit, sweet foods and drinks, potatoes, melons, fresh soybeans, mushrooms, tomatoes, eggplant, hot spices, coffee, alcohol.

NOSEBLEEDS

Anyone can have a nosebleed, but this condition is about twice as common in children as adults. Dark red blood indicates that the nosebleed is deeper in the nose, while a bright red color may indicate a nosebleed that is close to the nostril. Lightheadedness may result from the blood loss. Causes of nosebleeds vary greatly and include any injury to the nose, even a simple one caused by the act of picking one's nose; a foreign body in the nose; dry mucous membranes; and any number of disorders from nasal polyps and sinus infections to scarlet fever, high blood pressure, or atherosclerosis. Any of these causes or other disorders of the blood, liver diseases, the use of certain drugs such as aspirin, exposure to irritating chemicals, and high altitude or dry climates increase the risk of nosebleeds.

However, according to our macrobiotic understanding, there are two kinds of nosebleeds, yin and yang. The yin type of nosebleed is the one with which we are

---

CORNELLIA'S NATURAL HEALING AT WORK

Once at the French Meadows Summer Camp, a woman told me that she had been having a nosebleed. This woman was very yang so I asked her, "Do you have abnormal menstruations?" She said, "Yes." I recommended that she strike the back of ther neck at the base with the heel of her hand three times, but she had no success with this. I advised her to drink salt water and the nosebleeds stopped. The next morning she said that her menstruation had started. She admitted that she had not menstruated for one year.

My mother told me that my grandfather liked to eat one fertilized egg a day. When he was over 70 years old, he got a severe nosebleed. My mother called the doctor. The doctor said that the nosebleed had helped save my grandfather's life because he had high blood pressure (eating an egg every day caused a lot of blood to be made). The doctor said that in a case like that, he never would recommend stopping a nosebleed. ∎

NOSEBLEEDS

---

all familiar. It is caused by an overly yin condition of the membranes so that an irritant such as an attack of hay fever or severe sneezing accompanying a cold can result in a nosebleed. External remedies are offered for this condition. However, the yang type is caused by an excess of blood in the system such that it is advisable not to stop the bleeding.

Helpful Suggestions

If a person has just had a cerebral hemorrhage, or has chronic kidney disease, or is experiencing menopause, a nosebleed may be a natural, necessary process of the body protecting itself and there is no need to stop the bleeding at these times. Knowing when to stop and not to stop a nosebleed takes experience. If you are uncertain, it is best to consult a health-care advisor. Also, the underlying disorder needs to be treated.

OBJECTIVE	REMEDY
	FOR THE YIN TYPE
To deal with dark red blood	You do not need to stop the bleeding if the blood is dark red. If the blood changes color, stop the bleeding.
To stop bleeding when blood is light red or there is a change in blood color	Try using any of the following remedies 1 time only:
	Use a SALT BANCHA NASAL BATH solution; sit up with your head bent forward. It is advisable not to lie down or to tilt your head back such that blood goes down the throat causing you to swallow blood or to gag, resulting in the inhaling of blood. Dip a small cotton ball in the salted bancha tea and place a ball in each nostril. Clamp your nose between your thumb and index finger, closing it for 5 uninterrupted minutes. Breathe through your mouth during this time.
	or
	Drinking 1 cup of salty SHO-BAN TEA or SALT-WATER DRINK is also helpful. A middle-aged, strong person may use a more salty solution.
	or
	Striking the back of the neck with the heel of the hand 3 times may be helpful.
	or
	Use a MUSTARD PLASTER applied to the bottom of the feet for 10 minutes, or place 1 tablespoon of grated garlic in cheesecloth and apply to the bottom of the feet for 4 to 5 minutes. The blood will be drawn down to the feet and the nosebleed should stop.
	and

Lie back and rest after the bleeding stops.

and

Avoid strenuous exercise for a couple of days and don't blow your nose for at least 12 hours. If none of these remedies work and the bleeding persists, you had better consult a health-care advisor.

Dietary Recommendations

Following a macrobiotic dietary approach (see page 11) to keep the body in a strong (not overly yin) condition is the best preventative for nosebleeds

OSTEOMYELITIS

Osteomyelitis is an infection of the bone and bone marrow. According to Western medicine, the cause of osteomyelitis is basically a bacterial infection that invades the blood through the skin, respiratory organs, and digestive organs. Osteomyelitis is indicated when, after two or three days of inflammation, body temperature goes up quickly, there is pain in the bones, and an infection is indicated. It is most common among growing children from five to fourteen years of age, although any age may be affected. It is also more common among males, especially during periods of rapid growth.

According to our macrobiotic understanding, osteomyelitis is caused by eating too much animal protein, especially when combined with a high intake of sugary foods. Animal foods contain a higher percentage of protein than do vegetable foods and thus a greater possibility of contamination by bacteria from an outside source. However, more importantly, because of the high protein content, animal foods help microbes and other organisms develop by providing the building materials for their growth. Sugary foods accelerate the growth of microbes and provide an environment in which they thrive.

Helpful Suggestions

OBJECTIVE	REMEDY
To improve circulation and remove toxins	A GINGER COMPRESS applied on the affected area for 20 minutes followed by an ALBI PLASTER for up to 4 hours will help take toxins out of the area. Repeat both the compress and the plaster daily for a couple of weeks. The Ginger Compress also helps loosen the skin so the Albi Plaster is more effective.

To relieve itchiness	If the skin becomes itchy from the Albi Plaster, rub it lightly with a 1/4-inch-thick round piece of daikon.
To relieve pain	Try using an UMEBOSHI SAKÉ PLASTER applied to the affected area, changing it 3 times per day, until the pain stops.

Dietary Recommendations

All bone diseases can be helped by a diet high in sea vegetables with a small amount of Kombu Rolls with chuba iriko. Lotus root is the best vegetable for bone diseases. Use the following suggestions until the pain stops or for about one month. Then, widen your food choices using a macrobiotic dietary approach (see page 11). If the bone pain comes from the bacillus of tuberculosis (bone tubercle), refer to the tuberculosis section.

☐ Main foods: Brown Rice with Barley, Brown Rice, Azuki Rice served with Gomashio as a condiment. Chew each mouthful 200 times.

☐ Side dishes (one-fourth of main foods maximum): Ginger Miso, Sesame Miso, Wakame Nitsuke, Nori Nitsuke, Hijiki Lotus Root Nitsuke, Carp Soup, Burdock Carrot Nitsuke, Vegetable Tempura served with Grated Daikon, Eggplant Nitsuke with Miso, Takuan Pickles, Rice Bran Pickles, Kombu Rolls with Chuba Iriko, or Chuba Iriko Nitsuke.

☐ Miso soup ingredients: daikon, tofu, spinach, eggplant, carrots.

☐ Beverages: Bancha Tea, Brown Rice Bancha Tea, Brown Rice Tea, Grain Coffee.

☐ Avoid especially: all animal food including red-meat fish and shellfish (except for a small amount of white-meat fish), eggs, meat-based soups, all dairy foods (including ice cream); also sweet foods and drinks, hot spices.

See also OSTEOPOROSIS.

OSTEOPOROSIS

Osteoporosis is the gradual loss of bone mass and strength characterized by an increased risk of fractures, especially of the hip or arm, pain in the hip and back, loss of height, and spinal curvature. The risk of developing osteoporosis increases with age; it mostly affects post-menopausal women. A lack of calcium is thought to be the major cause of osteoporosis with estrogen deficiency as the leading contributing factor among postmenopausal women. Other causes that are often cited include a prolonged lack of adequate dietary calcium and protein, an inability to absorb sufficient amounts of calcium through the intestine, a calcium-phosphorus imbalance, the use of cortisone drugs, a lack of exercise, and prolonged disease such as alcoholism or cancer. One of the general recommendations commonly made is to eat a diet high in protein, calcium, and vitamin D.

However, no matter how much calcium is consumed, the fundamental cause of osteoporosis is eating too much protein-rich food. According to John McDougall in *The McDougall Plan*, when people consumed 75 grams of protein a day, even with daily intake of 1,400 milligrams of calcium, more calcium was lost in the urine than was absorbed into the body from the diet. In other words, if you consume more protein, you lose more calcium. This deficiency must be made up from the body's stores of calcium; namely, bones and teeth. This results in osteoporosis. In my opinion, the high consumption of proteins such as meats that contain a lot of nitrogen, phosphorous, and sulphur (all acid-forming elements), causes the bodily fluids to become acidic. The body uses calcium (an alkaline-forming element) from bones to help alkalize body- and nerve-cell fluids. Thus, any prolonged acidic condition of bodily fluids will eventually lead to osteoporosis. Therefore, eating a diet balanced with respect to acid-forming and alkaline-forming foods that are not too high in protein is the best preventative for osteoporosis.

Helpful Suggestions

OBJECTIVE	REMEDY
To improve kidney function	Each day, try applying a GINGER COMPRESS over the kidneys (see Figure 3.8 on page 176) for 20 minutes because the kidneys help make the bodily fluids alkaline.
To relieve pain	Use a GINGER COMPRESS on any painful area to help increase circulation to that area and thus reduce the pain.

Dietary Recommendations

Follow a macrobiotic dietary approach (see page 11) with lots of fresh vegetables and salads. Avoid high-protein foods, such as meat, chicken, fish, and eggs, and limit the intake of tofu and beans if you have osteoporosis. Eat only 25 to 50 grams of protein per day.

OVARIAN CYST

Ovarian cysts are sacs of fluid or semisolid material that develop in or on the ovary. They are rarely cancerous. Some ovarian cysts produce no symptoms. If there are symptoms, they include nonpainful swelling, painful intercourse, difficulty emptying the bladder completely, burning urination, irregular menstruation, and a brownish vaginal discharge. Fever, vomiting, and acute abdominal pain result if the cyst twists, bleeds, or breaks. The cause is thought to be a hormone disturbance and there is no known prevention.

However, according to our macrobiotic understanding, ovarian cysts are primarily caused by eating too much fatty, animal food, especially eggs, along with too many sugary foods and drinks, including fruit and fruit juices. This kind of diet can cause problems during the menstrual cycle, leading to the closure of the fallopian tubes. The end result is an ovarian cyst.

Helpful Suggestions

OBJECTIVE	REMEDY
To relieve pain	Apply a GINGER COMPRESS on the affected area for 20 minutes, followed by an ALBI PLASTER. Leave the plaster on for up to 4 hours. Then, repeat the compress and plaster as time permits until the pain subsides.
To dissolve cysts that are not accompanied by pain	Apply an ALBI PLASTER only until the cysts are dissolved.

Dietary Recommendations

Following a macrobiotic dietary approach (see page 11) that is low in protein, simple carbohydrates, and fat is the best preventative. Use good-quality sesame oil instead of animal fat.

OVARIAN INFLAMMATION

If the ovaries become enlarged from many small cysts or if the surface of the ovaries becomes too thick to allow ovulation, inflammation may result. Symptoms may include pain, often severe; fever; and constipation. According to our macrobiotic understanding, there are two types of ovarian inflammation, yin and yang. The cause of the yang type is continually eating too much meat and fish. In this case, the inflammation may lead to an infection. The cause of the yin type is the overeating of yin foods such as fruit, sugary foods, and coffee. However, in this case, the same suggestions are useful for either type.

Helpful Suggestions

OBJECTIVE	REMEDY
To relieve severe pain with fever	Never use an ice pack because it reduces circulation to the area. Instead, use a 1-inch-thick TOFU PLASTER applied to the lower abdomen so that it covers both ovaries (see Figure 3.8 on page 176). Change the plaster every 1 or 2 hours.
To relieve severe pain without fever	Place a ROASTED SALT PACK or a GINGER COMPRESS on the ovaries (see Figure 3.8 page 176) for 20 minutes, followed by drinking 1 cup of UMESHO BANCHA TEA. Repeat the compress and tea every 3 hours until the pain subsides.
To relieve mild fever and/or pain	Apply an ALBI PLASTER over the ovaries, changing it every 4 hours.
To relieve constipation	Use an ENEMA of warm salt water 1 time only if you have not had a bowel movement for 3 to 7 days.
To reduce inflammation/ pain	Take DAIKON or ARAME HIP BATHS for 20 minutes every evening until inflammation goes down. The bath helps increase circulation to the area, reducing pain and infection. If you have a yin constitution, add 1/3 to 1/2 cup of salt to the hip bath water.

Dietary Recommendations

Use the following dietary suggestions until the inflammation subsides or for one month. Then, widen your food choices using a macrobiotic dietary approach (see page 11).

☐ Main foods: Brown Rice, Azuki Rice.

☐ Side dishes (one-third of main foods): Scallion Miso, Nori Nitsuke, Hijiki Nitsuke, Carp Soup, Vegetable Stew, Natto with Soy Sauce and Scallions, Okara Nitsuke, Green Leafy Vegetables served with Homemade Agé, Azuki Beans with Kombu, Grated Daikon, Takuan Pickles, Kombu Rolls.

☐ Miso soup ingredients: wakame, arame, daikon, Chinese cabbage, tofu.

☐ Beverages: Brown Rice Tea, Brown Rice Bancha Tea, Bancha Tea, Mu Tea, Grain Coffee.

☐ Avoid especially: all animal foods (except carp), all sweet foods, all fruit, all drugs.

PAIN, FACIAL AND NERVE

Facial pain is sudden pain from the top of the head down the face, following the path of one or more nerves. Trigeminal neuralgia refers to pain in the fifth cranial nerve, which translates sensation from the brain to the face, scalp, teeth, nose, and mouth. This severe pain lasts only a few minutes and usually recurs for weeks or months at a time. Pain may be triggered by such simple acts as shaving, brushing teeth, chewing, touching the face, or feeling the wind. According to modern medicine, the cause of this pain is most often unknown, although sometimes it may result from pressure on the nerves from adjacent blood vessels. Anticonvulsant medications are often prescribed followed by major surgery if these aren't effective. However, even with surgery, the pain most often returns when the nerves regenerate in five to ten years. This is because the underlying cause is not dealt with.

Generally, according to our macrobiotic understanding, most pain is caused by an oxygen deficiency in the nerve cells resulting from bad circulation or a lack of red blood cells. Facial pain is due to an imbalance in the diet, that is to say, too much yin acid-forming food such as sugary foods, alcohol, most drugs and vinegar, and yin alkaline-forming food such as coffee, honey, and tree fruits along with a lack of yang alkaline-forming food such as salt and salt products. This kind of diet results in anemic, tired, and agitated people who have a tendency to get this condition. Also, an overly yin diet can cause muscles or blood vessels to become overly expanded resulting in pressure on surrounding nerve cells and thus pain. A high-fat diet contributes to nerve pain when fat deposits clog capillaries thus reducing the oxygen supply in the nerve cells.

Helpful Suggestions

OBJECTIVE	REMEDY
To relieve pain	Apply a GINGER COMPRESS on the affected area for 20 minutes. Keep warm. Apply an ALBI PLASTER after the ginger compress for up to 4 hours. Cover the area of pain with a flannel bandage over the plaster to keep it warm and out of contact with cold air. Repeat both the compress and the plaster as often as necessary.
To relieve severe nerve pain in areas other than the face	Use a very hot GINGER COMPRESS WITH SALT on the affected area for 20 minutes. *or* Use a MUSTARD PLASTER 1 to 3 times per day for 5 to 7 minutes each time until the skin turns red.

and/or
A GINGER SESAME OIL MASSAGE may be used.

Dietary Recommendations

The most helpful action is a change in dietary habits. Use the following dietary suggestions until the pain subsides or for about one month in serious cases. Then, widen your food choices using a macrobiotic dietary approach (see page 11).

FOR FACIAL PAIN

☐ Main foods: Brown Rice, Azuki Rice, Brown Rice Mochi, Fried Rice, and as much Gomashio as you want.

☐ Side dishes (one-third of main foods): Tekka Miso, Scallion Miso, Carp Soup, Hijiki Lotus Root Nitsuke, Hijiki Burdock Nitsuke, Hijiki Carrot Nitsuke, Hijiki Nitsuke, Burdock Carrot Nitsuke, Vegetable Tempura, Deep-Fried Kombu, Nori Roasted with Oil, Azuki Beans with Kombu and Winter Squash, Miso Pickles, Grated Daikon with Sesame Oil and Soy Sauce.

☐ Miso soup ingredients: wakame, scallions, onions, Homemade Agé, Brown Rice Mochi.

☐ Beverages: Sho-Ban Tea, Bancha Tea, Brown Rice Bancha Tea, Kombu Tea, Mu Tea. Drink less, a maximum of 2 cups per day.

☐ Avoid especially: all animal foods and fish, all dairy, soy milk, fruit, sugary foods, potatoes, melons, vinegar dishes, candy, sweet drinks, alcohol.

FOR NERVE PAIN OTHER THAN FACIAL PAIN

☐ Main foods: Brown Rice Balls, Azuki Rice Balls with Gomashio, Brown Rice Mochi, Baked Mochi with Soy Sauce, Buckwheat Noodles with Tempura.

☐ Side dishes (one-third of main foods): Tekka Miso, Burdock Carrot Nitsuke, Okara Nitsuke, Carp Soup, Grated Daikon with Sesame Oil and Soy Sauce, Vegetable Stew, Vegetable Stew with Fish, Takuan Pickles.

☐ Miso soup ingredients: wakame, scallions, spinach, tofu, daikon, snow peas, string beans.

☐ Beverages: Brown Rice Tea, Brown Rice Bancha Tea, Bancha Tea, Grain Coffee.

☐ Avoid especially: all overly yin and yang foods.

PARASITES

Parasites are organisms that live within or upon, and at the expense of other living organisms. Human parasites include disease-causing agents such as hookworms, pinworms, roundworms, or tapeworms that infect the digestive system, or fungi that live on the skin. Hookworms grow to half an inch in length and can be detected in excretion. In cases involving a large number of hookworms, symptoms include anemia, headache, dizziness, swelling of the entire body, kidney disorders, and pale complexion. Pinworms are an infestation of the intestines by very small worms (oxyuriasis). These worms cause the anal area to itch so severely that sleep may be impossible. If pinworms move to the vaginal opening, they can cause vaginal discharges, itching, and discomfort.

Roundworms are most common in children and are usually found in the gastrointestinal tract. They are round, like earthworms, and can reach one foot in length. They can be seen in excretion or in the child's bed. Symptoms indicating roundworms include irritability, loss of appetite, stomachaches, weight loss or no weight gain, and fatigue. Tapeworms are flat and look like a Japanese sash for a kimono. They develop in many sections of the body, usually in the abdomen of animal-food eaters. Symptoms of tapeworm presence can resemble stomach or intestinal diseases or psychological troubles. Some symptoms are chills, vomiting, sharp pains, hiccups, headache, dizziness, cramps, swelling, fast pulse, or fatigue. Causes of these symptoms are thought to be the parasites themselves.

These parasites are transmitted to the human body through contaminated water, food such as raw or spoiled meat, soil-contaminated hands, bare feet on contaminated ground, or the improper disposal of human waste. Yet many people come in contact with these parasites and have little or no adverse reaction. Why? Because, according to our macrobiotic understanding, the under-

lying cause of parasitic diseases is a diet high in sugar and/or fruit, a low salt level in the blood, and/or weak kidneys. These conditions create an internal environment conducive to the growth of parasites. Persons eating a balanced diet have little or no problem with parasites.

Helpful Suggestions

OBJECTIVE	REMEDY
To control hookworms	Eat 2 soybean-sized balls of UME EXTRACT before meals twice a day.
To control pinworms	Try taking a PYRETHRUM TEA ENEMA every day for 1 week if your condition allows it.
To relieve rash or itchiness	Once a day for 20 minutes, take a DAIKON or ARAME HIP BATH with 1/3 to 1/2 cup of salt added.
To control tapeworms	To bring quick results, and if you are strong, drink 1 cup of POMEGRANATE BARK TEA 3 times per day until tapeworms disappear. (If you are weak, this tea can make you tired because the pomegranate bark contains a small amount of a substance that is considered poisonous.) *and* Eating 1/4 cup of roasted winter squash seeds (shelled) 2 times per day for 1 week is beneficial.

Dietary Recommendations

Follow a macrobiotic dietary approach (see page 11) with the following variations: Drink Mugwort Tea instead of Bancha Tea. Every morning before breakfast (on an empty stomach) eat 1/3 cup of washed, raw brown rice and chew this very well. Eat Roasted Watermelon Seeds or Roasted Pumpkin Seeds, mugwort mochi (see Brown Rice Mochi), Buckwheat Noodles, Buckwheat Groats, and Mugwort Bread often. Eliminate fruit, candy, honey, and all sweeteners. Parasites like to live in sweet fluids.

CORNELLIA'S NATURAL HEALING AT WORK

During a visit, my friend told me, "My daughter has parasites." I asked her what kind of diet she was using for the child. She said that she was using a salt-free diet. I said, "No, George Ohsawa only recommended that diet until the child was more balanced, only about five to ten days." My friend had continued the diet for almost two months, so her daughter's body had not had enough salt, and parasites were starting. I recommended she give the child yang grains like buckwheat dishes and soba noodles seasoned with miso and soy sauce. She was better in one week—no more parasites.

If the body becomes salty, parasites cannot live. If you make a mistake and use too much salt, the remedy is easy; just cut down on salt. Parasites start because of eating too much sugar, fruit, and yin food. The bodily organs become expanded and yin. Then it takes time to heal. Even so, if all yin foods are avoided and the diet is balanced, then parasites cannot live and grow. ■

PARASITES

PENIS PAIN

The usual symptoms of penis pain are a burning sensation during urination or sexual intercourse, and a frequent urge to urinate. This may be caused by urethral infections usually stemming from gonorrhea. These problems can also be caused by an infection of the prostate gland. The penis has many blood vessels and is supplied with much blood. Nevertheless, an infection along the urethra can cause a shortage of oxygen, which is the cause of pain during urination or sexual intercourse.

According to our macrobiotic understanding, infection or the overgrowth of bacteria does cause a shortage of oxygen in the nerve cells of the painful area. However, the overgrowth of bacteria is the result of three conditions: one is the overeating of yin foods such as sugar, candy, fruits, ice cream, and other simple carbohydrates; another is weak kidneys resulting from an imbalanced diet or drinking too much liquids; and a third is a low- or no-salt diet.

Helpful Suggestions

OBJECTIVE	REMEDY
To relieve pain	Try applying a GINGER COMPRESS to the painful area for 20 minutes. Repeat every 2 hours or as necessary until pain subsides.

Dietary Recommendations

Use the following dietary suggestions during periods of pain or for one month. Then, widen your food choices using a macrobiotic dietary approach (see page 11).

☐ Main foods: Brown Rice, Azuki Rice, Gomashio with each meal.
☐ Side dishes (one-third of main foods): Carp Soup (2 cups per day), all sea vegetables, Shio Kombu, Burdock Carrot Nitsuke, Tekka Miso, Scallion Miso (scallions are the best vegetable for sexual organ problems).
☐ Miso soup ingredients: scallions, Brown Rice Mochi, Homemade Agé.
☐ Beverages: Grain Coffee, Brown Rice Tea, Brown Rice Bancha Tea, Bancha Tea, Sho-Ban Tea, Azuki Kombu Drink. Drink as much as possible for 3 days only. Since overdrinking can lead to weak kidneys resulting in an overgrowth of bacteria, after 3 days or as soon as pain subsides, drink a maximum of 2 cups of liquid per day.
☐ Avoid especially: all animal foods (except carp), alcohol, coffee, black tea, fruit, sweet foods and drinks.

PERICARDITIS

Pericarditis refers to an inflammation of the pericardium, the double membranous bag that encloses the heart, providing protection and lubrication for that rapidly beating muscle. There are many forms of pericarditis, and if the quantity of fluid in the layers of the pericardium is increased, it may cause pressure on the heart. This can be fatal if the fluid is not removed quickly. One of the signs of pericarditis is dull or sharp pain in the chest that increases with any movement of the body, even walking. Other indications include rapid breathing, cough-

ing, fever and chills, weakness, elevated white cell count, or an abnormal EKG. Sometimes the cause of pericarditis is unknown, but there are many known causes including a viral infection in the pericardium; chronic kidney failure; rheumatic fever; complications following a heart attack, heart surgery, or a chest injury; and the spread of cancer to this area. Heart problems can result from eating too much cholesterol and fatty food.

From our macrobiotic point of view, viral infection and rheumatic fever are caused by eating too much yin food or a low- or no-salt diet, or by weak kidneys. Kidney weakness is caused by too much salt intake, a low- or no-salt diet, and/or too much drinking of any liquids. Thus, the proper amount of salt, neither too much or too little, and a balanced diet are most important for the remedy or prevention of this condition.

Helpful Suggestions

The utmost care and careful monitoring should be employed since the most important signs of pericarditis are only apparent with medical examination and since quick action may be necessary to save your life. Consult your health-care advisor. The following suggestions are complementary.

OBJECTIVE	REMEDY
To strengthen a weak pulse	Drink the RANSHO DRINK prepared from 1 egg, once a day for 3 days before bedtime. If once a day is not enough, eat a second 1-egg preparation of ransho per day until the heart becomes stronger (shows a stronger pulse). *and/or* Eat 1 teaspoon of TEKKA MISO once a day at any meal for 1 week.
To improve circulation	Apply a MUSTARD PLASTER to the heart (see Figure 3.8 on page 176) until the skin turns a red color (about 15 minutes), then apply an ALBI PLASTER for up to 4 hours. Apply these plasters for 1 week. *and* Eat ½ teaspoon of EGG OIL 3 times per day for 1 week to help make the heart stronger.
To relieve chest pain	Apply an ALBI PLASTER on the painful area; change it every 4 hours as needed.
To relieve cough	Drink ½ to 1 cup of LOTUS ROOT TEA 2 or 3 times per day.
To eliminate (melt away) fat and crystalized salt	Take a FAR-INFRARED SAUNA several times per week.
To maintain a strong condition	Avoid hot baths. Short, warm showers are okay.

Dietary Recommendations

The following dietary suggestions may be used until your heart condition improves or for about one month. Then, widen your food choices based on a macrobiotic dietary approach (see page 11).

☐   Main foods: Brown Rice, Azuki Rice served with Gomashio, Fried Rice, Brown Rice Mochi. Chew each mouthful more than 100 times.

☐   Side dishes (one-fourth of main foods): Tekka Miso, Oily Miso, Hijiki Lotus Root Nitsuke, Burdock Carrot Nitsuke, Carp Soup, Vegetable Tempura, Nori Roasted with Oil, Miso Pickles. Slowly increase the amount of salt, measured by taste, in side dishes.

☐   Miso soup ingredients: wakame, scallions, onions, Brown Rice Mochi, tororo kombu.

☐   Beverages: Brown Rice Bancha Tea, Sho-Ban Tea, Kombu Tea, Mu Tea. Drink less than usual.

☐   Avoid especially: all animal foods including fish, shellfish, dairy foods (especially ice cream), and eggs; all fruit; sweet foods; alcoholic drinks; vinegar; mushrooms; melons; all beans except azuki beans.

PERIODONTAL DISEASE

Periodontal disease refers to any disorder of the gums or other structures that support the teeth. One of the earliest forms is gingivitis, an inflammation or infection of the gums. This condition is indicated by swollen, red gums that are soft around the teeth. Although the gums bleed easily and bad breath is present, there is no pain. If gingivitis is not remedied, periodontitis may result, causing a loss of supporting bone. In fact, periodontitis causes more tooth loss than dental caries (tooth decay). Bad breath, a loosening of teeth in their sockets, and aching pain when eating hot, cold, or sweet food signal periodontitis. Swelling, pain, fever, and tenderness occur if an abscess develops.

Pyorrhea is a term that is often used interchangeably with periodontitis, but actually refers to a pus-forming inflammation of the gums and is indicated by sore gums, large gum pockets, and the discharge of pus between the gums and teeth. The eroded gums bleed and the breath is foul.

Gingivitis is thought to be caused by a number of factors including poor nutrition such as vitamin deficiencies, the buildup of plaque (food, bacteria, and mucus trapped between or at the base of the teeth), any kind of blood disorder, and adverse reactions to certain drugs. If not treated, plaque continues to build up and periodontitis results. Since poor dental hygiene causes the accumulation of plaque, brushing and flossing the teeth properly are the best preventatives.

We do not disagree; however, according to our macrobiotic understanding, the main underlying cause of periodontal disease is the eating of too much sugary food and refined starches. Sometimes macrobiotic people, even though they do not eat these foods, have this disease. In such cases, they are not cleaning their teeth properly, especially in between the teeth. When starchy food remains on the teeth, it changes to sugar and increases the number of bacteria; the teeth decay and periodontal disease becomes likely. Swollen gums without other symptoms may occur as a result of eating too many yin sugary foods and not enough good-quality yang food such as miso, soy sauce, and sea salt. This condition may lead to gingivitis or other periodontal diseases.

Helpful Suggestions

In all cases, establishing good dental hygiene habits is a must. See your dentist if you have symptoms of periodontal disease; the following suggestions are complementary.

OBJECTIVE	REMEDY
To reduce swollen gums	Try using a WOOD ASH WATER TREATMENT for 30 minutes 3 times per day until the swelling goes down. This is a very effective treatment.
	and
	You can massage the gums with raw salt 3 times per day. The salt may cut the skin of the gums and cause temporary pain, but this is a quick method.
	or
	Three times per day, dentie powder can be gently worked into the gums using your index finger. This method is less painful than using salt.
To relieve pyorrhea	Gently rub the gums with dentie powder using your index finger and regularly use dentie to brush your teeth.

Dietary Recommendations

It is important to strengthen the whole body using a macrobiotic dietary approach (see page 11) since improper diet is one of the underlying causes of this condition. It is most important to eliminate all sugary foods and sweet foods, including fruits, when symptoms of periodontal disease are present. Make sure to include good-quality miso, soy sauce, and sea salt.

PERIOSTITIS

Periostitis is an inflammation of the connective tissues covering the bones. According to Western medicine, the cause of periostitis is basically a bacterial infection that invades the blood through the skin, respiratory organs, and digestive organs. In mild cases of periostitis, the inflammation is characterized by localized swelling of the affected tissue and mild pain, usually in the foot or knee. In severe cases there is a high temperature, pain, swelling, infections, constitutional disorders such as delirium, and death of tissues in a small localized area.

According to our macrobiotic understanding, the underlying cause of periostitis is eating too much animal protein, especially when combined with a high intake of sugary foods. Animal foods contain a higher percentage of protein than do vegetable foods and thus a greater possibility of contamination by bacteria from an outside source. However, more importantly, because of the high protein content, animal foods help microbes and other organisms develop by providing the building materials for their growth. Sugary foods accelerate the growth of microbes and provide an environment in which they thrive.

Helpful Suggestions

OBJECTIVE	REMEDY
To improve circulation and remove toxins	A GINGER COMPRESS applied on the affected area for 20 minutes followed by an ALBI PLASTER for up to 4 hours will help take toxins out of the area. Repeat both the compress and the plaster daily for a couple of weeks. The Ginger Compress also helps loosen the skin so the Albi Plaster is more effective.
To relieve itchiness	If the skin becomes itchy from the Albi Plaster, lightly rub the skin with a ¼-inch-thick round piece of daikon.
To relieve pain	Try using an UMEBOSHI SAKE PLASTER applied to the affected area, changing it 3 times per day, until the pain stops.

Dietary Recommendations

All bone diseases can be affected by a diet high in sea vegetables with a small number of Kombu Rolls with Chuba Iriko. Lotus root is the best vegetable for bone diseases. Use the following suggestions until the pain stops or for about one month. Then, widen your food choices using a macrobiotic dietary approach (see page

11). If the bone pain comes from the bacillus of tuberculosis (bone tubercle), refer to the tuberculosis section.

☐ Main foods: Brown Rice with Barley, Brown Rice, Azuki Rice served with Gomashio as a condiment. Chew each mouthful 200 times.

☐ Side dishes (one-fourth of main foods maximum): Ginger Miso, Sesame Miso, Wakame Nitsuke, Nori Nitsuke, Hijiki Lotus Root Nitsuke, Carp Soup, Burdock Carrot Nitsuke, Vegetable Tempura served with Grated Daikon, Eggplant Nitsuke with Miso, Takuan Pickles, Rice Bran Pickles, Kombu Rolls with Chuba Iriko, or Chuba Iriko Nitsuke.

☐ Miso soup ingredients: daikon, tofu, spinach, eggplant, carrots.

☐ Beverages: Bancha Tea, Brown Rice Bancha Tea, Brown Rice Tea, Grain Coffee.

☐ Avoid especially: all animal food including red-meat fish and shellfish (except for a small amount of white-meat fish), eggs, meat-based soups, all dairy foods (including ice cream); sweet foods and drinks and hot spices.

See also OSTEOPOROSIS.

PERITONITIS

The peritoneum is the serous membrane that covers the walls of the abdominal and pelvic cavities. Peritonitis is an infection or inflammation of part or all of the membrane lining the abdominal-pelvic walls. One symptom of peritonitis is pain in the abdomen that usually starts suddenly and becomes more severe. Other symptoms include shoulder pains, chills and fever, constipation, vomiting, rapid heart beat, thirst, high white blood cell count (10,000 to 50,000), dizziness, weakness, and low blood pressure. Inflammation is thought to occur when foreign material such as bacteria or gastrointestinal contents enter the abdominal cavity as a result of a rupture or perforation (as in peptic ulcer) of any organ in the abdomen such as an inflamed appendix or an infected gallbladder.

Such ruptures, according to our macrobiotic understanding, are caused by one's previous diet, which contained too much yin food, especially a high amount of simple carbohydrates, or too much yang protein food. The yang protein foods cause microbes to increase and result in a yin condition. Even though the overconsumption of both yin and yang foods results in an overly yin condition, there are still two types of peritonitis. The yin type is caused by the overconsumption of sugary foods or fruit, and the yang type is caused by the over-consumption of foods of animal origin including fish, cheese, and eggs. Also, there are chronic yin and yang types characterized by a longer lasting progression of illness and cure and an acute yang type characterized by more severe symptoms and rapid development. There is no acute yin type.

Helpful Suggestions

OBJECTIVE	REMEDY
	FOR THE ACUTE YANG TYPE
To relieve pain with fever	Use a GINGER COMPRESS for 20 minutes followed by a 3/4-inch-thick TOFU PLASTER over the entire stomach. Change the plaster every 1 to 2 hours for a period of 24 hours.
	and
	If there is no improvement after this treatment, then change to a BUCKWHEAT PLASTER, keeping it warm with a ROASTED SALT PACK on top. Change this plaster every 4 hours
To relieve pain with no fever	You do not need to use the Tofu Plaster, just try a BUCKWHEAT or ALBI PLASTER, changing either every 4 hours.
	or
	Try drinking 1 cup of SHO-BAN TEA up to 2 to 3 times per day.
To relieve persistent pain	Drink 1 cup of DAIKON TEA 2 to 4 times per day and eat 1/3 to 1/2 cup BROWN RICE CREAM (thick), or BROWN RICE as your 3 meals per day.
	and
	If you are still thirsty, try drinking 1 cup of BROWN RICE TEA.

Dietary Recommendations

If you have a persistent pain and eat only Brown Rice Cream at your daily meals, once the fever is down and there is less pain, expand your daily diet by adding one cup of Green Leafy Vegetables (using Chinese cabbage) with Homemade Agé, one to one and a half cups of Brown Rice Gruel with Miso, one cup of Green Leafy Vegetables with Homemade Agé, and one cup of Miso Soup with Mochi served with one tablespoon of Grated Daikon. Slowly change to the dietary suggestions for the yang type as described below.

The only real remedy for chronic yin or yang peritonitis is a change in dietary habits. You may try any of the "Helpful Suggestions" above for pain or fever. Follow the dietary suggestions listed above until your condition improves or for about one month. Then, widen your food choices using a macrobiotic dietary approach (see

page 11). If you are uncertain which type you have and whether your condition is acute, then use the suggestions for the yang type. If your condition is chronic, use the yin type suggestions.

FOR THE YANG TYPE

☐ Main foods: Brown Rice Balls (occasionally made with sweet brown rice) served with Gomashio, Brown Rice Cream, Brown Rice Gruel with Mochi. Chew each mouthful 200 times.

☐ Side dishes (one-third of main foods): Tekka Miso, wakame, Hijiki Burdock Nitsuke, Vegetable Stew, Carp Soup, Natto with Soy Sauce and Scallions served with Grated Daikon, Grated Daikon with Sesame Oil and Soy Sauce, Okara Nitsuke, Burdock Carrot Daikon Nitsuke, Cucumber with Kuzu Sauce, Umeboshi.

☐ Miso soup ingredients: daikon, burdock, Green Leafy Vegetables, winter squash, tofu, Homemade Agé, Brown Rice Mochi.

☐ Beverages: Brown Rice Tea, Brown Rice Bancha Tea, Bancha Tea, Vegetable Broth, Grain Coffee.

☐ Avoid especially: all animal foods (except carp), red-meat fish, shellfish, all dairy foods, eggs, meat-based soups, all sweet foods.

FOR THE YIN TYPE

☐ Main foods: Brown Rice Balls, Azuki Rice served with Gomashio (use Gomashio at each meal), Brown Rice Gruel with Miso and with Mochi, Baked Mochi with Soy Sauce, Brown Rice Cream. Chew each mouthful 200 times.

☐ Side dishes (one-fourth of main foods): Tekka Miso, Hijiki Nitsuke, Shio Kombu, Vegetable Tempura, Carp Soup, Chuba Iriko Nitsuke, Deep-Fried Kombu, Takuan Pickles, Miso Pickles.

☐ Miso soup ingredients: wakame, tororo kombu, scallions, onions, Homemade Agé, Brown Rice Mochi.

☐ Beverages: Brown Rice Tea, Brown Rice Bancha Tea, Bancha Tea, Sho-Ban Tea, Kombu Tea, Grain Milk.

☐ Avoid especially: all animal protein (except carp), red-meat fish, dairy foods (including ice cream), eggs, all sweet foods and drinks, alcohol, fruit, mushrooms, potatoes, tomatoes, eggplant, all beans.

PLEURISY

Pleurisy is an inflammation and irritation of the chest lining often accompanied by a buildup of fluid. There is sharp chest pain, worsened by breathing or coughing, and often displaced to the shoulder, abdomen, or neck. There is considerable shortness of breath and often fever.

As fluid accumulates or develops, the pain usually subsides while the breathlessness worsens. Pleurisy is thought to be caused by complications accompanying any number of diseases such as pneumonia, tuberculosis, or other lung or chest infections; kidney, liver, or heart disorders; injury to the chest or rib cage; collapse of part of the lung; or cancer in other parts of the body.

According to our macrobiotic understanding, the underlying cause of pleurisy is a long-time dietary imbalance. Yang pleurisy is caused by the presence of too much protein and/or salt (sodium) in the lung and chest area. This protein or salt usually comes from animal-origin foods that are high in protein and sodium. Thus, if you consume too much yang animal-origin foods such as red meat or too much salt, the result is yang pleurisy. If you consume too many simple carbohydrates such as yin sugary foods and fruits, then these carbohydrates oxidize (metabolize) and produce excess water. If the kidneys are weak and can't deal with the excess water, the result is yin pleurisy.

Helpful Suggestions

Refrain from sex and avoid taking hot baths until your condition improves.

OBJECTIVE	REMEDY
To reduce fever	Use a TOFU PLASTER applied to the forehead, changing it every 1 to 2 hours.
To relieve chest pain	Apply a GINGER COMPRESS to the chest for 20 minutes or a MUSTARD PLASTER to the chest for 5 to 7 minutes until the skin turns red. Then apply an ALBI PLASTER for up to 4 hours. Repeat both the compress and the plaster as often as possible until the pain is reduced.
	then
	When the pain is reduced and the fever is gone, continue applying Ginger Compresses and Albi Plasters twice a day for 2 to 3 weeks.
To improve circulation	Cleanse the body with GINGER BATH water as a sponge bath once a day.
To relieve cough	Drink 1 cup of *UME EXTRACT TEA* every 3 hours to help stop coughing.

Dietary Recommendations

Pleurisy is caused by a long-time dietary imbalance, so gradually change the condition of your whole body through a change in diet. Use the following dietary suggestions for about one month. Then, widen your food choices using a macrobiotic dietary approach (see page 11). If you are uncertain as to which type you have, use the suggestions for the yin type first.

FOR THE YANG TYPE

☐ Main foods: Brown Rice, Brown Rice with Barley served with a little Gomashio. Chew each mouthful 200 times.

☐ Side dishes (one-third of main foods): Tekka Miso (a little bit), Vegetable Tempura served with Grated Daikon, Eggplant Nitsuke with Miso, Burdock Lotus Root Nitsuke, Okara Nitsuke, Rice Bran Pickles. Cook these dishes with less salt.

☐ Miso soup ingredients: wakame, daikon, Chinese cabbage, tofu, Brown Rice Mochi.

☐ Beverages: Brown Rice Bancha Tea, Barley Tea, Vegetable Broth, Grain Coffee.

☐ Avoid especially: all animal food including red-meat fish and shellfish, dairy foods (including ice cream), sweet foods and drinks, cod liver oil.

FOR THE YIN TYPE

☐ Main foods: Brown Rice Balls with Gomashio, Azuki Rice, Brown Rice Gruel with mochi, Baked Mochi with Soy Sauce. Chew each mouthful 200 times.

☐ Side dishes (one-fourth of main foods): Tekka Miso, Oily Miso, Hijiki Nitsuke, Burdock Lotus Root Nitsuke, Burdock Carrot Nitsuke, Vegetable Tempura, Carp Soup, Takuan Pickles, Miso Pickles.

☐ Miso soup ingredients: wakame, onions, scallions, watercress, burdock, Brown Rice Mochi.

☐ Beverages: Brown Rice Bancha Tea, Sho-Ban Tea, Bancha Tea. Drink a maximum of 1½ cups of beverages per day.

☐ Avoid especially: all meat, red-meat fish, shellfish, all beans except azuki beans.

PNEUMONIA

Pneumonia is an acute inflammatory condition of the lung. It begins, like a cold, as an upper respiratory infection of the lung. The illness continues with sudden chills that may go on from several minutes to half an hour. This is followed by coughing, fever, a flushed face, the appearance of sweat on the forehead, and fast and labored breathing. The pulse rate may run from 100 to 130 beats per minute. Symptoms vary according to the type of pneumonia and causative agent.

According to modern medicine, pneumonia has more than fifty causes. The most significant and the most common causes are thought to be viral infections or bacterial organisms. Bacterial pneumonia is the most severe form as it usually results in a high fever over 102°F and a difficult cough with sputum that may contain blood. It may lead to greater disorders such as pleurisy or meningitis. The germs are usually spread by coughing, sneezing, or breathing; however, contact with the germs does not mean a person will automatically succumb to the disease. Your risk of getting pneumonia increases with smoking, poor general health or any illness that has lowered your resistance, the use of certain drugs such as anticancer drugs, stress, and crowded or unsanitary living conditions. There are dietary considerations as well.

According to our macrobiotic understanding, one of the underlying causes of any infection including pneumonia is a shortage of salt (sodium). If the bodily fluids contain less than 0.85 percent salt solution, microbes easily proliferate inside our bodies. Therefore, a salt-free or low-salt diet is the first cause of pneumonia. Reducing the percentage of sodium in bodily fluids by drinking too much liquid of any kind, especially fruit juice and sugary juices, is another cause. Thirdly, the kidneys control the amount of sodium in our bodily fluids. If the kidneys are weak, sufficient sodium isn't retained in our bodily fluids and we become vulnerable to all kinds of microbes and viruses. Since weakened kidneys can result from too much yin or yang food, there is a yin type and a yang type of pneumonia. The yang type of pneumonia is indicated when a person quickly develops a high fever. Usually the fever is high at night and lower in the morning, but with yang pneumonia there is a fever all day long. Yin pneumonia occurs when one has been sick a long time, or has had a cold from which he or she cannot recover. Then, suddenly, one has difficulty breathing, indicating pneumonia.

Helpful Suggestions

Avoid hot baths or showers and refrain from sex until your condition improves.

OBJECTIVE	REMEDY
FOR THE YANG TYPE	
To reduce fever	A CARP PLASTER is best. Leave the plaster on the chest until the body temperature returns to 98.6°F, about 2 to 3 hours. Check your temperature every 30 minutes by placing a thermometer in the armpit and stop using the plaster as soon as the temperature is normal.
	or
	If you have no carp, use a TOFU PLASTER on the chest; change it every hour until the fever returns to normal.
To remove toxins	Use an ALBI PLASTER on the chest; change it every 4 hours.
To improve lungs	Drinking 2 cups of *LOTUS ROOT DAIKON TEA* 3 times per day is very beneficial for the lungs.
To relieve headache	Apply a TOFU PLASTER on the forehead; change it every 1 or 2 hours.
	and
	Use a GINGER SESAME OIL MASSAGE on the neck.
To relieve thirst or dry mouth	Try drinking 1 cup of *BROWN RICE TEA WITH SHIITAKE MUSHROOMS* up to 4 times per day.
FOR THE YIN TYPE	
To reduce fever	Use only a TOFU PLASTER on the chest; change it every 1 or 2 hours until temperature returns to normal.
To remove toxins	Then change to an ALBI PLASTER; change it every 4 hours.
To relieve headache	Apply a TOFU PLASTER on the forehead and place a GREEN LEAVES APPLICATION on the back of the neck at the same time; change both every 2 hours.
To relieve thirst or dry mouth	Drink ½ to 1 cup of *BROWN RICE TEA WITH UMEBOSHI* or *LOTUS ROOT TEA* 2 to 3 times per day.

Dietary Recommendations

Use the following dietary suggestions until your condition improves or for about one month. Then, widen your food choices using a macrobiotic dietary approach (see page 11). If you are uncertain as to which type pneumonia you have, try the suggestions for the yin type first.

FOR THE YANG TYPE

☐ Main foods: Brown Rice Balls with a little Gomashio, Brown Rice Gruel served with Grated Daikon and Homemade Agé. Chew each mouthful 200 times. If you have no appetite, eat Brown Rice Cream (thick), Udon Noodles, Grain Milk, or Millet Rice.

☐ Side dishes (one-fourth of main foods): Sesame Miso, Daikon Nitsuke with Homemade Agé, Green Leafy Vegetables served with Homemade Agé, Grated Daikon, Umeboshi, Carp Soup (less salty taste).

☐ Miso soup ingredients: daikon, burdock, wakame, Chinese cabbage, Homemade Agé.

☐ Beverages: Brown Rice Tea, Brown Rice Bancha Tea, Bancha Tea, Grain Coffee, Vegetable Broth. Drink a maximum of 2 cups of beverages per day.

☐ Avoid especially: all animal food including fish (except carp) and shellfish, dairy foods, fruit, sweet foods and drinks, nightshade family vegetables, hot spices.

FOR THE YIN TYPE

Since this type of pneumonia is caused by a low-salt diet, eat Soy Sauce with Sesame Oil every day.

☐ Main foods: Brown Rice Kayu (made with brown rice or sweet brown rice), Brown Rice Cream served with Gomashio and Umeboshi for condiments. Chew very well.

☐ Side dishes (one-fourth of main foods): Tekka Miso, Shio Kombu, Burdock Carrot Nitsuke, Hijiki Lotus Root Nitsuke, Oysters Cooked with Miso, Poached Fish, Miso Pickles, Umeboshi.

☐ Miso soup ingredients: wakame, tororo kombu, scallions, onions, Homemade Agé, Brown Rice Mochi.

☐ Beverages: Brown Rice Tea, Sho-Ban Tea, Brown Rice Bancha Tea, Bancha Tea, Bancha Tea with Gomashio, Grain Milk.

☐ Avoid especially: all animal foods (except oysters, sole, and flounder), eggs, dairy foods, all fruit, sweet foods and drinks, nightshade family vegetables, beans, vinegar, salads, alcohol.

PRICKLY HEAT (HEAT RASH)

Prickly heat is a skin disorder characterized by a non-inflammatory, itchy rash resulting from sweat retention. All ages may be affected but it is most common in infants. The immediate cause of prickly heat is obstructed sweat-gland ducts. However, the reason for the obstruction is thought to be unknown. It is known that prickly heat is more common in hot, humid weather and that obesity, stress, and fair skin increase your chances of getting prickly heat. Oftentimes, people who have problems with prickly heat are advised to stay indoors in air-conditioned surroundings during hot, humid weather.

However, according to our macrobiotic understanding, the underlying cause of prickly heat is the over-consumption of fatty, animal foods such as meat and dairy products. Not only does this type of diet directly contribute to the obstruction of sweat-gland ducts, but over a period of time, it results in weak kidneys. Weakened kidneys cause many skin problems. The fact that recurrence is common, even following treatment, indicates that nothing would be more helpful than a change in dietary habits. If you are nursing your baby, a change in your diet should help the baby also. Note that cow's milk is a fatty food and is not recommended for babies.

Helpful Suggestions

OBJECTIVE	REMEDY
To induce sweating	Use a PEACH LEAVES BATH for 20 minutes twice a day until sweating begins. *then* Once this happens, take this bath for 20 minutes at a time as often as desired.
To relieve itchy rash	A CHESTNUT LEAVES BATH once a day for 20 minutes is also useful for itchy skin, skin abscesses, or other skin diseases.

Dietary Recommendations

The only real remedy for prickly heat is a change in diet to one that is low in fat such as a macrobiotoic dietary approach (see page 11).

See also SKIN, ITCHY.

PROSTATE PROBLEMS

The most significant of prostate disorders are prostatitis (inflammation or infection of the prostate gland), enlarged prostate, and prostate cancer. The most common symptoms of prostatitis and enlarged prostate are increased urgency and frequency of urination, burning urination, and straining and other problems in urinating. An abnormal urine color and weak urinary stream indicate an enlarged prostate. The presence of chills, and pain or muscle aches signals prostatitis. In cases of prostate cancer, there are usually no symptoms in the early stages. Later, urinary obstruction and lower back pain may result. The cause of prostatitis is thought to be bacterial infection; the cause of enlarged prostate is hormonal changes with aging and decreased sexual activity; and the cause of prostate cancer is unknown. While the risk factors for prostate cancer are thought to be unknown, stress, smoking, excess alcohol consumption, and the use of many drugs increase your risk of developing prostate problems.

According to our macrobiotic understanding, the underlying cause of prostate problems is a diet high in animal foods and sugary foods. The overproduction of male sex hormones—which is caused by eating too much animal food such as meat, chicken, pork, fish, cheese, and eggs—is the initiator of prostate cancer. Then, high simple carbohydrate and/or fruit consumption is the promoter of cancer and of enlarged prostate. Such a diet also weakens the body's natural immunity against infections. Thus, the macrobiotic approach is to change dietary habits both as a remedy and as a preventative for prostate problems.

The medical approach for prostatitis is the administration of antibiotics and pain relievers. Usually this results in relief of symptoms, but recurrence is common, showing that the cause has not been understood. Enlarged prostate is very common in men over fifty and this shows that the long-term effects of an inappropriate diet are at work. The same is true of prostate cancer. In both cases, surgery is the most common procedure, especially when the condition may lead to greater disorders. However, according to our macrobiotic understanding, removal of an organ should be done only after all other methods have failed, as a last resort to save a person's life.

Helpful Suggestions

Maintaining physical fitness (avoiding strenuous exercise in cases of cancer) and an active sex life are important.

OBJECTIVE	REMEDY
To relieve pain	Try applying a GINGER COMPRESS for 20 minutes followed by an ALBI PLASTER over the prostate gland area for 4 hours. Repeat as often as needed.
To reduce fever	Drink 1 cup of DAIKON GINGER TEA 3 or 4 times per day.

Dietary Recommendations

Following a macrobiotic dietary approach (see page 11) is the most beneficial procedure. In the case of cancer, eat beans only two to three times per month and avoid all fruits. Avoid foods that irritate the urethra such as spicy foods.

RASHES (POISON OAK OR POISON IVY)

Poison oak or ivy rash refers to an allergic reaction due to recent contact with the sap of either of these plants. Symptoms include an itchy rash, slight redness, swelling, and blistering. If symptoms last longer than one week or if there is fever or infection, a more serious disorder may be indicated. This should be determined and dealt with. There are many topical creams, ointments, or lotions that may be used to help reduce inflammation or preserve moisture. However, the macrobiotic approach is always to try the most natural forms of remedy first.

Helpful Suggestions

OBJECTIVE	REMEDY
To minimize rash after contact (before rash appears)	As soon as possible after you have come in contact with poison oak or ivy, take 1 heaping tablespoon of baking soda and add a little water to form a paste. Apply this paste over the total area that has been affected. This is very good because baking soda helps alkalize the skin.
To soothe symptoms after rash develops	An APPLICATION OF CRAB WATER directly on the rash is helpful. *or* Someone with a yin condition may crush the meat of a crab, shrimp, or crayfish and apply directly on the rash, changing it every 4 hours. *or* Someone with a yang condition may use a CHESTNUT LEAVES or ARAME BATH as a sponge bath on the rash area 3 times per day. *and/or* You may find it helpful to take a CHESTNUT LEAVES or ARAME BATH 3 times per day in lukewarm, not hot, water. In either case, pat the skin dry instead of rubbing it.

Dietary Recommendations

Following a macrobiotic dietary approach (see page 11) is helpful in preventing the development of infections or fever.

See also PRICKLY HEAT *and* CHICKENPOX.

RECTAL PROLAPSE

Rectal prolapse refers to a protrusion of the rectal mucous membrane through the anus. A firm mass of tissue can be felt at the anus after bowel movements. Rectal prolapse can be accompanied by a mucous discharge (sometimes with blood) from the rectum. According to modern medicine, this condition is caused by weak pelvic muscles or abdominal pressure as a result of a chronic cough, prolonged standing or walking, prolonged constipation, or straining to have bowel movements. Rectal prolapse mostly affects adults over sixty, usually women.

However, according to our macrobiotic understanding, the underlying cause of this condition is eating too much meat, cheese, chicken, pork, fish and other animal foods along with too much yin food such as sugary foods and drinks, coffee, and fruit. Often, disorders that primarily affect older persons are considered to be part of the aging process, and this is an accurate analysis for those eating a high-meat-and-sugar diet. But it doesn't have to be the case. A change in dietary habits is the best remedy and preventative for rectal prolapse.

Helpful Suggestions

It is best to avoid hot baths.

OBJECTIVE	REMEDY
To reduce protruding tissue	Lightly rub good-quality sesame oil on the outside, then gently push the protrusion back in.
	and
	If it comes out again, try placing a DAIKON PLASTER on the area 2 times per day for 20 minutes each time to keep it warm. After the compress, lightly rub again with sesame oil and gently push the protrusion back in.
	and
	If it comes out once more, apply a ½-inch thick ALBI PLASTER for 2 to 4 hours, and then lightly rub again with sesame oil and gently push it back in.
To alleviate more severe prolapsus	Try using a GINGER COMPRESS on the area for 20 minutes. Soak a piece of cotton in EGG OIL and apply it directly on the protrusion. Remain lying down for at least 20 minutes. Repeat both the compress and the egg oil application until your condition improves.

Dietary Recommendations

After starting a macrobiotic dietary approach, the body will become more flexible so you should not need an operation for this condition. However, if you do not have surgery and do not change your diet, the condition is likely to recur. Use the following suggestions until your condition improves or for about one month. Then, widen your food choices using a macrobiotic dietary approach (see page 11).

☐ Main foods: Brown Rice, Azuki Rice, Fried Rice served with Gomashio.
☐ Side dishes (one-third of main foods): Tekka Miso, Oily Miso, Hijiki Nitsuke, Shio Kombu, Burdock Carrot Nitsuke, Vegetable Stew, Carp Soup, Vegetable Tempura, Nori Roasted with Oil, Natural Caviar, Takuan Pickles, Miso Pickles.
☐ Miso soup ingredients: wakame, tororo kombu, Homemade Agé, seitan, Brown Rice Mochi.
☐ Beverages: Brown Rice Tea, Brown Rice Bancha Tea, Bancha Tea, Sho-Ban Tea, Kombu Tea, Grain Coffee.
☐ Avoid especially: all meats, red-meat fish, shellfish, eggs, dairy foods, milk, cheese, butter, ice cream, soy milk, all mushrooms, peanuts, hot spices, rice bran pickles.

RENAL FAILURE

See KIDNEY FAILURE.

RETINITIS

Retinitis is an inflammation or swelling of the retina, in one or both eyes, characterized by many symptoms including cloudiness, running tears, severe pains, ulcerations of the retina, mucus formation, eye discomfort, reduction of visual sharpness, and distortion of the form and size of objects. An infection that spreads to the eye from other body parts is the most common cause although the cause is unknown in many cases. An injury to the eye may also result in retinitis.

According to our macrobiotic understanding, there are two kinds of retinitis, that is to say, yin and yang retinitis. The yang type of retinitis is caused by syphilis or albuminuria (protein discharge in the urine), diseases that are caused by the overconsumption of animal foods. Yin retinitis is caused by leukemia or diabetes, which in turn is caused by the overconsumption of yin foods such as simple carbohydrates and/or fruit. After recovery from these major sicknesses, retinitis will disappear naturally.

Helpful Suggestions

OBJECTIVE	REMEDY
To reduce inflammation or swelling	Try using a SALT BANCHA EYE BATH on each affected eye 3 to 4 times per day.
	and
	Use a SESAME OIL EYE TREATMENT every night before sleeping.

Dietary Recommendations

A change in dietary habits is the best idea since this will help to control the underlying condition. Use the following dietary suggestions until your condition improves or for about one month. Then, widen your food choices using a macrobiotic dietary approach (see page 11). If you are uncertain which type retinitis you have, use the suggestions for the yin type first. If you have an underlying disorder, see also the appropriate section for additional suggestions.

FOR THE YANG TYPE

☐ Main foods: Brown Rice, Azuki Rice. Chew each teaspoon-sized mouthful 100 times.

☐ Side dishes (less than one-third of main foods): Ginger Miso, Miso Soup, Okara Nitsuke, Burdock Nitsuke, natto served with Grated Daikon, Boiled Daikon served with Lemon Miso, Tofu with Kuzu Sauce, Pressed Salad, Sour Cabbage, seasonal vegetables including tomatoes and eggplant in summer.

☐ Miso soup ingredients: wakame, daikon, Green Leafy Vegetables, and seasonal vegetables.

☐ Beverages: Bancha Tea, Brown Rice Tea, Grain Coffee. Drink a maximum of 1½ cups of beverages per day.

☐ Avoid especially: all meat, fish, shellfish, dairy foods, refined sugar, sweet foods, vinegar, coffee, alcohol.

FOR THE YIN TYPE

☐ Main foods: Brown Rice, Azuki Rice, Brown Rice Mochi, Brown Rice Gruel with Mochi.

☐ Side dishes (one-third of main foods): Tekka Miso, Oily Miso, Hijiki Burdock Nitsuke, Hijiki Lotus Root Nitsuke, Hijiki Carrot Nitsuke, Carp Soup, Burdock Carrot Nitsuke, Deep-Fried Kombu, Nori Roasted with Oil, Miso Pickles, Rice Bran Pickles, onions, scallions, and other seasonal yang vegetables.

☐ Miso soup ingredients: wakame, onions, carrots, Brown Rice Mochi, Chinese cabbage, daikon.

☐ Beverages: Bancha Tea, Brown Rice Tea, Grain Coffee. Drink a maximum of 1½ cups of beverages per day.

☐ Avoid especially: all meat, fish, shellfish, refined sugar, sweet foods, fruit, tomatoes, potatoes, eggplant, vinegar, dairy foods, coffee, alcohol, fruit drinks.

RHEUMATISM

Rheumatism is a general term referring to a variety of disorders characterized by inflammation, degeneration, or metabolic derangement of the joints and related structures such as muscles, tendons, and fibrous tissue. It can be very painful for the face, eyes, lips, nose, teeth, and tongue. There is pain in the ribs when breathing accompanies fever during periods of active flare-up. When pain occurs in the legs, it is usually on one side only; however, it can occur in both legs at the same time. Also, there may be pain in the hips, back of the thighs, knee caps, and feet. If rheumatism is confined to the joints only, it is classified as arthritis and often referred to as rheumatoid arthritis.

According to our macrobiotic understanding, the underlying cause of rheumatism is nerve damage, which is caused by a diet that is too yin and/or too yang. In the case of too many yin foods, whether acid-forming or alkaline-forming, red blood cells become more yin and carry less oxygen, resulting in a shortage of oxygen in the nerves around the joints and muscles. With an overly yang animal-food diet (more acid-forming), more oxygen is needed in the processing of animal foods, causing a shortage of oxygen in the nerves. In both cases, the result is pain. Also, acid-forming foods, whether yin or yang, cause pain because an overly acidic condition of the nerve cells damages nerve metabolism. Enzyme function, which is essential to nerve cell metabolism, is improved by maintaining a slightly alkaline condition.

Helpful Suggestions

For yin rheumatism, never get in a hot springs for treatment. See also the suggestions for fever and pain relief in the Arthritis section.

OBJECTIVE	REMEDY
To reduce high fever (yang condition)	Try drinking 1 cup of BROWN RICE TEA WITH SHIITAKE MUSHROOMS or DAIKON GINGER TEA every 3 hours, up to 4 cups per day.
To reduce high fever (yin condition)	Drink 1 cup of BROWN RICE TEA WITH DRIED PERSIMMON AND TANGERINE SKIN or BROWN RICE TEA WITH GINGER every 3 hours, up to 4 cups per day. If you cannot find persimmons, use dried dates or dried plums.
To relieve pain	Apply a GINGER or ARAME COMPRESS to the painful area for 20 minutes. *and* An UMEBOSHI PLASTER applied on the painful area 3 or 4 times per day is effective as well. *or* You may also apply a MUSTARD PLASTER until skin turns red or an ALBI PLASTER for up to 4 hours for pain relief. Repeat as necessary. *and* Using a GINGER SESAME OIL MASSAGE on the area is helpful also.

Dietary Recommendations:

Use the following dietary suggestions during periods of active flare-up or for about one month. Then, widen your food choices using a macrobiotic dietary approach (see page 11). If you have overeaten both yin and yang foods, try the suggestions for the yin type first.

FOR THE YANG TYPE

☐ Main foods: Brown Rice, Azuki Rice, Brown Rice with Barley, Brown Rice Mochi, Brown Rice Cream with Oil.

☐ Side dishes (one-fourth of main foods cooked with less salt than usual): Sesame Miso, Ginger Miso, Hijiki Burdock Nitsuke, Carp Soup, Grated Daikon with Soy Sauce, Vegetable Stew, Vegetable Stew with Fish, Okara

Nitsuke, Deep-Fried Kombu, Nori Nitsuke, Eggplant Nitsuke with Miso, Sour Cabbage, Takuan Pickles.

☐ Miso soup ingredients: daikon, sweet potatoes, tofu, spinach, eggplant, cucumber, Chinese cabbage, green leafy vegetables, Homemade Agé, Brown Rice Mochi.

☐ Beverages: Brown Rice Tea, Brown Rice Bancha Tea, Bancha Tea, Grain Coffee. Drink a maximum of 2½ cups of beverages per day.

☐ Avoid especially: all animal food, fish (except carp), shellfish, eggs, dairy foods, meat-based soups, sweet foods, hot spices, alcohol.

FOR THE YIN TYPE

☐ Main foods: Brown Rice, Azuki Rice, Azuki Millet Rice, Vegetable Fried Rice, Brown Rice Mochi, and Gomashio.

☐ Side dishes (one-third to one-half of main foods): Scallion Miso, Shio Kombu, Carp Soup, Hijiki Nitsuke, Burdock Carrot Nitsuke, Vegetable Stew with Fish, Vegetable Tempura, Nori Roasted with Oil, Deep-Fried Chuba Iriko, Takuan Pickles, Miso Pickles. For yin types of rheumatism, eating less of the side dishes is better. Eating less in general is better.

☐ Miso soup ingredients: wakame, tororo kombu, burdock, onions, scallions, dried seitan, Brown Rice Mochi.

☐ Beverages: Brown Rice Tea, Brown Rice Bancha Tea, Sho-Ban Tea, Bancha Tea, Kombu Tea, Grain Milk.

☐ Avoid especially: all animal foods, fish (except carp and fish in stew), shellfish, eggs, all dairy foods (including ice cream), sweet foods and drinks, fruit, black tea, tomatoes, eggplant, potatoes, melons, hot spices, peanuts.

RINGWORM

Ringworm refers to a group of fungal diseases and is identified by the formation of a ring of blisters on the skin. Lesions are red, circular, flat, and scaling when on the skin. When on the scalp, lesions cause spotty hair loss and scales. Ringworm of the feet is athlete's foot (see that section for more information). Ringworm may also affect the bearded area of the face, the nails, and the groin area. According to Western medicine, the cause of this skin disease is a fungus infection. All forms of ringworm are contagious. Ringworm can be carried by any animal such as cats, dogs, or horses, or may be transmitted by contact with infected surfaces such as towels, shoes, etc.

According to our macrobiotic understanding, a fungus infection is not the primary cause but is itself the result of overeating yang foods and having weak kidneys. Therefore, a change of diet is most helpful once

you have ringworm; it will also help minimize your susceptibility to the prevalent fungi that may lead to ringworm. Treat-ment of symptoms alone may lead to temporary relief, but recurrence is common. In fact, 20 percent of cases result in chronic ringworm, showing that symptomatic treatment does not deal with the primary cause.

Helpful Suggestions

OBJECTIVE	REMEDY
FOR RINGWORM ON THE BODY	
To alkalize the body	Try applying a DAIKON PLASTER WITH GINGER on the affected area for 20 minutes once a day. The plaster helps alkalize the body and causes sweating and increased circulation to the affected area.
To weaken the ringworm	Finely grate rhubarb and mix with white flour to form a paste. You may also add any good-quality vinegar using 2 parts of rhubarb to 1 part vinegar. Place either mixture directly on the ringworm for 20 to 30 minutes per day until the ringworm becomes weak.
	or
	Lightly rub the area with UME EXTRACT for 5 to 10 minutes once a day.
	and
	For ringworm around the sexual organs, mix 1 part UME EXTRACT with 10 parts water and apply.
To cleanse the body	Avoid soap; use a Rice Bran Bag (see BATHS) to wash with instead.
To care for the body	Fungus growth is increased in moist, warm environments, so keeping the skin dry is helpful. Wearing loose-fitting clothing and cotton underwear is always preferred.
To prevent the spread of ringworm	It is wise to sterilize all clothing, bedding, and towels that have come in contact with the affected area. If the groin area is affected, change underwear more than once a day.
FOR RINGWORM ON THE SCALP OR FACE	
To improve condition	Try washing the area with the water from a PEACH LEAVES, PINE NEEDLES, or CHESTNUT LEAVES BATH every day until your condition improves.
To cleanse hair	Avoid chemical shampoos. Short hair is best but there is no need to shave off all your hair.

Dietary Recommendations

Again, the best advice for any form of ringworm is to observe a macrobiotic dietary approach (see page 11).

☐ Avoid especially: all animal foods, fish, shellfish, especially shrimp and crab.

SCARLET FEVER

Scarlet fever is an acute contagious infection characterized by a bright red rash. Symptoms of scarlet fever usually follow a definite pattern although they may vary from person to person. The first day is usually marked with high fever, sore throat, cough, vomiting, and swollen tonsils and lymph glands in the neck. A bright red rash appears on the face on the second day. On the third day, the rash spreads to the entire body, looking like a sunburn with bumps. The tongue also becomes red. A shedding of the skin in scales or flakes begins on or about the sixth day and may last for up to another two weeks.

The specific cause of scarlet fever is a strep infection resulting from a certain type of streptococcal bacteria that produces a poisonous toxin. Not everyone is susceptible to this toxin; a person, therefore, may transmit the disease to others without being ill. Scarlet fever is not as prevalent as it once was and is rarely fatal. However, many complications may result if care is not taken.

According to our macrobiotic understanding, the underlying cause of this disease is overeating of animal foods such as meat, chicken, eggs, and fish. This kind of diet creates an environment in which infections thrive.

Helpful Suggestions

OBJECTIVE	REMEDY
To relieve sore throat	Apply a GINGER COMPRESS to the throat for 20 minutes, followed by an ALBI PLASTER for up to 4 hours. Repeat both the compress and plaster as often as possible until the sore throat is better. *and/or* GARGLE with 1 cup of BANCHA TEA WITH SALT or 1 cup of UME EXTRACT GARGLE 4 times per day.
To quench thirst	Try drinking 2 cups of *DAIKON GINGER TEA* each day. *and* This will help produce sweat, so cleanse the body with GINGER BATH water as a sponge bath.

To reduce high fever	Use a TOFU PLASTER on the forehead; change it every hour. *and* Use a GREEN LEAVES APPLICATION on the back of the neck; change the leaves every 2 hours.

Dietary Recommendations

Use the following dietary suggestions until the high fever and sore throat are gone, then follow a macrobiotic dietary approach (see page 11).

☐ Main foods: Brown Rice served with Gomashio. If the high fever or the sore throat continues, use Brown Rice Gruel with Shiitake Mushroom or Brown Rice Cream with Grated Daikon, 2½ cups maximum per day.
☐ Side dishes (less than one-fourth of main foods): Grated Daikon with Soy Sauce, Ginger Miso, Umeboshi, Eggplant Mustard Pickles, Takuan Pickles.
☐ Miso soup ingredients: daikon, Homemade Agé, scallions.
☐ Beverages: Brown Rice Tea, Brown Rice Bancha Tea, Bancha Tea, Grain Coffee.
☐ Avoid especially: overly yin or yang foods, especially meat and sugar.

SCIATICA

The sciatic nerve is a large nerve that begins at the base of the spine and passes through the buttocks down the back side of the thigh and down the leg. Specifically, sciatica is a syndrome characterized by pain that radiates from the back along the sciatic nerve extending down the back side of the leg; it is most commonly caused by prolapse of the intervertebral disk. "Sciatica" also is used to refer to any painful condition of any part of the sciatic nerve. According to our macrobiotic understanding, the underlying cause of sciatic nerve pain is almost always the overconsumption of yin foods such as simple carbohydrates—including the use of any sweetener in foods or drinks—vinegar, alcohol, coffee, and even fruit.

Helpful Suggestions

OBJECTIVE	REMEDY
To relieve mild pain	Try taking a DAIKON or ARAME HIP BATH WITH GRATED GINGER for 20 minutes. *then* Use a GINGER SESAME OIL MASSAGE on the painful area.

132

To relieve moderate pain	Try applying a GINGER COMPRESS to the spine for 20 minutes followed by an ALBI PLASTER for up to 4 hours. Repeat both the compress and the plaster as often as needed.
To relieve more severe pain	Apply a GINGER COMPRESS to the painful area for 20 minutes. *then* Use a GINGER SESAME OIL MASSAGE on the area. *then* Apply an ALBI PLASTER for up to 4 hours. Repeat the entire process as needed.

Dietary Recommendations

Following a macrobiotic dietary approach (see page 11) deals with the underlying cause and is the best remedy and preventative.

☐ Avoid especially: all animal protein, fish, shellfish, meat-based soups, dairy foods, eggs, all yin foods, fruit, soy milk, vinegar, peanuts, sweet foods and drinks.

SCOLIOSIS

See SPINAL CURVATURE.

SCROTUM SWELLING

In the male reproductive system, the scrotum is an organ that contains the testes and their accessory organs. Symptoms of scrotum swelling include reddening, swelling, pain, and fever in the scrotal area. There are chronic and acute types. According to Western medicine, the main cause of scrotum swelling is a gonorrhea infection or physical injury.

According to our macrobiotic understanding, swelling of the scrotum is caused by eating and drinking too much yin food such as simple carbohydrates (including sweeteners) and fruit, eggplant, tomatoes, potatoes, and coffee. These foods may themselves lead to a greater susceptibility to infections. In addition, they may lead to an excess of water in the body both because they contain a lot of water to begin with and because more water is produced in the oxidation process. Thus, this kind of diet, especially over a period of time, can weaken the kidneys, which may in turn lead to more infections. Also, a low-salt or no-salt diet can weaken kidneys so that they cannot produce enough diuretic hormone, leading to scrotum swelling.

Helpful Suggestions

OBJECTIVE	REMEDY
To relieve swelling and pain	Use a GINGER COMPRESS on the scrotum (see Figure 3.8 on page 176) for 20 minutes followed by an ALBI PLASTER for up to 4 hours. Repeat both the compress and the plaster as often as needed.

Dietary Recommendations

A change in dietary habits will produce the most long-lasting results. Use the following dietary suggestions until the swelling decreases or for one month. Then, widen your food choices following a macrobiotic dietary approach (see page 11).

☐ Main foods: Brown Rice served with Gomashio, Azuki Rice, Brown Rice Mochi served with Grated Daikon.
☐ Side dishes (one-third of main foods): Tekka Miso, Oily Miso, Hijiki Nitsuke, Takuan Pickles, Miso Pickles.
☐ Miso soup ingredients: wakame, tororo kombu, onions, scallions, Homemade Agé, Brown Rice Mochi.
☐ Beverages: Brown Rice Tea, Bancha Tea, Sho-Ban Tea.
☐ Avoid especially: all animal foods including fish, shellfish, eggs, all dairy foods, meat-based soups; all sweet foods and drinks; all fruit; eggplant; potatoes; tomatoes; mushrooms; vinegar; soy milk; alcohol; melons; coffee; cocoa; and all overly yin foods.

SEPTICEMIA

See BLOOD POISONING.

SHOULDER ACHE

A shoulder ache refers to mild pain that is continuous or fixed. This usually implies that a chronic inflammation is the specific initiator of pain, and it may signal the presence of bursitis or other nonserious problems. More serious conditions may be indicated if other symptoms such as swelling or fever are present, or if the pain comes on suddenly. According to our macrobiotic understanding, there are two kinds of shoulder aches, yin and yang. Usually an ache that is more apparent on the right side is caused by eating too much animal protein, which is yang. Pain on the left side is caused by eating too much sugar and fruit, which are yin. Pain in the joints of the shoulder is often caused by cold foods, especially iced drinks and ice cream. See also Arthritis for additional information on pain in the joints.

Helpful Suggestions:

OBJECTIVE	REMEDY
To relieve pain	The best remedy for pain in this case is a GINGER COMPRESS for 20 minutes on the affected shoulder area.

Dietary Recommendations:

Follow a macrobiotic dietary approach (see page 11) being careful to avoid those foods such as animal protein, sugar, fruits, and cold foods that are the specific cause of the pain in your case.

SINUS INFECTION

The sinuses are openings of ducts that pass secretions into the nasal cavity. They can become infected, resulting in inflammation (sinusitis). An infection of the sinuses may lead to inadequate drainage, resulting in congestion of the sinuses and finally polyps, a deviated septum, allergies, chronic rhinitis, or dental disorders.

Symptoms of sinus infections include nasal congestion with a greenish-yellow discharge, sometimes containing a small amount of blood; headache that is worse in the morning after lying down during the night; a feeling of increasing pressure inside the head; loss of the sense of smell; and pain around the eyes or cheeks. A complete blockage of the sinus openings results in ever-increasing pressure and pain. Sometimes there is fever, difficulty sleeping, a non-productive cough, and a swollen face. The discharge from the nose is thick and under a microscope is seen to contain many pus cells and bacteria. Sometimes when people have this condition, they swallow the pus and mucus, and this may weaken the intestines and the stomach.

The cause of sinus inflammation is considered to be an infection, usually started by a cold or other upper-respiratory disorder. Any illness that has lowered your resistance increases your risk of infections. Any irritation of the nasal passages such as allergies, smoking, or swimming may cause sinusitis as well. Nasal sprays, nose drops, and decongestants are available along with antibiotics if needed. However, these do nothing for the underlying causes of sinusitis and recurrence is common.

CORNELLIA'S NATURAL HEALING AT WORK

My father had a sinus operation but the congestion came back again. An operation doesn't work permanently if the diet is not changed. My mother's relative was a sinus doctor and he recommended that my father clean his nose with salt water (see the explanation for Salt Bancha Nasal Bath in the Remedies Section, page 174). I remember my father did this and it helped him.

In another case, I remember a country girl who came to stay at my house when I was young. She was awaiting a sinus operation. My parents advised her to use a salt water nasal wash. She tried this and lots of green pus came into the wash basin. She was surprised. After using this remedy, she did not need an operation. George Ohsawa recommended using a salt bancha nasal wash, but if you have no bancha tea, then plain salt water may be used. ■

SINUS INFECTION

According to our macrobiotic understanding, there are two underlying causes of sinus infections. One is the overconsumption of fatty foods such as milk and butter, which results in mucous congestion in the nasal cavity. The other underlying cause is an infection in the nasal cavity. This is caused by eating too many simple carbohydrates such as sugary foods, candy, snacks, sweet drinks, fruits, and alcoholic drinks and too many yin protein foods such as milk and beans. Too much yang protein food such as meat, chicken, fish, or eggs does not usually result in sinusitis directly because the nasal area is in the yin upper part of the body. However, these overly yang foods along with the yin foods mentioned above contribute to weakened kidneys; weak kidneys and/or a low- or no-salt diet contribute to a greater susceptibility to infections in general and sinus infections in particular.

Helpful Suggestions

OBJECTIVE	REMEDY
To remove congestion	Try using a SALT BANCHA NASAL BATH 3 to 4 times per day. and Use a LOTUS ROOT JUICE APPLICATION in each nostril every night. Put the soaked cotton ball in loosely and leave it in overnight. and Apply an ALBI PLASTER across the face under the eyes and covering the nose. Apply a second Albi Plaster on the forehead above the eyes. Neither plaster should cover the eyes. Leave both plasters on overnight. The Albi Plaster will help alleviate the sinus congestion more quickly than will other remedies.

Dietary Recommendations

A change in dietary habits is most helpful. Use the following dietary suggestions during periods of active flare-up or for about one month. Then, widen your food choices using a macrobiotic dietary approach (see page 11).

☐ Main foods: Brown Rice, Brown Rice Mochi, Gomashio as a condiment.

☐ Side dishes (one-fourth of main foods): Tekka Miso, Shio Kombu, Hijiki Burdock Nitsuke, Hijiki Lotus Root Nitsuke, Burdock Carrot Nitsuke, Deep-Fried Kombu, Nori Roasted with Oil, Miso Pickles, Carp Soup.

☐ Miso soup ingredients: wakame, tororo kombu, burdock, scallions, onions, Homemade Agé, Brown Rice Mochi.

☐ Beverages: Brown Rice Tea, Sho-Ban Tea, Bancha Tea, Grain Milk, Kombu Tea. Less drinking is better, a total of about 1 cup per day. Drinking more is usually recommended to help thin secretions. However, drinking more may further adversely affect the kidneys; thus according to our macrobiotic understanding, it is best is to drink less. Note that drinking less is possible with a grain-and-vegetable diet, but should not be tried with a meat-and-sugar approach.

☐ Avoid especially: overly yin or yang foods, all fatty foods, overeating.

SKIN, ITCHY

Itching may result from any number of disorders, especially when there are other symptoms and/or a general ill feeling. It may also happen because of allergic or chemical reactions. According to our macrobiotic understanding, itching skin is primarily caused by eating too much animal food, including fish. Overeating these foods produces excess acids and/or weakens kidneys so that acid normally eliminated by urination is instead expelled through the skin.

Helpful Suggestions

OBJECTIVE	REMEDY
To relieve itchiness	Try drinking 1 cup of DAIKON GINGER TEA 3 times per day, or taking a GINGER, DAIKON, or RICE BRAN BATH for 20 minutes once a day. *or* A DAIKON GINGER COMPRESS or RICE BRAN COMPRESS may be applied to the itchy area for 20 minutes once a day. *then*

	Lightly rub the area with good-quality sesame oil or use a GINGER SESAME OIL MASSAGE after the compress. *and* Before going to bed try a WOOD ASH WATER TREATMENT to help relieve itching that is hindering your sleep.
To control itchiness	Try not to scratch; instead, rub the area with a slice of daikon. *and* You can place a thin straw mat on top of your sheet at night; this should help keep you cooler and less itchy. Using linen pajamas is helpful. Avoid the use of soap; wash with a Rice Bran Bag (see page 173) instead.

Dietary Recommendations

Use the following special dietary suggestions until your condition improves or for one month. Then select foods from a variety of choices using a macrobiotic dietary approach (see page 11).

☐ Main foods: Brown Rice with Soybeans. Chew each mouthful 100 times.

☐ Side dishes (one-fourth to one-third of main foods): Burdock Nitsuke, Boiled Daikon, Shiitake Tea, Wakame Nitsuke, Arame Nitsuke, Eggplant Nishime, Cucumber with Kuzu Sauce, Baked Yams or Sweet Potatoes, Grated Daikon. Eat fresh fruit once a day.

☐ Miso soup ingredients: daikon, Chinese cabbage, tofu, scallions, wakame.

☐ Beverages: Brown Rice Tea, Brown Rice Bancha Tea, Bancha Tea, Grain Coffee.

☐ Avoid especially: all animal foods.

SKIN, MOISTURE PROBLEMS

According to our macrobiotic understanding, all skin problems are seen as a result of weak kidneys. Basically, the underlying causes of weak kidneys are a diet too high in fatty (oily) foods and drinks; drinking too much water, coffee, juice, or other liquids; and ingesting too many chemicals from medicines, chemicalized foods, or other sources. Too little or too much salt may also result in weakened kidneys. The proper amount and use of salt is one of the most important aspects of one's dietary approach.

Dry skin is the result of a hormonal imbalance due to the effects of an overly yang diet. It can also be due to malfunctioning of the intestines and stomach. Contact with cold water or cleaning products, or ovary or testicle diseases can lead to chapped skin. In cases of ovary or testicle disorders, the underlying cause is eating too much animal food and a lack of good-quality vegetable oil in the diet. You must remedy the ovary or testicle disorders first. See the appropriate sections.

George Ohsawa has said not to use commercial external medications because the poison of the medications goes into the body and affects the internal organs. This can be the cause of disease, especially kidney diseases. For all skin problems avoid the use of soap; wash with a Rice Bran Bag (see Baths, page 173) instead. See the secton on Kidney Failure for ideas to improve the overall condition of the kidneys.

Helpful Suggestions

OBJECTIVE	REMEDY
To deal with dryness such as dry eczema	MASSAGE the dry-skin area with CHLOROPHYLL JUICE for 20 minutes once a day.
	and
	If the hands or feet are affected, try using a GINGER BATH, soaking the hands or feet directly in the water for 10 minutes once a day. Hands and feet will become red, which shows that blood is circulating and is a good sign.
	then
	MASSAGE the dry-skin area with GINGER SESAME OIL.
To relieve chapped skin	Finely grate several young green turnips and squeeze out the juice. Mix the turnip juice with 1/3 the equivalent of lemon juice and heat slightly. Lightly rubbing this liquid on the chapped places may be helpful.
To aid rough skin	Try gently rubbing the rough skin with the most natural sesame oil.

Dietary Recommendations

In all cases of skin problems, the best approach is a change in dietary habits. Select foods from a variety of choices using a macrobiotic dietary approach (see page 11).

☐ Avoid especially: all animal food, particularly red meat, tuna, bonita, salmon, sardines, mackerel, shrimp, crab, shellfish, abalone; buckwheat groats; eggs; alcohol; ice cream; cocoa; coffee; black tea; all fruit; sweet foods; hot spices; vinegar dishes; eggplant; tomatoes; potatoes.

See also ACNE.

SKIN ABSCESSES

When pus collects in a small, localized cavity formed by the disintegration of tissues, an abscess results. Abscesses on the skin may occur in one area or all over the body. According to our macrobiotic understanding, all surface conditions indicate an underlying susceptibility to greater disorders. This is because all skin problems are seen as a result of weak kidneys. Basically, the underlying causes of weak kidneys are a diet too high in fatty (oily) foods and drinks; drinking too much water, coffee, juice, or other liquids; and ingesting too many chemicals from medicines, chemicalized foods, or other sources. Too little or too much salt may also result in weakened kidneys. The proper amount and use of salt is one of the most important aspects of one's dietary approach. The specific cause of skin abscesses is overeating animal foods that are also high in fat. Too much yang food results in pus and pain, while too much yin food is indicated by skin eruptions or pimples all over the body.

Helpful Suggestions

George Ohsawa has said not to use commercial external medications because the poison of the medications goes into the body and affects the internal organs. This can be the cause of disease, especially kidney diseases. (See the secton on Kidney Failure for ideas to improve the overall condition of the kidneys.) For all skin problems avoid the use of soap; wash with a Rice Bran Bag (see Baths, page 173) instead.

OBJECTIVE	REMEDY
To control skin abscesses	Try taking a DAIKON BATH WITH GRATED GINGER.
	or
	Apply a DAIKON GINGER COMPRESS over the affected area for 20 minutes followed by an ALBI PLASTER for up to 4 hours. Work on the most troublesome areas first if large areas or the whole body is affected. Repeat as necessary.
	and/or
	The best remedy is to change your diet, to FAST, or to eat less.
To control a child's spreading abscesses	Finely grate potatoes and apply directly on the rash. Secure with bandages.
	and/or
	You can use a TOFU APPLICATION; change it every 1 or 2 hours.
	or
	Lightly rub UME EXTRACT directly on the abscess for 5 to 10 minutes.

136

Dietary Recommendations

In all cases of skin problems, the best approach is a change in dietary habits. Select a variety of foods using a macrobiotic dietary approach (see page 11).

☐ Avoid especially: all animal food, particularly red meat, tuna, bonita, salmon, sardines, mackerel, shrimp, crab, shellfish, abalone; buckwheat groats; eggs; alcohol; ice cream; cocoa; coffee; black tea; all fruit; sweet foods; hot spices; vinegar dishes; eggplant; tomatoes; potatoes.

SKIN CANCER

There are several forms of skin cancer depending on the layer of skin affected. A malignant growth of the external surface of the skin is characterized by a small, scaling bump that doesn't hurt or itch and is called squamous-cell skin cancer. A small cut in the skin that doesn't heal in three weeks is indicative of cancer affecting the inner, basal layer (the fifth layer) and is called basal-cell skin cancer. The cut slowly grows larger but doesn't hurt or itch. Malignant melanoma is the name of a skin cancer that spreads to other areas of the body. A melanoma of this type usually begins with a mole or with some other pre-existing skin lesion and is characterized by a flat or slightly raised skin lesion with irregular borders that may bleed. These melanomas develop in a variety of colors.

Excessive exposure to sunlight is thought to be responsible for most skin cancers. In the case of cancer affecting the skin's basal layer, the skin damage from the sun occurs many years before the cancer appears. Also, overexposure to x-rays may cause skin cancer on the external surface of the skin. Skin cancer mostly affects adults over forty. A dark lump, a new mole, or a change in a mole that a person over twelve has had since childhood may signal a malignant melanoma. In my opinion, overexposure to ultraviolet rays along with a diet high in animal protein is the cause. Animal protein contains elements such as sulfur that produce strong acid when exposed to ultraviolet rays. These elements and acids have a tendency to damage the genetic material (DNA) in the skin cells, resulting in skin cancer.

Helpful Suggestions

Skin cancer responds well to surgical treatment. However, the macrobiotic approach is to try natural remedies first.

OBJECTIVE	REMEDY
To prevent skin cancer	Limiting your exposure to the sun is a good idea.
To relieve irritated skin	Try taking a 1 percent SALT BATH every other day for 30 minutes to 1 hour.
To remove toxins	Apply an ALBI PLASTER over the cancerous area, changing it every 4 hours, to help remove toxins from the cancer site.
To strengthen system	Apply a GINGER COMPRESS over the kidneys (see Figure 3.8 on page 176) for 20 minutes several times a week.

Dietary Recommendations

Use the following dietary suggestions for about one month. Then, widen your food choices using a macrobiotic dietary approach (see page 11).

☐ Main foods: Brown Rice Balls, Azuki Rice Balls. Chew each mouthful 200 times. Use a little Gomashio as a condiment.
☐ Side dishes (one-third of main foods): Tekka Miso, Grated Daikon, Burdock Carrot Nitsuke, burdock dishes, Eggplant Nitsuke with Miso, Soybeans with Kombu, Rice Bran Pickles, Pressed Salad, Sour Cabbage, Umeboshi.
☐ Miso soup ingredients: daikon, albi, green leafy vegetables, eggplant, spinach, tofu.
☐ Beverages: Brown Rice Tea, Brown Rice Bancha Tea, Bancha Tea, Vegetable Broth, Grain Coffee. Drink a maximum of 2½ cups of beverages per day.
☐ Avoid especially: all animal foods including eggs and meat-based soups.

SKIN INFECTION

Some examples of skin infections are boils, carbuncles, impetigo, and tinea versicolor (a kind of ringworm). Skin infections that affect the face result in skin that is painful and warm. A rash usually appears and may be accompanied by chills, fever, and headache. Also, the face and lymph nodes may become swollen.

A boil is actually a painful bacterial infection of a hair follicle. Symptoms include domed nodules that are very painful and red with pus on the surface, fever, and swelling of the nearest lymph glands. A carbuncle is an infection of the skin causing the death of tissues and composed of a cluster of boils. Impetigo refers to a bacterial skin infection of the upper (superficial) layers of the skin. Symptoms include a red rash with many blisters—some of which contain pus, rupture, and form yellow crusts. Sometimes, there is a slight fever. The blisters may itch but are not painful. Tinea versicolor is a yeast infection of the skin resulting in lesions that are white on exposed skin or brownish on covered areas. These lesions are flat and small although they may join together to form large patches.

The agent most commonly involved in bacterial skin infection is staphylococci bacteria, although in impetigo, streptococci bacteria may also be involved. A developing stage of the yeast, pityrosborum orbiculare, is the known cause of tinea versicolor. Like other bacterial infections, skin infections are more likely with poor nutrition, any illness that lowers your resistance, or the use of certain drugs. Sensitive skin, poor hygiene, and warm, moist weather increase your risk of surface skin infections, too. Exposure to heat and humidity also helps yeast infections develop.

According to our macrobiotic understanding, the underlying cause of all skin infections is the long-term overeating of animal foods such as red meat, chicken, fish, and eggs that contain high percentages of protein and fat. This kind of diet helps promote bacterial growth. Boils and carbuncles may also come from liver trouble, and it is wise to avoid all foods that cause liver trouble such as animal foods and overly yin foods, including sugary foods and alcohol.

Helpful Suggestions

OBJECTIVE	REMEDY
To reduce high fever	Try drinking 1 cup of DAIKON GINGER TEA or BROWN RICE TEA WITH SHIITAKE MUSHROOMS 3 times per day at a hot-to-warm temperature. Stop drinking these teas when your temperature returns to normal. and Use a GINGER COMPRESS on the affected area for 20 minutes.

FOR FACIAL INFECTIONS

To relieve pain	Apply a TOFU PLASTER to the forehead and another to the heart area at the same time to help protect the heart. Change the plasters every 1 or 2 hours. and A GREEN LEAFY VEGETABLES APPLICATION for 1 hour as often as needed and/or a WOOD ASH FACIAL TREATMENT once a day are very effective.

FOR SKIN INFECTIONS ON OTHER PARTS OF THE BODY

To relieve pain	Use a GINGER COMPRESS on the affected area for 20 minutes followed by either an ALBI PLASTER for up to 4 hours, or a GREEN PLASTER

	for up to 2 hours. Repeat both the compress and either plaster as needed.
To control boils	It is generally not wise to squeeze a boil or a carbuncle since the infection usually affects many layers of skin, and opening the surface layers may result in bacteria penetrating into the deeper layers. and If you can find burdock seeds, drinking 1 to 1½ cups of BURDOCK SEED TEA or using a BURDOCK SEEDS APPLICATION may be effective.

Dietary Recommendations

Use the following special dietary suggestions until your condition improves or for about one month. Then, widen your food choices using a macrobiotic dietary approach (see page 11).

FOR FACIAL SKIN INFECTIONS

Don't eat cold food or iced drinks or use cold treatments on the face. Even after the infection is gone, cut down on meat and eggs or a relapse may occur.

☐ Main foods: Brown Rice with Barley, Brown Rice, Azuki Rice.

☐ Side dishes (one-fourth of main foods cooked with less salt): Ginger Miso, Soybean Soup, Okara Nitsuke, Natto with Soy Sauce and Scallions served with Grated Daikon, Eggplant Pressed Salad, Shiitake Nitsuke, Hijiki Nitsuke.

☐ Miso soup ingredients: potatoes, eggplant, sweet potatoes, spinach, tofu, burdock, daikon.

☐ Beverages: Brown Rice Tea, Brown Rice Bancha Tea, Bancha Tea, Vegetable Broth, Grain Milk.

☐ Avoid especially: all animal foods including meat-based soups, eggs, dairy; and sweet foods.

FOR SKIN INFECTIONS ON THE BODY

This is a very yang disease, so after your condition improves, avoid animal proteins and buckwheat for several years as these foods can cause a relapse.

☐ Main foods: Brown Rice, Brown Rice with Barley, Udon Noodles, whole-wheat spaghetti.

☐ Side dishes (one-third to one-half of main foods): The vegetables recommended for a macrobiotic dietary approach are fine for this conditon. Sea vegetables and Carp Soup are very good for eliminating toxins.

☐ Miso soup ingredients: daikon, Chinese cabbage, tofu, potatoes, eggplant, scallions.

☐ Beverages: Bancha Tea, Brown Rice Bancha Tea, Vegetable Broth, Grain Coffee.

☐ Avoid especially: all animal protein including fish (except carp), shellfish, eggs.

SMALL INTESTINE CANCER

Small intestine tumors are abnormal new cell growths in the small intestines. They are cancerous in only 10 percent of cases. Sometimes there are no symptoms. However, tiredness, pale color, anemic condition, unexplained blood loss, and blood in stools or black-colored stools may indicate small-intestine cancer.

The cause of the tumors, whether cancerous or not, is considered to be unknown although inflammatory disorders of the small intestine such as Crohn's disease are known to increase your risk of developing tumors. The major complication is the possibility of intestinal obstruction and, for this reason, most tumors are removed surgically. However, the macrobiotic approach is to try dietary changes first.

According to our macrobiotic understanding, there are yin and yang types of small intestine tumors or cancer. The underlying cause of tumors is a diet high in fatty, animal foods. These foods are also high in protein, contributing to the tumor's growth. All tumors (excess growths) are a yin condition but may have a yin or a yang cause resulting in a yin or a yang type of cancer. The overconsumption of yang animal foods such as red meat, cheese, chicken, and eggs results in a yang type of tumor. The overconsumption of yin animal (fatty) foods such as cow's milk, other dairy foods, and beans results in a yin type.

Furthermore, yang small-intestine cancer is caused by eating too much meat, pork, chicken, eggs, and fish. These foods all produce an overly acidic condition of bodily fluids. Yin small-intestine cancer is caused by overeating yin foods such as fruit and sugary cakes and by drinking too many sugary drinks and alcoholic beverages once either type of tumor is present. Yin small-intestine cancer grows more slowly than yang small intestine cancer.

Helpful Suggestions

OBJECTIVE	REMEDY
To relieve pain	Try applying a GINGER COMPRESS over the intestines (see Figure 3.8 on page 176) for 20 minutes followed by an ALBI PLASTER for up to 4 hours to help remove excess toxins. Repeat both the compress and the plaster as often as needed.

Dietary Recommendations

The best remedy and preventative is a change in dietary habits. Use the following dietary suggestions for about one month. Then, widen your food choices using a macrobiotic dietary approach (see page 11).

FOR THE YANG TYPE

☐ Main foods: Brown Rice or Azuki Rice with a little Gomashio. Chew each mouthful 200 times.

☐ Side dishes (less than one-third of main foods cooked to a less salty taste than usual): a little Tekka Miso, Ginger Miso, Grated Daikon (about 2 tablespoons) with Soy Sauce, Burdock Carrot Nitsuke, Carp Soup, Rice Bran Pickles, Umeboshi.

☐ Miso soup ingredients: daikon, albi, Green Leafy Vegetables, Chinese cabbage, spinach, tofu, eggplant.

☐ Beverages: Brown Rice Tea, Brown Rice Bancha Tea, Bancha Tea, Grain Coffee, Vegetable Broth. Drink a maximum of 2½ cups of beverages per day.

☐ Avoid especially: all animal foods including fish (except carp), shellfish, eggs, meat-based soups; all alcohol; all sweet foods and drinks; fruit; and ice cream.

FOR THE YIN TYPE

☐ Main foods: Brown Rice Balls and Brown Rice Mochi. Use a little Gomashio at each meal. Chew each mouthful 200 times.

☐ Side dishes (one-third to one-half of main foods cooked to a salty taste): Tekka Miso, Hijiki Nitsuke, Burdock Carrot Nitsuke, Shio Kombu, Carp Soup, Natural Caviar, Takuan Pickles, Miso Pickles.

☐ Miso soup ingredients: wakame, tororo kombu, onions, scallions, Homemade Agé, Brown Rice Mochi.

☐ Beverages: Sho-Ban Tea, Brown Rice Tea, Brown Rice Bancha Tea, Bancha Tea, Mu tea. Drink a maximum of 2 cups of beverages per day.

☐ Avoid especially: all animal foods (except carp), dairy foods (including ice cream), soy milk, eggs, all alcohol, fruit, sweet foods, vinegar, hot spices, tomatoes, mushrooms, melons, peanuts, rice bran pickles (except Takuan Pickles), rice gruel.

SORE THROAT

A sore throat is not a disease but rather a symptom of many disorders from the common cold, influenza, and hay fever to tonsilitis, strep throat, and diphtheria. A sore throat that doesn't go away and/or is accompanied by fever, cough, swelling, or other symptoms should be checked in order to determine the underlying cause. See the appropriate section for additional suggestions.

According to our macrobiotic understanding, sore throat problems are almost always due to eating and drinking too much yin food, especially sugary foods, fruit, and sweet drinks.

Helpful Suggestions

These suggestions may be used for a sore throat with no other symptoms or as additional remedies in cases of underlying disorders.

OBJECTIVE	REMEDY
To relieve a sore throat	A SALT PLASTER used all night is very effective. The plaster can be used for children as well as adults who are suffering from a sore throat or sore tonsils. *and* GARGLE with ½ to 1 cup of HOT BANCHA TEA WITH SALT 3 times per day. *also* Drinking ½ to 1 cup of *SHIITAKE DAIKON LOTUS ROOT TEA* 3 times per day is very effective.
To eliminate excess phlegm in the throat	Sip 1 to 2 tablespoons of BURDOCK JUICE 2 times per day and the mucus should dissolve or be expelled.
To prevent sore throat	Keeping the throat warm by wearing a turtleneck or scarf is helpful.

Dietary Recommendations

Following a macrobiotic dietary approach (see page 11), reducing all yin foods, is the most effective step.

SPINAL CORD INFLAMMATION

Inflammation of the spinal cord, called myelitis, has symptoms that vary with the location of the inflammation. In general, myelitis involves pain in the back, a girdling sensation, increased sensitivity of the reflexes to stimuli, the sensation of ants crawling on the body, paralysis of the sphincter muscles, and spasmodic contractions of the paralyzed limbs. According to modern pathology, any physical inflammation is caused by bacterial or viral infection, heat or cold, mechanical crushing or cutting, acid or alkaline damage, or irradiation. The specific cause of myelitis is thought to be hereditary or the result of syphilis. This is half true according to our macrobiotic thinking. In any event, leakage of plasma protein and/or glucose (blood sugar) into the tissues causes inflammation because protein and/or glucose holds water.

According to our macrobiotic understanding, the underlying cause of spinal cord infection is eating too much yin food such as sugar, candy, sugary drinks, ice cream, and fruit. Also, a low- or no-salt diet and weak kidneys (which cannot maintain the proper amount of sodium in the intercellular fluid) can result in an infection of the spinal cord.

Helpful Suggestions

OBJECTIVE	REMEDY
To relieve pain	Apply a GINGER COMPRESS to the painful area for 20 minutes followed by an ALBI PLASTER for up to 4 hours. Repeat both the compress and the plasters as often as necessary.
To relieve numb legs	Try applying a GINGER COMPRESS on the legs for 20 minutes followed by a GINGER SESAME OIL MASSAGE of the area. *or* Use a DAIKON or ARAME HIP BATH WITH GRATED GINGER for 20 minutes followed by a GINGER SESAME OIL MASSAGE.
To save energy	Men in particular should refrain from sex until the condition improves because ejaculations involve the loss of protein and energy.

Dietary Recommendations

Use the following special dietary suggestions until your condition improves or for about one month. Then, widen your food choices using a macrobiotic dietary approach (see page 11).

☐ Main foods: Brown Rice served with Gomashio, Azuki Rice, Millet Rice, Brown Rice Cream, Brown Rice Gruel, Mochi Soup, Baked Mochi with Soy Sauce.

☐ Side dishes (one-third of main foods maximum): Tekka Miso, Oily Miso, Shio Kombu, Hijiki Nitsuke, Vegetable Stew, Vegetable Stew with Fish, Carp Soup (very beneficial for this condition), Kombu Rolls with Chuba Iriko, Deep-Fried Kombu, Vegetable Tempura, Takuan Pickles, Miso Pickles.

☐ Miso soup ingredients: wakame, tororo kombu, scallions, onions, Homemade Agé, Brown Rice Mochi. Every morning, eat miso soup with mochi for energy and always eat sea vegetables at every meal to help cleanse the blood.

☐ Beverages: Brown Rice Tea, Brown Rice Bancha Tea, Bancha Tea, Kombu Tea, Grain Milk.

☐ Avoid especially: all meats, fish (except carp), shellfish, all dairy foods (including ice cream), all eggs, sweet foods and drinks, alcohol, fruit, potatoes, tomatoes, vinegar, cider, pressed salads.

CORNELLIA'S NATURAL HEALING AT WORK

A young boy had a very bad spine. He went to a chiropractor to correct his spine, but in vain. Then the boy's mother was taught to massage his spine with ginger sesame oil before bed every night. After one year of this massage, the child's bad spine was completely straight. In this case, an important curing factor was the love of the mother. So, love may be the greatest remedy. But right action such as good diet or massage may accelerate the healing process. Macrobiotic thinking says that the most important way to cure disease is with love and devotion; secondly, good diet; then, natural external remedies; and lastly, medical treatment and medications. ■

SPINAL CURVATURE

SPINAL CURVATURE

Spinal curvature, known as scoliosis, is a progressive bending and twisting of the spinal column. It is usually painless with no obvious symptoms or signs in the early stages. Eventually, the spine becomes S-shaped and the chest and back may be distorted. The condition is most common among boys and girls between the ages of twelve and fifteen. The cause is generally unknown although diseases of the central nervous system or congenital defects of the spine may result in scoliosis. It is best to correct the curvature since it may lead to breathing difficulties, lung infections, or congestive heart failure.

According to our macrobiotic understanding, animals walking on four legs have no spinal curvature problems. It is because humans walk upright that they have such trouble. Bad posture may contribute to spinal curvature but is more likely to be the result and not the cause. Spinal curvature is probably caused by a poor diet that leads to an overly acidic condition. Then, calcium, an alkaline element used to balance excess acidity, is lost from the bones and the bones become weak. In order to support the head, which is heavy, the spine begins to curve and can become progressively more curved unless corrective measures such as a change in diet are taken.

Helpful Suggestions

Usually, the spine is corrected naturally as one is sleeping, but if the spine is curved too much, sleeping is not enough to correct it naturally.

OBJECTIVE	REMEDY
To correct spine naturally	Use a GINGER SESAME OIL SPINAL MASSAGE every night before going to bed for as long as needed; months or years are often required. It is also important not to sleep on too soft a mattress. (We use a cotton futon on a 1/2-inch-thick piece of hardwood.)
To correct difficult cases	More severe cases or those that don't respond to these suggestions may require the temporary, daily use of a back brace and restricted sports activities.

Dietary Recommendations

A balanced diet such as a macrobiotic dietary approach (see page 11) is helpful.

SPRAINS

A sprain is a stretched and torn ligament with accompanying pain and tenderness, bruising, swelling, and loss of normal mobility in the injured joint, although the joint can still function with pain. A ligament that is only stretched results in a strain. Sprains result from overuse or an abnormal stress on a ligament around a joint. Any joint can be sprained, but sprains occur most often in ankles, knees, and fingers.

According to our macrobiotic understanding, a diet high in acid-forming foods such as meat and other animal products and refined sugar is a major contributor to sprains. When the blood is acidic from eating too much acid-forming food, then calcium in the blood and connective tissues is lost, weakening the joints and making them more vulnerable to sprains.

Helpful Suggestions

Ice is usually recommended for the first twenty-four hours followed by heat. However, in the macrobiotic approach, cooling plasters are used first to help prevent swelling, and heat is used if swelling has already begun.

CORNELLIA'S NATURAL HEALING AT WORK

Once while traveling on a summer lecture tour around Michigan, I twisted my ankle. I couldn't stand. I applied a green plaster only one time and the pain was gone. This is a very helpful plaster that Mr. Muramoto, author of *Healing Ourselves*, taught me to use in emergency cases. ■

SPRAINS

OBJECTIVE	REMEDY
To minimize swelling	Try applying a cooling plaster such as an ALBI PLASTER for up to 4 hours, a TOFU PLASTER for up to 1 or 2 hours, or a GREEN PLASTER for up to 2 hours. Repeat until swelling begins.
To reduce swelling	Apply a BUCKWHEAT PLASTER for 1 to 4 hours, a GINGER COMPRESS for 20 minutes followed by an ALBI PLASTER for up to 4 hours, or a GREEN PLASTER for up to 2 hours. Repeat as often as needed and as time allows.
	and
	Elevating the joint whenever possible is beneficial to help reduce swelling.
	and
	Until the swelling subsides, avoid soaking a sprain in warm or hot water.
To relieve pain	An UMEBOSHI PLASTER can be applied directly to the sprain for 1 to 2 hours with good results.
	and
	Rest the joint for 1 to 2 days and then begin to exercise it gently without putting weight on it.
To relieve pain accompanying a twisted ankle	A RICE PLASTER is the traditional Japanese folk remedy. Change the plaster every 4 hours.

Dietary Recommendations

Following a macrobiotic dietary approach (see page 11) is recommended to help reduce your vulnerability to sprains.

STOMACH, DOWNWARD DISPLACEMENT OF

Downward displacement of the stomach is a condition in which the stomach, which normally expands and contracts, loses its power of contraction, remains expanded, and hangs down. Symptoms include pain, nausea, abnormal appetite—either loss of appetite or ravenous hunger—and diarrhea. According to our macrobiotic understanding, the stomach muscles are weakened by always eating yin potassium-rich foods, especially when accompanied by a lack of salt (sodium). The human body is regenerated daily, but without enough sodium and too much potassium, the body loses its contracting power and stays expanded.

Helpful Suggestions

OBJECTIVE	REMEDY
To relieve pain	Try applying a GINGER COMPRESS on the stomach for 20 minutes.
To relieve nausea	Drink 1 cup of UMESHO BANCHA TEA or SHO-BAN TEA up to 3 times per day.
To stimulate appetite	Eating up to 1 cup of thick BROWN RICE CREAM (SPECIAL) cooked with a pinch of salt 3 times per day is helpful.
To control diarrhea	Try keeping the stomach warm with a GINGER COMPRESS or ROASTED SALT PACK for 20 minutes and drink 1 cup of UMESHO BANCHA TEA 3 to 4 times per day until diarrhea stops.
To curb overeating	Control this mentally and chew each mouthful of food 200 times.
	or
	Eat less, but in several small meals per day.

Dietary Recommendations

Dietary changes are most beneficial for stomach disorders. Use the following special dietary suggestions for about one month. Then, widen your food choices using a macrobiotic dietary approach (see page 11). If you have been on a salt-free diet, slowly add more salt to your cooking, cook foods longer, and eat a little more yang food. Note that salt is added in cooking, not at the table. Also, eat and drink less. It is better to slowly change one's condition to more yang because if you change quickly, you may be attracted to too much yin food and you may end up yin instead of yang.

☐ Main foods: Brown Rice Balls with Gomashio at each meal, Brown Rice Mochi.

☐ Side dishes (one-third of main foods): Tekka Miso, Oily Miso, Shio Kombu, Burdock Carrot Nitsuke, Vegetable Tempura, Kombu Rolls with Chuba Iriko, Miso Pickles, Takuan Pickles.

☐ Miso soup ingredients: wakame, tororo kombu, onions, scallions, winter squash, string beans.

☐ Beverages: Sho-Ban Tea, Bancha Tea, Brown Rice Bancha Tea. Drink less.

☐ Avoid especially: all animal food (except small dried fish), red-meat fish, shellfish, all fruit, sweet foods, potatoes, eggplant, tomatoes, melons, all dairy foods (including ice cream), sweet drinks, all alcohol, vinegar, rice gruel.

STOMACH CANCER

Stomach cancer is uncontrolled (malignant) cell growth in the stomach, characterized in the later stages by upper abdominal pain, frequent fatigue and weight loss, vomiting of blood, black stools, anemia, loss of appetite, and the inability to eat much. In the early stages, there are vague symptoms of indigestion that may include burping, nausea, poor appetite, or a feeling of fullness. If these symptoms last more than a few days and don't respond to remedies, do not ignore these warning signals.

Although the incidence of stomach cancer remains high in some countries such as Japan and Austria, it has decreased significantly in the United States. The cause of stomach cancer is considered to be unknown, yet many factors such as having type-A blood, pernicious anemia, the absence of normal stomach acid for whatever reason, a diet high in smoked or salted meats, and excess alcohol consumption along with a family history of this disorder or being over sixty-five all increase your risk of getting stomach cancer. It is currently considered incurable even with surgery or radiation treatments.

According to our macrobiotic understanding, there are yin and yang types of stomach cancer. Yang stomach cancer is caused by eating too much yang food such as pork, chicken, eggs, and fish. Yin stomach cancer is caused by overeating yin foods such as fruit and sugary cakes and by the overconsumption of sugary drinks and alcoholic beverages. All these foods, whether yin or yang, help produce an acidic condition of bodily fluids. Thus, both yin and yang stomach cancer are initiated by excess acidity of cell fluid, which damages the DNA of a cell and makes it a malignant cell. The growth of a malignant cell is promoted by the consumption of too much simple carbohydrate (yin) food such as refined sugar along with excess protein. Yin stomach cancer grows more slowly than yang stomach cancer.

Helpful Suggestions

OBJECTIVE	REMEDY
To relieve pain	Use a GINGER COMPRESS for 20 minutes followed by an ALBI PLASTER for up to 4 hours. Repeat both the compress and the plaster as often as necessary and as time allows. *or* Add 1 CHARCOALED UMEBOSHI to the Albi Plaster to help remove toxins more quickly.

Dietary Recommendations

A change in dietary habits is most beneficial. Use the following special dietary suggestions while there is pain or symptoms of stomach cancer or for about one month. Then, widen your food choices using a macrobiotic dietary approach (see page 11).

FOR THE YANG TYPE

☐ Main foods: Brown Rice or Azuki Rice served with a little Gomashio. Chew each mouthful 200 times.

☐ Side dishes (less than one-third of main foods cooked to a less salty taste than usual): a little Tekka Miso, Ginger Miso, Grated Daikon (about 2 tablespoons) with Soy Sauce, Burdock Carrot Nitsuke, Carp Soup, Rice Bran Pickles, Umeboshi.

☐ Miso soup ingredients: daikon, albi, Green Leafy Vegetables, Chinese cabbage, spinach, tofu, eggplant.

☐ Beverages: Brown Rice Tea, Brown Rice Bancha Tea, Bancha Tea, Grain Coffee, Vegetable Broth. Drink a maximum of 2½ cups beverages per day.

☐ Avoid especially: all animal foods including fish (except carp), shellfish, eggs, meat-based soups, all alcohol, all sweet foods and drinks, fruit, and ice cream.

FOR THE YIN TYPE

☐ Main foods: Brown Rice Balls and Brown Rice Mochi. Use a little Gomashio at each meal. Chew each mouthful 200 times.

☐ Side dishes (one-third to one-half of main foods cooked to a salty taste): Tekka Miso, Hijiki Nitsuke, Burdock Carrot Nitsuke, Shio Kombu, Carp Soup, natural caviar, Takuan Pickles, Miso Pickles.

☐ Miso soup ingredients: wakame, tororo kombu, onions, scallions, Homemade Agé, Brown Rice Mochi.

☐ Beverages: Sho-Ban Tea, Brown Rice Tea, Brown

CORNELLIA'S NATURAL HEALING AT WORK

When I was a child in Japan, my dentist was a very strong-willed man, like a samurai. He had stomach cancer, which he cured by eating only buckwheat for three years.

Buckwheat noodles were sold in a noodle shop near his house. These noodles were handmade using only buckwheat flour. He used these noodles to make scrambled buckwheat and buckwheat cream. He was completely cured in three years.

Buckwheat is very yang. Holy men who live in the mountains meditating and chanting every day eat buckwheat flour mixed only with a little cold water. If you are healthy, you can digest it this way, but, of course, sick people should cook it for a long time so it becomes more yangized and digestible. ∎

STOMACH CANCER

Rice Bancha Tea, Bancha Tea, Mu Tea. Drink a maximum of 2 cups of beverages per day.

☐ Avoid especially: all animal foods (except carp), dairy foods (including ice cream), soy milk, eggs, all alcohol, fruit, sweet foods, vinegar, hot spices, tomatoes, mushrooms, melons, peanuts, rice bran pickles (except Takuan Pickles), rice gruel.

STOMACH CRAMPS

According to our macrobiotic understanding, the underlying cause of stomach cramps is the overconsumption of acid-forming foods such as animal foods, cheese, eggs, chicken, fish, sugary foods, alcohol, and sugary drinks. These foods make the blood overly acidic, a condition that draws calcium (an alkaline element) out of stomach-muscle cells, makes the muscles contract, and inhibits relaxation of the stomach muscles.

Helpful Suggestions

OBJECTIVE	REMEDY
To relieve stomach cramps	Lay down and relax. Apply a HOT TOWEL COMPRESS on the stomach (see Figure 3.8 on page 176) for 20 minutes followed by a MUSTARD PLASTER until the skin turns red.
	or
	Apply a GINGER COMPRESS for 20 minutes followed by an ALBI PLASTER with a ROASTED SALT PACK on top of the Albi Plaster to keep the plaster a little warm. Leave the Albi Plaster on for up to 4 hours. Repeat both the compress (either kind) and its corresponding plaster as needed for relief of stomach cramps.
To induce vomiting (if needed)	Try drinking ½ cup of strong SALT WATER DRINK or 1 cup of specially prepared SHO-BAN TEA 1 time only.

Dietary Recommendations

Since this is usually an acute condition, after the remedies and special dietary suggestions are used for a couple of days and you are feeling better, return to a macrobiotic dietary approach (see page 11).

☐ Main foods: after the pain is gone, eat Brown Rice Balls with Gomashio. Chew each mouthful 200 times.
☐ Side dishes (one-third of main foods): Tekka Miso, Takuan Pickles, Umeboshi with Soy Sauce.
☐ Miso soup ingredients: wakame, onions, scallions.
☐ Beverages: Umesho Bancha Tea, Sho-Ban Tea, Bancha Tea.

☐ Avoid especially: all animal food, fish, eggs, shellfish, all sweet foods and drinks, ice cream, all fruit, melons, potatoes, vinegar, hot spices, all alcohol, tomatoes, eggplant, and pressed salads or commercial pickles.

STOMACH ULCER

An ulcer is an open sore or lesion on the surface of an organ or tissue and can occur any place in the body. The three main types of ulcers in the stomach area are esophageal, gastric, and duodenal. The most common symptom is a very strong gnawing pain in the abdomen.* Pain may occur one-half hour to many hours after eating because the pain is caused by the oversecretion of stomach acids and a certain amount of time lapses before the acids reach and affect the site of the ulcer. These acids cause a local erosion of the intestinal or stomach wall,

---

CORNELLIA'S NATURAL HEALING AT WORK

A couple of years ago, a former Vega Study Center student came back because she had a stomach ulcer. She said that she had tried everything and that nothing had worked. I taught her how to chew well and explained about thoroughly digesting food before going to bed. I also gave her George Ohsawa's remedy of baked rice balls with soy sauce: Toast both sides of a rice ball on top of the stove using a Japanese metal toaster until both sides are crispy and then sprinkle with a small amount of soy sauce on each side. People with stomach ulcers are afraid to eat this because the rice ball is so hard. However, the trick is to cut the ball into 10 or more small pieces and to chew each small bite at least 200 times. Even though the skins of the rice remain, the saliva helps protect the stomach lining. The student was completely better after a short time of chewing her food thoroughly and abstaining from eating just before going to bed.

To another victim of stomach ulcer, I recommended dried codfish. He tried it and said it worked very well. The Japanese macrobiotic healer Mr. Ohmori recommends pressure-cooked brown rice with gomashio and side dishes of burdock carrot lotus root nitsuke sautéed with soy sauce, and hijiki lotus root nitsuke. Avoiding all fruit is important. These are the basic food recommendations for a quick recovery.   ■

STOMACH ULCER

---

* Important note: A sudden, agonizing pain in the abdomen accompanied by a rise in pulse rate and temperature, a decrease in blood pressure, a paled face, or the vomiting of blood, may indicate a perforation in the stomach. Consult a medical doctor immediately.

and the pain becomes worse. It takes even longer for duodenal ulcer pain to start.

Other symptoms of stomach ulcers typically include anemia, loss of appetite, weight loss, and occasional vomiting. The specific cause of stomach ulcers is considered to be unknown although irregular life-style and tension are suspected because the risk of developing a stomach ulcer increases with stress, poor diet, irregular eating patterns, smoking, excess alcohol or coffee consumption, and the use of certain drugs including aspirin.

According to our macrobiotic understanding, the underlying cause of stomach ulcers is eating fatty food too much and/or too often. This slows down reproduction of the stomach lining. After this happens, foods enter the stomach and the stomach juice is produced without the protection of an adequate lining. This causes pain or an ulcer. If you have an ulcer and a yang condition, stop eating all high-protein foods such as animal foods and completely stop consuming alcohol. Stomach ulcers result in an overly acidic condition, thus it is important to eat more alkaline-forming foods such as salt and salt products—miso, soy sauce, and umeboshi.

Helpful Suggestions

OBJECTIVE	REMEDY
To alkalize the system	Eating ½ cup of POTATO CONCENTRATE once a day is effective for all stomach and duodenal ulcers because it helps alkalize the body.
To maintain a more alkaline condition	Avoid hot baths; short, warm showers are okay.
To control occasional vomiting of blood	Try drinking 1 cup of warm, strong BANCHA TEA WITH SALT. (If you are hemorrhaging from the stomach or if the vomiting of blood doesn't stop, consult a physician immediately for emergency procedures.) *then* Lie down and apply a GINGER COMPRESS to the stomach area for 20 minutes. Then apply an ALBI PLASTER for up to 4 hours to help increase circulation and promote faster healing.
To relieve extreme pain	This may be relieved temporarily by eating or drinking bland food with a coating-like quality such as cooked kuzu.

Dietary Recommendations

Use the following dietary suggestions for four to five weeks, then slowly change to the gastritis suggestions, and then to a macrobiotic dietary approach (see page 11) after another month or two. Do not fast, since in this condition, you might become too weak. Alternately eat three

mouthfuls of brown rice, then one mouthful of vegetables. For all stomach diseases, it is important to chew very well (200 times) to mix the food with saliva and make it more alkaline-forming. Chewing well means putting pressure on both the upper and lower teeth. This also stimulates the brain. Of equal importance is to digest your food completely before sleeping. This means it is best to stay up for three to four hours after eating and to avoid snacking before going to bed. Stomach acids can be balanced with salt (alkaline-forming), so use a moderate amount of salt in your cooking. For all stomach diseases, I recommend kuzu for cooking because kuzu makes the stomach and intestines strong.

☐ Main foods: Brown Rice Balls with Gomashio; chew 200 times until rice is really soft, then swallow.
☐ Side dishes (one-fourth or one-fifth of main foods): Tekka Miso, Umeboshi, Takuan Pickles, Miso Pickles.
☐ Miso soup ingredients: wakame, tororo kombu, onions, scallions.
☐ Beverages: Brown Rice Tea, Brown Rice Bancha Tea, Bancha Tea. Drink less than 2 cups per day. If you have no appetite but are thirsty, try thick Brown Rice Cream (Special), mix well with saliva in the mouth and then swallow.
☐ Avoid especially: all meat, eggs, meat-based soups, dairy foods (including ice cream), all alcohol, soy milk, sweet foods and drinks, fruit, vinegar, hot spices, tomatoes, potatoes, pressed salads, white bread.

STOMACHACHE

Pain in the stomach is a common symptom of many sicknesses. In fact, with the exception of the common cold, troubles with the digestive organs are the most common problems. Since one of the functions of the stomach and other digestive organs is the handling of food, these organs are prone to sicknesses that are caused mainly by foods. However, the stomach's function is very much influenced by emotions. Therefore, the best care for the digestive organs is to eat moderately, chew well, abstain from eating just before sleeping, avoid too much of any condiment or seasoning, and maintain peace of mind—do not be angry.

Here, we discuss stomachaches that occur after eating. Eating heavy, oily food, especially in hot weather, may cause a stomachache by creating too much acid. The overconsumption of protein-rich animal foods and oily or fatty foods places an extra burden on the stomach and the intestines. Even those persons following a macrobiotic dietary approach can get a stomachache from eating fish cooked with lots of oil. For stomachaches as part of other disorders, see those sections.

Helpful Suggestions

If you have a severe stomachache after eating, you may need to vomit the food you ate.

OBJECTIVE	REMEDY
To induce vomiting (if needed)	Try drinking 1 cup of strong *SALTWATER DRINK* to induce vomiting within 2 hours after eating.
	or
	Adults may try putting two fingers on top of the tongue and pressing down deeply to induce vomiting.
To relieve pain from an over-acidic condition	Drinking 1 cup of *DAIKON GINGER TEA* up to 3 times per day is helpful.
	or
	Drinking 1 cup of very good-quality green tea up to 3 times per day is beneficial because green tea has lots of vitamin C. Vitamin C is good for digesting protein and alkalizing acidity. Drink a maximum of 3 cups of tea per day.

Dietary Recommendations

Fish or oily foods should be balanced with natural, non-chemicalized vinegar or lemon juice, grapefruit juice, or ume vinegar because these contain citric acid. Grated Daikon is also good. Following a macrobiotic dietary approach (see page 11) is the best preventative, especially being careful to avoid too much heavy oily food in the summertime.

See also GASTRITIS.

CORNELLIA'S NATURAL HEALING AT WORK

My son Jiro once had a stomachache that was caused by overeating. It was May 5—Boys' Day—a traditional Japanese holiday. We had a party in my front yard, and I served mugwort mochi (two per person) and a snack with shaved ice and apple juice. All the kids—and adults—enjoyed the food very much; Jiro ate too much shaved ice. When the guests left, he developed a stomachache. I gave him saltwater. He drank only about three mouthfuls. I kept his stomach warm with my palms for about 10 minutes. Then, he vomited all the shaved ice he had eaten. He learned something he could not do. Even for grown-ups, overeating or drinking can cause stomachaches. ∎

STOMACHACHE

STROKE

Stroke refers to a sudden decrease in the blood supply to part of the brain, such that it cannot function normally. There are three general types of stroke: cerebral hemorrhage, cerebral thrombosis, and cerebral embolism. A cerebral hemorrhage occurs when a blood vessel to the brain ruptures and bleeds into the brain or under its covering membranes. Cerebral thrombosis results when blood flow is blocked by the formation of a blood clot or by other narrowing in the cerebral arteries. A cerebral embolism occurs when a piece of clot (or other debris) is carried by the blood stream from the place it was formed to another place where it lodges, in this case, in the cerebral arteries. Cerebral thrombosis and cerebral embolism are very dangerous because they may cause the death of brain cells.

Symptoms of cerebral hemorrhage, in most cases, begin with a sudden loss of consciousness. After losing consciousness, the victim exhibits slow pulse, loud snoring, slow breathing, cold feet, loss of control of bowel movements and urination. Half of the body becomes numb or paralyzed. The symptoms of cerebral thrombosis and cerebral embolism are somewhat similar to those of cerebral hemorrhage and include: a loss of speech, confusion, paralysis of one side of the body (hemiplegia), paralysis of one side of the face, paralysis of movement of the eyes, staggering and loss of coordination, loss of sensation in parts of the body, headaches, nausea, vomiting, and loss of consciousness. If the person falls down, usually coldness and numbness come more slowly than in the case of cerebral hemorrhage. Also, the feet are warm instead of cold, the eyeballs are big and open, and there is no snoring.

The causes of stroke are usually thought to be hardening of the arteries or high blood pressure. The rupture of an aneurysm in a small artery to the brain can also lead to a stroke. Macrobiotic thinking agrees on one level, but looks further to find the cause of hardening of the arteries and high blood pressure. Thus, according to our macrobiotic understanding, the underlying cause of a cerebral hemorrhage is the overconsumption of animal foods such as meat, chicken, fish, and eggs. These foods are high in fat and cause high blood pressure. In addition, alcohol and/or eating too much fruit or sweet foods make the blood vessels weak until they finally rupture. Contributing factors for persons who have high blood pressure or who drink heavily are too many hot baths or suddenly becoming too cold from a sudden change of temperature.

In the case of cerebral thrombosis or embolism, there are several causes of obstruction-forming blood clots.

One is an acidic condition of the blood that withdraws calcium (an alkaline element) from the bone into the blood stream. Excess calcium in the blood stream crystalizes and produces sharp edges. Fat and/or cholesterol are then captured by the calcium crystals, forming obstructing clots. Thus, the underlying cause of obstruction-causing blood clots is the overconsumption of fatty foods because these foods increase fat and cholesterol in the blood stream and also cause an acidic condition of the blood. Also, an excess of sugary foods and fruits is transformed into fat by the liver. Furthermore, sugar causes an acidic condition of the blood and too much fruit, although alkaline-forming, will produce a cooling of the blood that contributes to the production of obstructing clots.

Helpful Suggestions

Two-thirds of all stroke cases result in death or permanent damage or disability. As with all life-threatening conditions, there is no substitute for proper medical attention. The suggestions here are offered to help you understand macrobiotic thinking and are complementary to medical treatment.

OBJECTIVE	REMEDY
FOR CEREBRAL HEMORRHAGE	
To help control bleeding	The following are helpful: A TOFU PLASTER on the head, changed every hour; a MUSTARD PLASTER on the feet until the skin turns red; if needed, you may drink up to 4 cups per day of SHIITAKE DAIKON TEA.
To relieve headache or the feeling of a heavy head	MASSAGE the head all over with APPLE JUICE every hour as needed to help relieve pain.
To ease numb or paralyzed body parts	Apply a GINGER COMPRESS to the numb or paralyzed area for 20 minutes 3 to 4 times per day. *and* Use a GINGER SESAME OIL MASSAGE on the side of the head that is opposite the numb or paralyzed side 3 or 4 times per day.
To improve blood circulation	After a stroke, drink 1 cup of DAIKON JUICE WITH RICE SYRUP AND GINGER. You may drink up to 3 or 4 cups per day for up to 3 or 4 days.
FOR CEREBRAL THROMBOSIS OR CEREBRAL EMBOLISM	
To ease numbness	If the right side of the body is numb, MASSAGE the left side of the head strongly with GINGER SESAME OIL, and vice versa. Do this massage 3 or 4 times per day.
To relieve head pain	Wash the head with HOT GINGER BATH water 2 times per day.
To relieve other pain	Use a GINGER COMPRESS on the arms and feet for 20 minutes, and MASSAGE them with GINGER SESAME OIL up to 3 times per day. Because they are the result of an acidic condition and an excess of fat, cerebral thrombosis and cerebral embolism are yin conditions. Therefore, a yang treatment such as a Ginger Compress (hot) is used as opposed to a Tofu Plaster (cold) which is recommended for a cerebral hemorrhage. *and* Improving blood circulation would also be beneficial.

Dietary Recommendations

Use the following special dietary suggestions for about one month. Then, widen your food choices using a macrobiotic dietary approach (see page 11).

FOR CEREBRAL HEMORRHAGE

☐ Main foods: Azuki Rice, Brown Rice with Barley, a little Gomashio as a condiment.

☐ Side dishes (one-third of main foods): Azuki Beans with Kombu and Winter Squash, Eggplant Nitsuke with Miso, Vegetable Tempura, Pressed Salad, Cucumber Pressed Salad, seasonal green vegetables such as cabbage. Eat sea vegetables every day because they are high in minerals and will help alkalize the blood.

☐ Miso soup ingredients: daikon, cabbage, Chinese cabbage, scallions, onions.

☐ Beverages: Vegetable Broth, Kombu Tea, Brown Rice Tea, Bancha Tea.

☐ Avoid especially: all animal foods including meat, fish, eggs, dairy foods; all sweet foods; hot spices; coffee; alcohol.

FOR CEREBRAL THROMBOSIS OR CEREBRAL EMBOLISM

☐ Main foods: Brown Rice, Azuki Rice, Brown Rice Mochi, Gomashio as a condiment.

☐ Side dishes (one-third of main foods): Burdock Nitsuke, Burdock Carrot Lotus Root Nitsuke, Lotus Root Nitsuke, Burdock Carrot Nitsuke, azuki kombu dishes, Deep-Fried Kombu, Vegetable Tempura, Miso Pickles, Rice Bran Pickles.

☐ Miso soup ingredients: wakame, tororo kombu, scallions, onions, Brown Rice Mochi.

☐ Beverages: Sho-Ban Tea, Kombu Tea, Bancha Tea, Grain Milk.

☐ Avoid especially: all yin foods including sugary foods, fruit, alcohol, vinegar, potatoes, melons, mushrooms, tomatoes, eggplant, ice cream, and coffee.

See also ANEURYSM *and* ARTERIOSCLEROSIS.

STUTTERING

This speech problem is characterized by the repetition of words or parts of words, the prolongation of sounds or pauses, and the interjection of sounds or words. It is a common temporary condition among children just learning to speak, and it should take care of itself after a period of time.

According to our macrobiotic understanding, the cause of stuttering is usually the overeating of animal protein, which causes an overly yang condition. More specifically, animal protein makes the right side of the brain too yang. The right side of the brain controls the speaking muscles. When the right side of the brain is too yang, the muscles move too fast and stuttering results.

Dietary Recommendations

Following a macrobiotic dietary approach (see page 11), avoiding food that is too yang for your condition, is most helpful. If this doesn't work, then contact your health-care advisor.

STY

A sty is a localized, inflammatory bacterial infection of one of the glands of the eyelid margin. Symptoms include redness, swelling, and pain or tenderness in the top or bottom eyelid; increased sensitivity to bright light; increased tear production; and a gritty feeling in the eye. Squeezing open the sty may spread the infection to other parts of the eyes or into the blood stream. As with all infections, stress, poor dietary habits, unsanitary living conditions, or any illness that has lowered resistance increases the chances of getting a sty. Irritation from smoking and exposure to chemicals or environmental irritants are also contributing factors.

According to our macrobiotic understanding, these factors do increase the risk, but the underlying cause of the infection is weakened kidneys, which result from an improper diet that is excessively high in fatty animal foods, especially dairy foods such as milk and butter, salty foods, sugary (sweetened) foods and drinks, and/or fruits. Overeating or overdrinking, a low- or no-salt diet, and the use of chemicals or drugs also contribute to weakened kidneys. Since the eyes are connected with the liver according to Far Eastern medicine, something harmful to the liver is also harmful to the eyes. See the Jaundice or Liver Cancer sections for ideas on improv-

---

CORNELLIA'S NATURAL HEALING AT WORK

My friend had a four-year-old boy who had eaten a standard American diet for the first three years of his life. Then his mother suddenly changed him to a macrobiotic diet and served gomashio to him at every meal. When I visited her, the boy was crying and refusing gomashio and also stuttering. I advised her to stop giving him gomashio if he didn't want it.

The next time I visited her, the boy was not stuttering. Of course, gomashio does not *cause* stuttering but this boy had a lot of animal foods for the first three years of his life and they were still in his body. Therefore, the gomashio was too yang for his condition. As a result, his mouth muscles moved too fast and without coordination. ∎

STUTTERING

---

ing the liver, and the Kidney Failure section for ideas on improving the condition of the kidneys.

Helpful Suggestions

OBJECTIVE	REMEDY
To relieve a sty	Rub the back of a smooth wooden implement (a spoon or comb) on a carpet or other object to make it very hot by friction. Then, slowly place the back of the implement on the swelling (sty). When the implement cools, heat it up again in the same way and reapply to the sty. Repeat the process 5 to 6 times per treatment once a day for 2 to 3 days. When it is small, a sty improves quickly.

Dietary Recommendations

Following a macrobiotic dietary approach (see page 11) is very helpful. Chew well.

☐ Avoid especially: overly yang foods such as red meat, fish, eggs, and overly yin foods such as fruits and sweeteners. Also avoid oily foods, all animal foods, overeating, and overdrinking.

See also CORNEAL INFLAMMATION.

SUNSTROKE

Sunstroke results from overexposure to the sun and is similar to heat stroke. Symptoms include headache, general weakness, sudden dizziness or faintness, hot and dry

148

skin, high body temperature, and rapid heartbeat. If untreated, it may lead to symptoms of shock such as hallucination, convulsions, high skin temperature, weak pulse, and finally unconsciousness.

According to our macrobiotic understanding, those eating an overly yin diet high in simple carbohydrates are more likely to suffer severe symptoms of sunstroke. Overheating in the head and/or heart consumes more oxygen; the less oxygen available, the more pronounced the symptoms. Simple carbohydrates burn (oxidize) quickly while complex carbohydrates such as whole grains provide a longer-lasting oxygen supply.

Helpful Suggestions

Sunstroke and heat exhaustion are potentially dangerous conditions, especially if the person who has symptoms of sunstroke is very hot and is not sweating. This is an emergency; arrange transportation to the nearest hospital. Also, never force food or water on a person who is unconscious or feels faint. The following suggestions are offered for milder cases or for cases when help is unavailable.

OBJECTIVE	REMEDY
FOR MILD CASES	
To aid the victim to regain consciousness	Move the unconscious person to the shade; make sure the area is well ventilated. Loosen clothing. Use a GINGER SESAME OIL MASSAGE on the person's head. *then* Massage the head and feet with cold water. *and* Finely grate a piece of fresh ginger and squeeze out the juice. Lightly rub the victim's throat with this juice to wake the person up.
To strengthen the victim's system	When the victim is awake, give 1 cup only of *SHO-BAN TEA* as a stimulant.
FOR MORE SEVERE SUNSTROKE	
To aid the victim to regain consciousness	Apply a TOFU PLASTER to the victim's head and one to the breast area to cool the person down. Change the plasters every 1 or 2 hours until the person regains consciousness. *and/or* Apply a MUSTARD PLASTER behind the ears and to the back of the neck for 5 to 7 minutes to help wake the person up.

To cool the head	After regaining consciousness, the victim should take a MUSTARD POWDER FOOT or GINGER FOOT BATH until the feet are a red color. This cools the head by drawing blood to the feet.

Dietary Recommendations

After awakening from an unconscious condition, following a macrobiotic dietary approach (see page 11) is helpful.

SYPHILIS

Syphilis is a venereal disease that leads to widespread tissue destruction. There are two forms of syphilis. The contagious form is spread by intimate sexual contact with someone who has syphilis in the first or second stages, while the congenital form is spread to the fetus through the blood stream. If a mother is infected before or during pregnancy, the baby may contract syphilis also. In such cases, the baby is usually stillborn or lost during pregnancy, or dies within a month after birth. If the child lives beyond two to three months, the sickness appears later in its life.

Syphilis is divided into three distinct stages. The first stage is characterized by a painless, raised, red hard spot (chancre) on the genitals, lips, pharnyx, or rectum. The second stage, occurring about six weeks to three months after the primary stage, has the following symptoms: fever; enlarged lymph glands in the neck, armpit or groin; headache; rash on the skin and mucous membranes of the penis, vagina, or mouth; white tumor appearing on the lips; coarse throat and voice; weakened eyesight; ringing in the ears; loss of head hair; bone infections; arthritis; loss of appetite; and general weakness. The third stage is noncontagious and may appear years after the first and second stages and may last for decades. In this stage, all body structures such as bones, skin, muscles, and internal organs such as the heart start to deteriorate. Mental deterioration and sexual impotence also may result. The cause of both forms of syphilis is considered to be infection from the bacteria *Treponema pallidum*.

However, according to our macrobiotic understanding, the bacteria is the initiator but not the underlying cause. The real cause is a diet that contains too much fat and protein, and too many simple carbohydrates. Protein is the material of the bacteria's growth, and fat and simple carbohydrates supply energy for that growth. Thus, a diet high in protein, fat, and simple carbohydrates increases the number of syphilis bacteria in the system. This kind of diet also weakens the body's immune system leading to greater susceptibility to syphilis.

Helpful Suggestions

OBJECTIVE	REMEDY
To control sexual lesions (chancres)	Use a DAIKON PLASTER on the affected area for 20 minutes twice a day. *then* After the compress, use a GINGER SESAME OIL MASSAGE on the area 3 times per day.
To relieve swelling or pain	Use a DAIKON GINGER or GINGER COMPRESS on the affected area for 20 minutes followed by an ALBI PLASTER for up to 4 hours. Repeat both the compress and the plaster as often as needed until swelling goes down or until your condition improves.

Dietary Recommendations

Changing your diet to help clean out all the toxins is the most effective remedy for this condition. Use the following dietary suggestions for several months or until your condition improves. Then, widen your food choices using a macrobiotic dietary approach (see page 11).

☐ Main foods: Brown Rice, Brown Rice with Barley, Brown Rice Cream, Brown Rice Gruel with Grated Daikon, Gomashio with each meal.

☐ Side dishes (one-fourth of main foods): Sesame Miso, Hijiki Burdock Nitsuke, Carp Soup, Okara Nitsuke, Eggplant Nitsuke with Miso and Ginger, Burdock Carrot Nitsuke, Vegetable Tempura served with Grated Daikon, Azuki Beans with Kombu and Winter Squash, Takuan Pickles, raw organic apples, raw persimmons.

☐ Miso soup ingredients: daikon, burdock, eggplant, spinach.

☐ Beverages: Bancha Tea, Habucha Tea, Grain Coffee, Vegetable Broth.

☐ Avoid especially: all animal foods (except freshwater fish), eggs, meat-based soups, all dairy foods (including ice cream), all sweet foods and drinks, vinegar, alcohol, black tea.

See also TESTICULAR INFLAMMATION.

TACHYCARDIA

See HEARTBEAT, RAPID

TEARS, EXCESSIVE

Excessive tearing is a common and disturbing disorder in infants although not generally a sight-threatening problem. The tear ducts drain through a connection into the nose, the nasolacrimal duct, which in an infant is a very small passageway. Not infrequently, the duct does not function properly for weeks or even months after birth so that the eyes stream steadily. Almost always, this trouble is caused by the overconsumption of yin foods and is caused very rarely by an overconsumption of yang foods. The overconsumption of yin foods and drinks can lead to watery eyes in adults, too.

Helpful Suggestions

OBJECTIVE	REMEDY
To improve circulation	Use a SALT BANCHA EYE BATH 3 times per day to help improve blood circulation to the area.

Dietary Recommendations

Mothers who are breastfeeding infants with this problem or adults with watery eyes may use the following special dietary suggestions until the condition improves or for about one month. Then, widen your food choices using a macrobiotic dietary approach (see page 11).

☐ Main foods: Brown Rice, Azuki Rice, Brown Rice with Soybeans (using black soybeans), Fried Rice, Brown Rice Mochi and a little Gomashio as a condiment. Chew very well.

☐ Side dishes (one-fourth of main foods): Tekka Miso, Sesame Miso, Shio Kombu, Hijiki Nitsuke, Azuki Beans with Kombu and Winter Squash, Vegetable Tempura, Rice Bran Pickles.

☐ Miso soup ingredients: wakame, onions, Homemade Agé.

☐ Beverages: Bancha Tea, Sho-Ban Tea, Brown Rice Tea, Grain Coffee. Drink a maximum of about 1 cup of beverages per day.

☐ Avoid especially: all fruit, sweet drinks, sugary foods, alcohol, overeating.

TESTICULAR INFLAMMATION

Testicular inflammation is a characteristic of several diseases. Symptoms include pain, heat, redness, and swelling. According to our macrobiotic understanding, an underlying yin cause of inflammation of the testicles is gonorrhea and the cause of gonorrhea is eating too much yin (both alkaline- and acid-forming) food, which weakens the immune system. Therefore, one's diet must be changed first. Another yin cause is tuberculosis. A yang cause is syphilis, which is the result of an excess of yin simple carbohydrates and yang protein foods.

Helpful Suggestions

OBJECTIVE	REMEDY
To reduce testicular heat	Use a TOFU PLASTER on the testicles (see Figure 3.8 on page 176), holding the plaster in place with a cheese cloth and changing it every 1 to 2 hours, until the heat subsides.
To relieve pain with swelling	Apply a GINGER COMPRESS for 20 minutes to help relieve pain; follow with an ALBI PLASTER for up to 4 hours to help reduce swelling.
To relieve pain	Lie down and elevate the testicles by gently tying a cloth around them.
	and
	If you go outside on a hot day, protect the testicles with 2 to 3 leaves from any green leafy vegetable to keep them cool.
	and
	MASSAGING the testicles with GINGER SESAME OIL is helpful.

Dietary Recommendations

If you have no appetite, eat Brown Rice Cream (thick) and Miso Soup. If the inflammation comes from tuberculosis (less common), use the dietary suggestions in the Tuberculosis section. Use the following special dietary suggestions until the inflammation subsides. Then, widen your food choices using a macrobiotic dietary approach (see page 11).

FOR THE YANG TYPE (SYPHILIS)

☐ Main foods: Brown Rice, Azuki Rice, Brown Rice Cream, Brown Rice Gruel with Mochi, whole-wheat spaghetti, Udon Noodles.

☐ Side dishes (one-third of main foods cooked with less salt than usual): Sesame Miso, Hijiki Nitsuke, Natto with Soy Sauce and Scallions served with Grated Daikon, Okara Nitsuke, Burdock Carrot Nitsuke, Azuki Beans with Kombu, Carp Soup, steamed vegetables, Vegetable Tempura served with Grated Daikon, Eggplant Nitsuke with Miso served with ginger, Sour Cabbage, Pressed Salad.

☐ Miso soup ingredients: daikon, daikon greens, Chinese cabbage, burdock, eggplant, green leafy vegetables, Brown Rice Mochi.

☐ Beverages: Brown Rice Tea, Brown Rice Bancha Tea, Bancha Tea, Grain Coffee. Drink as much as possible for 3 days only to help cleanse the body.

☐ Avoid especially: all red meat, fish (except carp), shellfish, eggs, dairy foods, alcohol, sweet foods, hot spices, black tea.

FOR THE YIN TYPE (GONORRHEA)

☐ Main foods: Brown Rice, Azuki Rice, Millet Rice, Brown Rice Mochi, all served with Gomashio at each meal.

☐ Side dishes (one-fourth of main foods): Tekka Miso, Scallion Miso, Shio Kombu, Hijiki Nitsuke, Vegetable Stew, Vegetable Stew with Fish, Carp Soup, Azuki Beans with Kombu and Winter Squash, Vegetable Tempura, Deep-Fried Kombu, Takuan Pickles, Miso Pickles.

☐ Miso soup ingredients: wakame, tororo kombu, scallions, onions, dried daikon, Brown Rice Mochi.

☐ Beverages: Bancha Tea, Brown Rice Tea, Brown Rice Bancha Tea, Sho-Ban Tea, Kombu Tea.

☐ Avoid especially: all yin foods especially alcohol.

TETANUS

Tetanus (lockjaw) refers to an infectious disease in a traumatized (wounded or injured) area of the body that causes severe muscle spasms and pain. In addition, difficulty in opening the mouth, chewing, and swallowing because of spasms in jaw and neck area can occur. Later, spasms advance to the spine and abdomen (making it difficult to breathe), arms, and legs. Temperature often reaches 104°F or more and seizures are common. According to Western medicine, the cause of tetanus is bacterial *(colostridium tetani)*. This bacteria is present almost everywhere, especially in soil, manure, or dust. When one is injured, these bacteria enter through wounds. Toxins made by this bacteria reach the nerves that control muscle contraction and the result is spasms. Tetanus is not contagious from person to person.

According to our macrobiotic understanding, the reason bacteria reaches toxic levels is a diet that contains too much animal food, leading to putrefaction and the overgrowth of anaerobic bacteria. Thus, a change in dietary habits is a good preventative and useful for lessening the effects of tetanus. Health departments strongly recommend tetanus immunizations as the best preventative. However, according to our thinking, immunizations adversely affect the body's natural immune system, and a proper diet provides the best immunity by keeping the immune system strong. On the other hand, immune-system and other problems can occur if a person who was once eating a balanced diet changes back to a high meat and animal food diet, especially in cases of women who then become pregant. Before deciding for or against immunization, you should carefully consider the options, and fully understand the necessary level of commitment to proper habits.

Helpful Suggestions

Tetanus is considered a highly fatal disease with a death rate of 50 percent. Seek proper medical attention if needed; the remedies and dietary suggestions offered here are complementary.

OBJECTIVE	REMEDY
To increase circulation	Apply a GINGER COMPRESS above the liver (see Figure 3.8 on page 176) and all down the spine for 20 minutes 3 times per day to help fight the infection through increased circulation. and/or Take an ARAME or DAIKON BATH for 20 minutes 1 to 2 times per day and/or a GINGER or MUSTARD POWDER BATH for 20 minutes once a day for better circulation.
To reduce fever	Try drinking 3 to 5 cups of DAIKON GINGER TEA per day until the fever is gone and to help clean up animal toxins.

Dietary Recommendations

Use the following dietary suggestions until your condition improves or for one month. Then, widen your food choices using a macrobiotic dietary approach (see page 11).

☐ Main foods: Brown Rice Cream with Grated Daikon with soy sauce.
☐ Side dishes (one-fourth of main foods): Cucumber Salad with Rice Vinegar, Eggplant Nitsuke with Miso served with ginger, Shiitake Nitsuke, Azuki Beans with Kombu flavored with a little yinnie syrup or maple syrup for a sweet taste.
☐ Miso soup ingredients: daikon, scallions, wakame, Chinese cabbage, onions.
☐ Beverages: Barley Tea, Brown Rice Tea, Brown Rice Bancha Tea, Grain Coffee.
☐ Avoid especially: all animal food.

THROMBOSIS

Thrombosis refers to formation of a blood clot. A blood clot that forms inside a vein is called deep vein thrombosis. While any veins in the body may be affected, those in the lower legs (calves) or lower abdomen are most often involved. The problem with these clots is that they may break off and travel to the lung, resulting in the death of lung tissue. This is called a pulmonary embolism. Symptoms of deep vein thrombosis commonly include swelling and pain in the area normally drained by the blocked vein with the swelling extending from the clot to the toes, tenderness, redness, and soreness when walking. There may also be fever or increased heartbeat.

Blood-clot formation in an artery is called arterial thrombosis. If the clot forms in one place and then breaks off and travels to a distant artery or organ, it is called an embolus. Any of the large or medium arteries in the body may be affected. Clots in the brain result in a stroke (see pages 146-147) and are very dangerous. Clots in the kidneys or intestines are also life-threatening. Clots in the extremities are easier to deal with but must be cared for since they may break off and travel to a more dangerous location. Symptoms of clots in the extremities, including pain, weakness, numbness, or tingling sensations in the arms or calves, usually become manifest after exercise and subside with rest.

The cause of deep vein thrombosis is considered to be the pooling of blood in a vein due to prolonged bed rest or a major illness. The cause of arterial thrombosis is any condition, including hardening of the arteries or injury, that damages the smooth lining of a blood vessel. However, according to our macrobiotic understanding, the underlying cause of clots in the veins or arteries is the overconsumption of cholesterol-rich foods. Actually, anything that contributes to hardening of the arteries (see Arteriosclerosis) increases the risk of thrombosis.

Helpful Suggestions

OBJECTIVE	REMEDY
To relieve pain and swelling	Use a GINGER COMPRESS on the area nearest the clot for 20 minutes followed by an ALBI PLASTER for up to 4 hours. Repeat both the compress (to help reduce pain by increasing circulation) and the plaster (to help reduce swelling by removing toxins) as often as needed.
To reduce high fever	Try applying a TOFU PLASTER on the head; change it every hour until the fever goes down. and

A GREEN LEAVES APPLICATION at the back of the neck is helpful.

To improve circulation — Move your lower limbs as soon as possible and often after an illness requiring prolonged bed rest. Elevating the feet higher than the hips when sitting for long periods of time is also beneficial.

Dietary Recommendations

The following dietary suggestions may be used until your heart condition improves or for about one month. Then, widen your food choices based on a macrobiotic dietary approach (see page 11).

FOR THE YANG TYPE

☐ Main foods: Brown Rice (or any whole grains) served with Gomashio, Brown Rice Mochi.

☐ Side dishes (one-third of the main foods): Tekka Miso, Hijiki Nitsuke, Nori Nitsuke, Shio Kombu, Vegetable Tempura, Azuki Beans with Kombu and Winter Squash, Burdock Carrot Nitsuke. Use less salt than usual in the cooking of side dishes.

☐ Miso soup ingredients: wakame, tororo kombu, daikon, burdock.

☐ Beverages: Brown Rice Tea, Bancha Tea, Grain Coffee.

☐ Avoid especially: all animal foods including fish and shell fish, all sweet foods and drinks, ice cream, all fruit, all alcohol.

See also STROKE AND ARTERIOSCLEROSIS.

THRUSH

Thrush is a common fungus infection of the mouth mostly affecting newborns and infants although older children and adults may also be affected. Patches of slightly raised milky bumps that can't be wiped off the lips, tongue, and palette signal the presence of thrush. These patches are not painful until or unless they are rubbed off, which results in small, painful ulcers. Thus, this disease may create a sore, inflamed mouth in infants.

The cause of thrush is thought to be a fungus, *Candida albicans*, which develops at birth during the baby's passage through the birth canal, especially if the mother has a vaginal yeast infection at the time of delivery. In older persons, thrush may be the result of treatment with antibiotics that upset the body's natural balance, or the effects of aging whereby a person has a lower natural resistence. According to our macrobiotic understanding, thrush usually starts when the infant drinks formula and not mother's milk. While thrush in adults may result

from the previously stated causes, it indicates an improper diet over a long time.

Helpful Suggestions

OBJECTIVE	REMEDY
To soothe ulcers inside the mouth	Tie a cotton ball onto a chopstick and soak the ball in *HABUCHA TEA* or *BANCHA TEA WITH SALT*. Gently swab and clean the mouth. Wait 10 minutes and swab again. Do this 2 to 3 times per day for up to 2 to 3 days.

Dietary Recommendations

The pain usually is gone in one day and the baby can drink mother's or grain milk again. If you are feeding the baby formula and if mother's milk is unavailable, gradually reduce the amount of formula and feed the baby rice milk sweetened with yinnie syrup or amasake.

See also CANDIDIASIS.

THYROIDITIS

Thyroiditis is an inflammation of the thyroid gland. Symptoms include a thyroid gland that is enlarged, painful, and tender. The overlying skin is often red and warm, and there may be fever. When the gland is acutely inflamed, large amounts of thyroid hormone may be released into the blood stream, causing a temporary form of hyperthyroidism (overactivity of the thyroid gland). Later, the thyroid gland becomes weak (yin) and may cause hypothyroidism (underactivity of the thyroid resulting in a deficiency of thyroid hormone). The cause of thyroiditis is generally considered to be a malfunctioning of the autoimmune system along with the presence of various viruses such as mumps or the flu, rheumatoid arthritis, or—more rarely—a bacterial infection (staphylococcic or streptococcic) of the thyroid gland.

However, according to our macrobiotic understanding, the underlying cause of any enlargement of the thyroid gland is the result of long-time overconsumption of yin foods such as potatoes, tomatoes, eggplant, bananas, and other foods high in potassium; and simple carbohydrates including fruits, honey, molasses, and any sweeteners. In addition, the overconsumption of liquids contributes to the expansion. These dietary excesses also lead to greater susceptibility to autoimmune system disorders.

Helpful Suggestions

OBJECTIVE	REMEDY
To relieve throat pain	Apply a GINGER COMPRESS on the throat for 20 minutes followed by an ALBI PLASTER for up to 4 hours. Repeat both the compress and the plaster as often as needed.
To alleviate protruding eyes	Use a warm SALT BANCHA EYE BATH 3 times per day. *or* Place a 1/8-inch-thick slice of any red meat on each eyelid; change it every 2 hours for 2 days.
To reduce excess perspiration and to cool the body	Try eating 1 to 2 cups of MISO SOUP WITH MOCHI 1 or 2 times per day, 1/2 cup of OYSTERS AND TOFU WITH MISO 1 or 2 times per day, or 1 cup of CARP SOUP once a day.
To relieve dizziness	Drink the RANSHO DRINK from 1 egg once per day only for 3 days maximum.
To relieve headache	MASSAGE the scalp with GINGER SESAME OIL or APPLE JUICE as often as needed.
To relieve heart palpitations	The heart may be affected by this disease. If you are experiencing heart palpitations, drink 1/2 to 1 cup of SHO-BAN TEA or drink the RANSHO DRINK from 1 egg when palpitations start. Use ransho only if it's not being used for dizziness.
To reduce heart pain	Try an ALBI PLASTER on the heart (see Figure 3.8 on page 176), changing it every 4 hours until pain stops. This will also serve to strengthen the heart.
To strengthen the heart	Eat 1/3 teaspoon of EGG OIL 3 times per day to strengthen the heart.

Dietary Recommendations

Use the following dietary suggestions until your condition improves or for one month. Then, widen your food choices using a macrobiotic dietary approach (see page 11).

☐ Main foods: Brown Rice served with Gomashio, Azuki Rice, Brown Rice Kayu, Brown Rice Cream. Chew each mouthful 200 times. Eat Brown Rice Kayu or Brown Rice Cream only when you have no appetite because these dishes contain so much water.

☐ Side dishes (less than one-half of main foods): Tekka Miso, Oily Miso, Shio Kombu, Hijiki Carrot Nitsuke, Burdock Carrot Nitsuke, Azuki Beans with Kombu, Vegetable Tempura, natural caviar.

☐ Miso soup ingredients: wakame, onions, scallions, Homemade Agé, Brown Rice Mochi.

☐ Beverages: Brown Rice Tea, Brown Rice Bancha Tea, Sho-Ban Tea, Bancha Tea with Gomashio, Grain Milk. Drink less, a maximum of 1½ cups per day.

☐ Avoid especially: all animal foods (except carp and caviar), eggs, dairy foods (including ice cream), all fruit, all sweet foods and drinks, potatoes, melons, hot spices, salads, black tea, coffee.

TONGUE PROBLEMS

If the tongue is painful or swollen, it may be a sign of overeating. Tongue inflammation is also associated with several greater disorders. These include infections; poor dental habits and health; allergies; burns or other injury; excessive consumption of hot, spicy foods, alcohol, or tobacco; and an adverse reaction to certain drugs and medications.

According to our macrobiotic understanding, the condition of the tongue reflects your overall health. The tongue should be uniformly pink. A white coating on the front of the tongue shows stomach and intestinal trouble and on the back of the tongue shows that the kidneys are weak. A yellow color on the tongue signals liver trouble. A black color on the tongue is a very bad sign indicating a serious health problem. Change your diet immediately to a macrobiotic approach with no animal protein, no fruit or refined sugar, and not too much salt either.

Helpful Suggestions

Good oral hygiene is most important. Consult your dentist. In the case of the tongue's signaling an organ or other disorder, see the related section for helpful suggestions.

Dietary Recommendations

If the color of the tongue changes and there is less appetite, don't force food. Drink light KUZU BANCHA TEA, BROWN RICE CREAM (thin), BANCHA TEA, BROWN RICE TEA, or BARLEY TEA if you desire something. These teas help your internal organs quickly by allowing the body to rest and the organs to restore themselves naturally. Once the trouble stops and your appetite returns, use a macrobiotic dietary approach (see page 11).

See also PERIODONTAL DISEASE.

Tonsillitis

Tonsils and adenoids are protective organs of lymph tissue that help prevent infections of the sinuses, mouth, and throat from spreading to other parts of the body. Tonsillitis is an inflammation of the tonsils and is common during early childhood. Chills, high fever (over 104°F), and extreme pain in the tonsil area appear at the onset of tonsillitis. Headache, pain in the back of the jaw and in the neck, and a stiff neck also occur. Swallowing is painful and difficult, and the tonsils are enlarged and red. Chronic tonsillitis is characterized by colds, fatigue, and bad breath (which in our macrobiotic understanding are all signs of poorly functioning kidneys), greatly enlarged tonsils, and frequent sore throats. Tonsillitis is considered to be caused by a viral or bacterial infection.

However, according to our macrobiotic understanding, the underlying cause of tonsillitis is the heavy consumption of sweets, fruit, and sweet drinks combined with a high protein diet. The long-term effect of such a diet is that the body's immune system is weakened and the tonsils and adenoids become easily infected and often enlarged, resulting in altered speech and breathing. In such cases, modern medical practitioners often suggest surgery to remove these organs. However, according to our macrobiotic understanding, the tonsils and adenoids have a function thoughout life and should not be removed routinely. A dietary change is much more appropriate and should be tried first.

Helpful Suggestions

If the tonsil infection comes from a cold, try the remedies for colds.

OBJECTIVE	REMEDY
To reduce high fever	Try drinking 1 cup of DAIKON GINGER TEA (if needed, you may drink up to 3 or 4 cups per day); applying a TOFU PLASTER on the forehead, changing it every hour; and placing a GREEN LEAVES APPLICATION at the back of the neck to be left on while you sleep. *or* In addition to the above suggestions, try drinking 1 cup of KUZU TEA or 1 cup of BROWN RICE TEA WITH DRIED PERSIMMON AND TANGERINE SKIN. You may drink up to 3 cups per day.
To control infection	GARGLE with 1 cup of SHO-BAN TEA or 1 cup of DENTIE WATER 4 times per day. *then*
	After gargling, tie a piece of cotton to the large end of a chopstick and dip it into the dentie water. Swab the tonsils.
To remove toxins	Apply an ALBI PLASTER externally to the throat to help draw out the toxins; change the plaster every 4 hours.

Dietary Recommendations

Use the following dietary suggestions until your condition improves or for one month. Then, widen your food choices using a macrobiotic dietary approach (see page 11).

☐ Main foods: Brown Rice Gruel with Miso and Scallions, Mochi Soup, Brown Rice Cream. If you cannot swallow food, it is all right to fast for a short time.

☐ Side dishes (one-fourth or less of main foods): Tekka Miso, Shio Kombu, Hijiki Nitsuke, Oysters Cooked with Miso, Burdock Carrot Nitsuke, Vegetable Tempura, Nori Roasted with Oil, Miso Pickles.

☐ Miso soup ingredients: wakame, scallions, daikon, Brown Rice Mochi.

☐ Beverages: less drinking is better once the throat is no longer very sore. If you are thirsty, drink Brown Rice Bancha Tea, Mu Tea, Sho-Ban Tea, or Grain milk.

☐ Avoid especially: soy milk, all fruit, all sweet foods and drinks, all vinegar dishes, hot spices, tomatoes, eggplant, potatoes, melons, all meats, red-meat fish, shellfish, dairy foods.

Tooth Pain

See DENTAL CARIES.

Trachoma

Trachoma refers to a chronic inflammatory disease of the eye caused by an organism that is a strain of the bacteria *Chlamydia trachomatis*. The first symptoms of trachoma appear after about a one-week incubation period. There is swelling of the eyelids and the eyes become bloodshot. The membranes lining the eyelids and covering the eyeball become thickened and roughened; as a result, part of the eyelid's edge may turn inward. In a few weeks, corneal ulceration and swelling obstruct vision. Permanent scar tissue may form on the inner eyelids.

According to our macrobiotic understanding, this disease is primarily caused by the overconsumption of yin foods such as candy, cake, ice cream, soft drinks, and fruits along with a low- or no-salt diet, resulting in an overly yin condition. These yin foods contain a lot of simple carbohydrates that promote the growth of microbes, leading to trachoma and other infectious diseases. A low- or no-salt diet leads to a weakened immune system that allows the overgrowth of microbes and greater susceptibility to infections.

Helpful Suggestions

OBJECTIVE	REMEDY
To reduce swelling	Use a SALT BANCHA EYE BATH 4 times per day until swelling goes down.
	and
	After an eye bath and just before going to bed, use a SESAME OIL EYE TREATMENT.
	then
	Apply an UMEBOSHI EYE PLASTER and sleep with it on overnight.

Dietary Recommendations

A change in dietary habits is most beneficial. Use the following dietary suggestions until your condition improves or for one month. Then, widen your food choices using a macrobiotic dietary approach (see page 11).

☐ Main foods: Brown Rice with a little Gomashio as a condiment. Chew each mouthful 200 times.

☐ Side dishes (one-fourth of main foods): Hijiki Nitsuke, Hijiki Burdock Nitsuke, Burdock Nitsuke, Carp Soup, Okara Nitsuke, Grated Daikon with Soy Sauce, Waterless Cooked Vegetables, Deep-Fried Kombu, Nori Roasted with Oil, Rice Bran Pickles.

☐ Miso soup ingredients: daikon, tofu, Homemade Agé, scallions, onions.

☐ Beverages: Brown Rice Tea, Bancha Tea, Vegetable Broth. Drink a maximum of 3 cups of beverages per day.

☐ Avoid especially: all meats, fish (except carp), shellfish, all dairy foods, eggs, all sweet foods, all fruit, alcoholic drinks.

TUBERCULOSIS

Tuberculosis refers to an acute or chronic, contagious, bacterial infection of the lungs and to a lesser extent other parts of the body. It is characterized by the formation of small, rounded nodules (tubercles) and the localized death of tissues. Childhood tuberculosis usu-

ally occurs in the middle parts of the lungs, while adult tuberculosis usually affects the top parts of the lungs. In the early stages, there are either no symptoms or symptoms that resemble those of the flu. In the second stage, symptoms include fever, weight loss, chronic fatigue, and/or heavy sweating at night. In the later stages, the person has a pale face, a cough with bloody sputum, chest pains, shortness of breath, and reddish urine.

The cause of tuberculosis is considered to be infection by the germ *Mycobacterium tuberculosis*. This germ is usually transmitted in the air from person to person and is usually spread before the disease is diagnosed. A tuberculin skin test is often given in schools, and vaccination and preventive treatment is recommended to those determined to be at risk because of their reaction or the reactions of their schoolmates. Those living in or traveling to places where tuberculosis is prevalent are also advised to be vaccinated.

However, according to our macrobiotic understanding, germs are not the true cause of the disease because many people do not acquire tuberculosis even though they may have tuberculosis germs in their bodies. Germs are one of the environmental factors, but the underlying cause is a yin physical and psychological condition, which can result from heavy consumption of sugary foods and fruits and/or a low- or no-salt diet. The long-term effect of such a diet is an overly yin condition that leads to severe fatigue, weakened kidneys, and a greater susceptibility to tuberculosis germs.

Once considered to be controlled, tuberculosis has rebounded with vaccination- and medication-resistant strains that are most troublesome. This has caused much concern among health officials and the general public. According to our macrobiotic understanding, this is yet another signal that people need to take greater responsibility for their own health by eating in a way that promotes a healthy immune system, properly functioning kidneys and other organs, and a positive (non-fearful) outlook on life. Then, vaccinations, which are detrimental to one's immune system, are not needed.

Helpful Suggestions

If you change to a macrobiotic dietary approach when you have tuberculosis, your temperature may go up and your condition may initially appear to be getting worse. This shows that your body is being cleansed and there is no reason for worry unless your temperature does not return to normal soon. The temperature should return to normal within three days after your change to a macrobiotic dietary approach. Refrain from sex until your condition improves.

OBJECTIVE	REMEDY
To reduce high fever	Try applying a TOFU PLASTER on the chest, changing it every hour.
To reduce fever that lasts longer than 3 days	Try drinking 1 cup of BROWN RICE TEA WITH DRIED PERSIMMON AND TANGERINE SKIN 2 to 3 times per day.
To control sweating at night	Before you sleep, cleanse your body with warm GINGER BATH water as a sponge bath to help improve circulation. *and* A recipe that is helpful for night sweating is OYSTERS AND TOFU WITH MISO. Try eating ½ to 1 cup once a day until you are no longer sweating at night.
To relieve cough	Drink ½ cup LOTUS ROOT TEA 2 to 3 times per day. *and* Eating 1 to 2 tablespoons of BURDOCK CARROT LOTUS ROOT NITSUKE or LOTUS ROOT NISHIME once a day is helpful for a cough.
To control coughing up blood	Drink ½ cup of strong SALTWATER DRINK 1 time only. *then* Lie down slowly and apply a 1-inch-thick TOFU PLASTER to the chest; change it every 2 hours. Repeat until you are no longer coughing up blood. *and* Slowly sipping 1 tablespoon of LOTUS ROOT JUICE 2 to 3 times per day is helpful.
To relieve chest pain	Use a GINGER COMPRESS on the chest for 20 minutes followed by an ALBI PLASTER for up to 4 hours. You may repeat the Ginger Compress and Albi Plaster sequence as often as needed. *or* Use a MUSTARD PLASTER once only until the skin turns red, followed by an ALBI PLASTER for up to 4 hours.
To strengthen a weak heart	Try drinking 1 cup of SHO-BAN TEA 3 times per day, or the RANSHO DRINK from 1 egg once a day for 3 days, or 1 cup of BROWN RICE TEA WITH SOY SAUCE 3 times per day until the heart becomes strong.
To relieve insomnia with fever	Eat supper earlier and eat less. Drink no beverages after 4:00 P.M. *and* To help you sleep, before going to bed, take 1 teaspoon of GOMASHIO or ⅓ to ½ cup SHO-BAN TEA, place a GREEN LEAVES APPLICATION at the back of the neck, and place a TOFU PLASTER on the forehead for 1 hour. You may leave the green leaves at the back of the neck overnight.
To relieve intestinal trouble or constipation	Eat ½ cup of GREEN LEAFY VEGETABLES WITH HOMEMADE AGÉ and ¼ to ½ cup of AZUKI BEANS WITH KOMBU once a day.
To control diarrhea	Eat 1 cup of MISO SOUP WITH MOCHI (with 1 to 2 mochi) or 1 to 1½ cups of BROWN RICE GRUEL WITH MISO AND SCALLIONS 1 or 2 times per day, and drink 1 cup of KUZU BANCHA TEA or 1 cup of UMESHO BANCHA TEA 1 or 2 times per day.
To stimulate appetite	Eat 1 cup of thin BROWN RICE CREAM 1 or 2 times per day.
To control anemia	Drink 1 cup of SHO-BAN TEA and eat 1 cup of MISO SOUP using hatcho or barley miso 1 or 2 times per day. *and* Eating 1 tablespoon of SOY SAUCE WITH SESAME OIL AND GINGER JUICE 1 to 2 times a day is helpful in strengthening your whole body. *and* Use natural sesame oil and soy sauce in your side dishes. It should not be necessary to take iron pills or other supplements if a balanced diet of whole foods is maintained.

Dietary Recommendations

Use the following dietary suggestions for about one month to help improve your condition. Then, widen your food choices using a macrobiotic dietary approach (see page 11).

☐ Main foods: Brown Rice Balls with Gomashio, Azuki Rice, Brown Rice Gruel with Mochi, Baked Mochi with Soy Sauce. Chew each mouthful 200 times.

☐ Side dishes (one-fourth of main foods): Tekka Miso, Oily Miso, Sesame Miso, Shio Kombu, Hijiki Burdock Nitsuke, Burdock Carrot Nitsuke, Carp Soup, Oysters Cooked with Miso, Oyster Tempura, Small Fish Tempura served with Grated Daikon, Miso Pickles, Umeboshi.

☐ Miso soup ingredients: wakame, onions, scallions, tororo kombu, Homemade Agé, Brown Rice Mochi.

☐ Beverages: Brown Rice Tea, Brown Rice Bancha Tea, Sho-Ban Tea, Bancha Tea, Grain Coffee, Bancha Tea with Gomashio.

☐ Avoid especially: all meat (except oysters, small fish, and carp soup), dairy foods (including ice cream), soy milk, all fruit, all sweet foods and drinks, potatoes, tomatoes, eggplant, vinegar, melons, coffee, alcohol.

TUBERCULOSIS OF THE INTESTINES

According to modern medicine, intestinal tuberculosis is caused by tuberculosis germs moving from the lungs to the intestines, or by infectious germs from milk or milk products. Often there are no symptoms. Sometimes, one has random, very severe, abdominal pain, constipation or diarrhea, weakness, anemia, or intestinal hemorrhaging.

According to our macrobiotic understanding, intestinal tuberculosis is caused by a lack of sodium in the bodily fluids that results from insufficient salt in the diet or from weak kidneys that cannot control the amount of sodium and other minerals in the body. Too much sugary food in the diet can also result in a lack of sodium in the bodily fluids.

Helpful Suggestions

OBJECTIVE	REMEDY
To control diarrhea	Take a DAIKON or ARAME HIP BATH WITH GRATED GINGER for 20 minutes once a day. *and/or* Drinking 2/3 cup of KUZU BANCHA TEA, UMESHO BANCHA TEA, or UMESHO KUZU TEA 2 or 3 times per day is helpful.
To relieve intestinal pain	Drink 2/3 cup of UMESHO BANCHA tea 2 or 3 times per day. *and* Use a ROASTED SALT PACK for 20 minutes, or a DAIKON or ARAME HIP BATH WITH MUSTARD POWDER for only 7 to 8 minutes, to warm the intestinal area.
To reduce fever	Place a TOFU PLASTER on the forehead; change it every hour.
To relieve constipation	Swallow 2 to 3 tablespoons of sesame oil once only.
To contract weak intestines	Eating 1/4 to 1/2 cup of AZUKI BEANS WITH KOMBU or 1/2 cup of GREEN LEAFY VEGETABLES WITH HOMEMADE AGÉ once a day is useful.

Dietary Recommendations

Until the diarrhea stops, use these special dietary suggestions, eating 80 to 90 percent grains and only 10 to 20 percent side dishes. When you change your diet, you may experience a temporary worsening of the diarrhea. Don't worry; it should gradually decrease and eventually stop. After the diarrhea stops, follow the remedies and dietary suggestions for tuberculosis.

☐ Main foods: Brown Rice Balls (occasionally using sweet brown rice) served with Gomashio, Mochi Soup with Miso. It is very important to chew each bite 200 times.

☐ Side dishes (if desired, eat only very small quantities): Ginger Miso, Miso Pickles, Takuan Pickles, Tekka Miso.

☐ Miso soup ingredients: wakame, Homemade Agé, Brown Rice Mochi.

☐ Beverages: Brown Rice Tea, Brown Rice Bancha Tea, Umesho Bancha.

TUBERCULOSIS OF THE SPINE

Tuberculosis of the spine is seen as a complication of tuberculosis of the lungs; it occurs when the tuberculosis germ infects the spine. Symptoms include stiffness, back pain during motion, tenderness, abscess formation, paralysis, and, occasionally, abdominal pain. According to our macrobiotic understanding, the specific cause of this disease is overeating sugary foods.

Helpful Suggestions

OBJECTIVE	REMEDY
To remove toxins	Use an ALBI PLASTER on the spine and on the hips, changing it every 4 hours. The albi will help cause the skin pores to enlarge and the pus to come out. If the pus goes into the hips, one may not be able to walk so it is important to apply an Albi Plaster in order to draw out the pus.
To maintain circulation	Avoid the use of a corset because it can cause poor blood circulation.

Dietary Recommendations

Dietary changes are most helpful. Use the dietary suggestions under Tuberculosis. Also, use the most natural sesame oil and soy sauce you can find. Cook vegetables and sea vegetables longer than usual so that they become more yang. Especially use sea vegetables, burdock, and lotus root. Sea vegetables are good for calcium, burdock for detoxification, and lotus root for helping reduce the number of tuberculosis germs.

See also TUBERCULOSIS.

TYPHOID FEVER

Typhoid fever is a bacterial infection of the gastrointestinal tract, mainly the small intestine. The first signs of typhoid fever are fatigue, loss of appetite, pain in the legs, and difficulty sleeping, followed by chills, fever, dry mouth, constipation or diarrhea, low temperature in the morning and high temperature at night. After one to three weeks, a rash appears on the chest and abdomen and body temperature rises. The body temperature remains high for three or four weeks and is followed by heavy sweating after which one usually starts to feel better. A characteristic of this sickness is dry skin. If there is sweating before the characteristic heavy sweating that breaks the fever, it is probably not typhoid fever. Typhoid fever often causes hearing problems.

The cause of typhoid fever is considered to be infection with the bacteria *Salmonella typhosa*. The bacteria is transmitted from animals to persons through contaminated meat or milk, or from person to person because of improper hand-washing after bowel movements and before handling food. However, according to our macrobiotic understanding, the underlying cause of typhoid fever—and the reason some people infected with the bacteria develop the disease while others do not—is excessive consumption of overly yin or overly yang foods, contributing to a weakened immune system. If the immune system lacks sodium, that system cannot prevent infections by bacteria or viruses. In the macrobiotic view, the following dietary habits lead to a lack of sodium in the cells that the immune system needs to function at its best: the excessive consumption of overly yin foods such as sugary foods and drinks, vinegar, fruits, alcohol, and fatty foods; a low- or no-salt diet or too much salt, leading to kidney weakness; the overconsumption of yang animal foods such as meat, eggs, cheese, and fish that, even though they are high in sodium, weaken the kidneys because they are acid-forming; and/or the overconsumption of beverages such as water and tea, and especially those fluids that are both sugary and acid-forming.

Helpful Suggestions

OBJECTIVE	REMEDY
To reduce high fever	Apply a TOFU PLASTER on the forehead and another on the lower abdomen, changing each plaster every hour. *and* Place a GREEN LEAVES APPLICATION on a pillow and lie down with the pillow at the back of your neck. Change the leaves every 2 hours.
To quench thirst	Try drinking 1 to 3 cups per day of BROWN RICE TEA WITH UMEBOSHI.
To relieve stomach pain	Take DAIKON or ARAME HIP BATH WITH GRATED GINGER for 20 minutes as often as needed.
To relieve chills	Placing a ROASTED SALT PACK on top of the intestines (see Figure 3.8 on page 176) for 20 minutes is helpful.
To weaken the microbes	Drink ½ to 1 cup of UMESHO BANCHA TEA 2 to 3 times per day.
To control diarrhea	Try drinking ½ cup of UMESHO KUZU TEA up to 3 times per day.
To relieve bed sores	Apply a RICE BRAN COMPRESS to the sores for 5 to 6 hours once a day to help heal broken skin. The sores should disappear after a couple of applications. *and* The cause of bed sores is too much watery food, so cut down your liquid intake if you have bed sores.

Dietary Recommendations

Use the following dietary suggestions until the symptoms subside or for one month. Then, widen your food choices using a macrobiotic dietary approach (see page 11).

☐ Main foods: Brown Rice Balls, Brown Rice Gruel with Grated Daikon, Brown Rice Mochi with Homemade Agé cooked with less salt, Brown Rice Gruel with Mochi or with Miso. When there is lack of appetite, serve Brown Rice Cream (thick) only.

☐ Side dishes (less than one-fourth of main foods): Grated Daikon with Soy Sauce, Ginger Miso, Umeboshi, Eggplant Mustard Pickles, Takuan Pickles.

☐ Miso soup ingredients: daikon, Homemade Agé, scallions.

☐ Beverages: Brown Rice Tea, Brown Rice Bancha Tea, Bancha Tea, Grain Coffee.

☐ Avoid especially: overly yin or yang foods, especially meat and sugar.

TYPHUS, EPIDEMIC

Epidemic typhus is an infectious disease of the gastrointestinal tract. There is a short incubation period, and then the victim displays symptoms including severe headache, pain in arms and legs, fatigue, loss of appetite, vomiting, and sleepiness. However, the disease can start with the following symptoms without an incubation period: sustained high fever over 104°F, fast pulse, severe headache, dizziness, and loss of consciousness. Approximately five days after the onset of these symptoms, many rashes appear all over the body for three to seven days. In mild cases, one can recover after two weeks of sickness. Severe cases may result in delirium and coma, ending in death in 20 percent of untreated cases.

The cause of epidemic typhus is considered to be infection by the bacteria *Rickettsia prowazekii*, which is transmitted from person to person by lice. According to our macrobiotic understanding, the underlying cause of typhus and the reason for greater susceptibility of some people is a diet that consists of too much animal food such as red meat, chicken, eggs, cheese, and fish. This bacteria is very yin so it is attracted to yang protein such as meat. The very first stage of infection with symptoms such as high body temperature (such as 104°F), fast pulse, and severe headache damages the kidneys, resulting in the rashes that appear as the yang foods are discharged. These symptoms appear quite fast indicating that this is a very yang disease.

Helpful Suggestions

Use the same remedial suggestions for symptoms of epidemic typhus as listed under Typhoid Fever.

OBJECTIVE	REMEDY
To remove excess salts	GINGER, ARAME, or DAIKON BATHS are very helpful to take out excess salts if necessary. Take these baths for 20 minutes at a time 1 or 2 times per day.

Dietary Recommendations

Use the following special dietary suggestions until your condition improves or for one month. Then, widen your food choices using a macrobiotic dietary approach (see page 11).

☐ Main foods: Brown Rice Gruel with Grated Daikon served with Homemade Agé, Mochi Soup, Brown Rice Cream cooked to a less salty taste than usual.
☐ Side dishes (one-fifth of main foods): Sesame Miso, Ginger Miso, plenty of Grated Daikon with Soy Sauce, Takuan Pickles.
☐ Miso soup ingredients: daikon, Homemade Agé, burdock, Brown Rice Mochi.
☐ Beverages: Brown Rice Tea, Bancha Tea, Grain Coffee, Vegetable Broth.
☐ Avoid especially: all animal foods including fish, shellfish, meat-based soups, dairy foods, sweet foods, sweet drinks, fruit, vinegar, tomatoes, beans, mushrooms, ice water.

Uremia

Uremia is a toxic condition that occurs when excessive amounts of urea and other waste products of protein metabolism are retained in the blood. Uremia usually develops gradually but can come on unexpectedly. In its acute state, it is very dangerous. In the beginning, the symptoms include dizziness, ringing in the ears, insomnia, excessive worry, depression, and irritability. If the condition continues further, chronic uremia symptoms are general fatigue, mental disturbance, breathing difficulties, digestion difficulties, loss of appetite, vomiting, and constipation or diarrhea. Chronic uremia may lead to severe uremia, which may result in cramps, and, eventually, in death. Seek proper medical attention in such cases.

According to our macrobiotic understanding, poor kidney function is the main cause of uremia, and one of the main reasons for weakened kidneys is an excess of salt in the diet. However, taking medication or consuming too many foods and drinks that weaken the kidneys and prevent normal urination are also contributing factors.

Helpful Suggestions

OBJECTIVE	REMEDY
FOR THE ACUTE TYPE	
To reduce fever and chills	Try drinking 4 to 8 cups of DAIKON TEA per day for 2 to 3 days. This tea may cause sweating, diarrhea, or vomiting while helping to remove excess toxins from the body.
To improve circulation	Use a MUSTARD POWDER FOOT BATH or cleanse the entire body with MUSTARD POWDER BATH water as a sponge bath until the skin turns red; this helps regenerate the body. *and* Eating ¼ cup of AZUKI BEANS WITH KOMBU once a day, using less salt than usual, is helpful for this condition.
FOR THE CHRONIC TYPE	
To control abnormal urination	Try drinking ½ cup of DAIKON TEA WITH SOY SAUCE 2 times per day until urination becomes normal.
To increase urination	Eat ½ cup of ccoked daikon (boiled or in soup) once a day, every day.
To relieve headache	Wash the head with warm water and MASSAGE the head with GINGER SESAME OIL or APPLE JUICE.

To reduce fever	Apply a TOFU PLASTER on the forehead; change it every hour.
To relieve nausea	Apply a MUSTARD PLASTER to the solar plexus region (see Figure 3.8 on page 176) for 5 to 6 minutes until the skin becomes a red color. Remove this plaster and then apply an ALBI PLASTER for up to 4 hours. Repeat both plasters as often as needed until no longer nauseated.

Dietary Recommendations

Initially, the main food for both acute and chronic cases is Brown Rice Broth. For side-dish vegetables use daikon, scallions, and burdock only until the fever and chills have stopped. Then use the following suggestions until your condition improves or for one month. Later, widen your food choices using a macrobiotic dietary approach (see page 11).

☐ Main foods: Brown Rice Balls, Azuki Rice. Chew each mouthful 200 times. For severe cases, use Brown Rice Cream (thick) with Grated Daikon.

☐ Side dishes (one-fourth of main foods): Sesame Miso, Hijiki Nitsuke, Burdock Nitsuke, Natto with Soy Sauce and Scallions, Okara Nitsuke served with Grated Daikon, Vegetable Tempura served with Grated Daikon, Azuki Beans with Kombu and Winter Squash (2/3–1 cup every day), Eggplant Nitsuke with Miso served with ginger, Cucumber with Kuzu Sauce, Daikon Nitsuke with Homemade Agé, Chinese Cabbage Pickles, Mustard Green Pickles, Watermelon Syrup, Carp Soup.

☐ Miso soup ingredients: daikon, tofu, eggplant, Chinese cabbage, green leafy vegetables.

☐ Beverages: Brown Rice Tea, Brown Rice Bancha Tea, Bancha Tea, Grain Coffee, Azuki Kombu Juice. Don't drink cold drinks; drink warm drinks only.

☐ Avoid especially: all animal food including meat-based soups (except Carp Soup), eggs, dairy foods, sweet foods and drinks, and hot spices.

See also KIDNEY FAILURE.

UTERINE BLEEDING

Uterine bleeding is painful, prolonged, or irregular bleeding through the vagina that is not related to a woman's normal menstrual pattern. There are many causes of uterine bleeding including disorders of the liver, blood cells, lymphatic system, or heart; hormonal imbalances; use of certain drugs; tumors or other problems of the uterus or cervix; and the inability to return to normal conditions after giving birth.

According to our macrobiotic understanding, one cause of uterine bleeding is the overeating of very yang food such as meat, which also produces an overly acidic condition. This results in a yang type of illness. The consumption of very yin food such as sugary foods, fruit (especially tropical), alcoholic drinks, and vinegar, and the use of drugs containing hormones, anticoagulants, or aspirin also lead to an overly acidic condition and cause a yin type of uterine bleeding. Whether yin or yang foods are the initiator, the overly acid condition damages capillary walls, which in turn causes bleeding.

Helpful Suggestions

If you have overeaten both yin and yang foods in the past and are uncertain which type of uterine bleeding you have, use the suggestions for the yin type first. If you bleed after any change in diet, it may be the result of a discharge. You may choose to let it flow for a few days if it is not excessive, but do not let bleeding continue more than three days without treatment. If the bleeding continues for more than three days or if you are concerned about it before then, use the following remedies.

OBJECTIVE	REMEDY
To control bleeding (yang type)	Sip 1 tablespoon of LOTUS ROOT JUICE 1 or 2 times per day until bleeding stops. *and* Drinking ¼ teaspoon CHARCOALED HAIR TEA 3 times per day is effective. This is strongly contracting and should stop the bleeding.
To control bleeding (yin type)	Drink 2 cups of SHO-BAN TEA per day. *and* Eat ½ teaspoon CHARCOALED HAIR with a swallow of water 2 to 3 times per day until bleeding stops.
To alleviate any uterine problem	The most effective treatment for uterine problems is a DAIKON or ARAME HIP BATH for 20 minutes 1 or 2 times per day for 1 week. If your condition is yin, add ⅓ to ½ cup of salt to the hip bath. The best time to take a hip bath is just before going to bed. *and* It is good for a weak person to drink ½ to 1 cup of SHO-BAN TEA before taking a hip bath. Taking hip baths for 1 week should clear up any discharge, and you should feel and smell good. *and* Abstain from sex until your condition improves.

To improve circulation and remove excess toxins	A GINGER COMPRESS applied over the ovaries (see Figure 3.8 on page 176) for 20 minutes followed by an ALBI PLASTER for up to 4 hours is helpful. Repeat both the compress and plaster as often as needed.
To reduce fever	A TOFU PLASTER can be applied to the center of the belly; change it every 1 or 2 hours. *and* If the belly is cold, a ROASTED SALT PACK can be applied on top of the tofu plaster to provide warmth.
To control excessive bleeding during menstruation	At the time of menstruation, there may be hemorrhaging or an abnormally heavy flow of blood. This may result from a tumor or cancer. CHARCOALED HAIR, as used above for bleeding, may be used in this case.

Dietary Recommendations

Use the following dietary suggestions until the bleeding stops or for one month. Then, widen your food choices using a macrobiotic dietary approach (see page 11).

FOR THE YANG TYPE

☐ Main foods: Brown Rice, Azuki Rice, Brown Rice Gruel with Mochi.

☐ Side dishes (one-third of main foods cooked with less salt): Sesame Miso, Hijiki Nitsuke, Shio Kombu, Nori Nitsuke, Wakame Miso Soup, Okara Nitsuke, Carp Soup, Grated Daikon, Boiled Daikon (cut in thick pieces) served with Ginger Miso, Azuki Beans with Kombu, Vegetable Tempura, Cucumber with Kuzu Sauce, Pressed Salad.

☐ Miso soup ingredients: daikon, wakame, tofu, tororo kombu, Chinese cabbage, snow peas, string beans, Green Leafy Vegetables.

☐ Beverages: Brown Rice Tea, Brown Rice Bancha Tea, Sho-Ban Tea, Mu Tea. Drink less.

☐ Avoid especially: all animal protein including fish (except carp), shellfish, eggs, dairy foods, meat-based soups, sweet foods and drinks, and hot spices.

FOR THE YIN TYPE

☐ Main foods: Brown Rice, Millet Rice, Azuki Rice, Fried Rice, all served with a little Gomashio.

☐ Side dishes (one-fourth of main foods): Tekka Miso, Scallion Miso, Hijiki Nitsuke, Vegetable Stew, Vegetable Stew with Fish, Carp Soup, Azuki Beans with Kombu, Shio Kombu, Burdock Carrot Nitsuke, Vegetable Tempura, Deep-Fried Kombu, Nori Roasted with Oil, Takuan Pickles, Miso Pickles.

☐ Miso soup ingredients: wakame, tororo kombu, scallions, onions, Homemade Agé, Brown Rice Mochi.

☐ Beverages: Bancha Tea, Brown Rice Bancha Tea, Sho-Ban Tea, Mu Tea. Drink less.

☐ Avoid especially: all animal foods (except carp), shellfish, red-meat fish, dairy foods (including ice cream), eggs, meat-based soups, sweet foods and drinks, all fruit, potatoes, eggplant, tomatoes, peanuts, all mushrooms, black tea, pressed salads.

UTERINE TUMORS

A tumor is a swelling or a growth of useless cells and tissues. Uterine tumors are often benign (non-cancerous) fibroid growths that show no symptoms other than the growth. Sometimes, however, there is abnormal bleeding during menstruation or slight discomfort when the tumor presses against other organs. Many uterine tumors are cancerous with some 40,000 new cases reported each year.

According to our macrobiotic understanding, tumors, whether cancerous or not, thrive in an overly acidic environment, which can be created by a diet high in protein, especially when combined with a low- or no-salt regime. Thus, the underlying cause of a tumor's growth is the overconsumption of high-protein foods such as animal foods, including dairy products. But, there is another way that the uterus becomes overly acidic. After sexual intercourse, most of the sperm are left in the uterine cavity or around the cervix. These sperm may become acidic and damage the surface of the uterus, the mucous lining of the uterus, or the uterine wall. Also, from the vagina to the ovary there is a 90° curved tube that has a tendency to hold broken eggs (protein) and sperm (protein), leading to an overly acidic condition. This acidic condition can cause tumors and ultimately cancer in the uterus, cervix, and ovaries.

Helpful Suggestions

Many, many women have hysterectomies because of uterine tumors. However, according to our macrobiotic understanding, all parts of the body are useful and should only be removed or altered as a last resort if natural remedies and dietary suggestions do not improve the situation.

OBJECTIVE	REMEDY
To improve circulation	Apply a GINGER COMPRESS on the skin over the uterus (see Figure 3.8 on page 176) for 20 minutes once a day. These compresses may be applied several times per week.
To improve condition	Take a DAIKON or ARAME HIP BATH each night for 20 minutes before sleeping. *and*

A 1-percent SALT BATH for 20 minutes is helpful and may be alternated with the ginger compresses.

To reduce acidity	After sexual intercourse, wash away sperm with warm water. Using a condom avoids the problem.

Dietary Recommendations

Use the following dietary suggestions until your condition improves or for one month. Then, widen your food choices using a macrobiotic dietary approach (see page 11).

☐ Main foods: Brown Rice or Azuki Rice served with a little Gomashio. Chew each mouthful 200 times.

☐ Side dishes (less than one-third of main foods cooked to a less salty taste than usual): a little Tekka Miso, Ginger Miso, Grated Daikon (raw, about 2 tablespoons) with Soy Sauce, Burdock Carrot Nitsuke, Carp Soup, Rice Bran Pickles, Umeboshi.

☐ Miso soup ingredients: daikon, albi, green leafy vegetables, Chinese cabbage, spinach, nigari tofu, eggplant.

☐ Beverages: Brown Rice Tea, Brown Rice Bancha Tea, Bancha Tea, Grain Coffee, Vegetable Broth. Drink a maximum of 2½ cups of beverages per day.

☐ Avoid especially: all animal foods including fish (except carp), shellfish, eggs, meat-based soups; all alcohol; all sweet foods and drinks; fruit; and ice cream.

VAGINITIS

Vaginitis refers to an infection or inflammation of the vagina. There are several forms depending on the causative agent, but all are similar in their symptoms. Symptoms vary between women and from time to time in the same woman. These include an itchy discharge with an unpleasant odor; general vaginal discomfort and pain, especially during sexual intercourse; and a change in vaginal color from pale pink to red. Swelling and burning urination may be present as well.

Vaginitis occurs when germs (organisms) that normally inhabit the vagina multiply and cause infection because the pH and hormone balance in the vagina is upset. (Since one of these organisms is *Candida albicans*, see also Candidiasis.) Bacteria normally found in the rectum, or parasites that enter the vagina during sexual intercourse may also cause vaginitis. Poor health, hot weather, non-ventilating underwear, and any condition that increases moisture, warmth, or darkness in the genital area increase your chances of vaginitis.

According to our macrobiotic understanding, the underlying cause of vaginitis is the overconsumption of fatty foods such as cheese and simple carbohydrates including fruit. People believe that fruit is a good, natural food and that cheese is part of a balanced vegetarian diet. However, fatty foods, especially dairy foods, make the bodily fluids acidic and simple carbohydrates allow bacteria to grow more easily. These conditions create a favorable environment for infections and can result in itchy discharges.

Helpful Suggestions

OBJECTIVE	REMEDY
To relieve discomfort and pain	Use a DAIKON or ARAME HIP BATH for 20 minutes once a day until recovered. If you don't have any daikon or arame, use a SALT-WATER HIP BATH.
	and
	For all cases, showers are preferable to tub baths. Avoid chemicalized and scented soaps. Wearing cotton underwear is a good idea. Also, avoid sitting around in a wet bathing suit or other wet clothing.
To improve condition	After each meal, a drink of UME EXTRACT TEA —made with 3 soybean-sized extract balls with ½ cup warm water—is effective.
	and
	Refrain from sex until your condition improves. Avoiding overexertion, heat, and excessive sweating is also beneficial.
To relieve infection	Mix 1 teaspoon of UME EXTRACT with ⅔ cup of boiling water. Let cool. Soak a tampon in this liquid and insert it into the vagina before going to bed. Leave it in overnight and discard in the morning. Repeat each night until the infection is gone.

Dietary Recommendations

Following a macrobiotic dietary approach (see page 11), avoiding fruit and cheese completely, is most helpful.

VARICOSE VEINS

Varicose veins are permanently dilated and twisted veins, usually in the legs. Symptoms include enlarged, bluish veins visible under the skin when a person is standing, fatigue, aching legs, and a feeling of heaviness in the legs. Varicose veins are the result of the failure of the veins' valves, which help blood return to the heart against gravity. If the valves do not work properly, blood does not drain but accumulates in the veins. Also, weakness of the vein walls can cause varicose veins. Other contributing factors are a lack of exercise and anything that contributes to lack of circulation. Constipation may lead to varicose veins since it often requires straining during bowel movements, and the straining blocks off veins used for the return of blood from the legs.

However, according to our macrobotic understanding, the underlying cause of varicose veins is a diet high in fat, cholesterol, sugar, and fruit, and yin proteins such as tofu, tempeh, and beans without enough salt, miso, or soy sauce. Such a diet causes poor circulation, constipation, and weakness in the veins and in valves inside the veins. When blood in the veins becomes sluggish or slow-moving, swelling results; this is similar to a river's slowing down and becoming wider.

Helpful Suggestions

OBJECTIVE	REMEDY
To reduce vein swelling	Exercise daily and take hot baths or SAUNAS at a temperature of 110° to 115°F once a day. (This is also ideal for those who have high blood pressure.)
To relieve pain	Apply a GINGER COMPRESS on the affected area for 20 minutes. Repeat 3 or 4 times a day if necessary. This will also help improve circulation to the area.
To promote good circulation	Walking is a good daily exercise to help keep the leg muscles and circulation functioning well. Avoid prolonged standing and sitting with your legs crossed. Elevating the legs slightly helps promote good circulation.

Dietary Recommendations

Following a macrobiotic dietary approach (see page 11) without dairy products, fruits, or beans (other than miso and soy sauce) is the most effective way to change this condition.

WARTS

Warts are benign, noncancerous tumors in the outer skin layer. A wart appears as a very small, raised bump on the skin and grows larger. Warts are often found in clusters and are the same color or slightly darker than the surrounding skin. They are painless and don't itch. Warts are contagious both from one area of the body to another and from person to person.

Venereal warts are warts in the genital area. These, like other warts, will probably disappear eventually. However, because they may be a signal of cancer, it is

best to consult with your health-care advisor. Plantar warts are warts that appear on the sole of the feet. These pinhead-sized bumps cause pain when the afflicted person walks.

According to Western medicine, warts are caused by a virus. According to our macrobiotic understanding, warts are the result of overeating animal foods including shellfish, which contain large amounts of phosphorus.

Helpful Suggestions

Be careful with medications for warts, especially if you are pregnant. To avoid spreading warts, don't scratch them.

OBJECTIVE	REMEDY
To remove warts	Use a MOXA TREATMENT once a day for 2 or 3 days. *and* Drinking 1 cup of HATOMUGI TEA 2 to 3 times per day, eating 1 serving of HATOMUGI every other day, or eating 1 serving of BROWN RICE WITH HATOMUGI every day until the warts are gone may be helpful.
To remove plantar warts	Place an 1/8-inch-thick slice of fresh garlic (organic is best) on the sole of the foot with the cut part touching the skin; attach with a bandage. Change periodically and apply until the wart disappears, usually in 3 to 10 days.

Dietary Recommendations

Changing to a macrobiotic dietary approach (see page 11), avoiding all animal foods until the warts are gone, is the best remedy. It is also the best preventative.

WHOOPING COUGH

Whooping cough is a contagious, bacterial infection of the bronchial tubes and lungs. This infection primarily affects infants and children although all ages may be affected. There is a five- to seven-day incubation period, after which the early stages are manifest as a runny nose, a slight fever, and a dry cough that eventually produces a thick sputum. After coughing for one to two weeks, a person starts coughing so severely that when a breath is taken, it produces a whooping sound. Periodic attacks last from two to three weeks. There may also be diarrhea and fever. This can be a very serious infection in the first six months of an infant's life. The condition climaxes with periodic sudden attacks that are so long and fierce that the cougher turns blue and vomits.

The cause of whooping cough is considered to be infection by the bacteria, *Bordetalla pertussis*. The disease may be transmitted by direct or indirect contact with contagious persons. Immunizations are recommended by health professionals and are credited with greatly reducing the incidence of whooping cough throughout the world. While many doctors recommend immunizations, there are many others who do not. In my opinion, immunizations are not natural and are harmful to the body's immune system. In other words, injecting an animal's antibody into human beings causes a degeneration contrary to the natural biological order. The macrobiotic approach always seeks to follow the natural order rather than to oppose it. On the other hand, if you are not committed to following the natural order and to ensuring that your children eat well, immunizations should be thoughtfully considered. Consult with your health-care advisor if you decide to be immunized and if you are pregnant or plan to become pregnant within three to four months of immunization.

According to our macrobiotic understanding, the real cause of this sickness is the poor condition of the child's immune system, which in turn is caused by the mother's unbalanced diet of too much yin food such as sugary foods and drinks, milk and other dairy products (other than salted cheeses), and fruit; or too much yang food such as meat, chicken, fish, eggs, and cheese.

Helpful Suggestions

OBJECTIVE	REMEDY
To relieve mild cough	Drink any of the following 2 or 3 times a day: ½ to 1 cup of *LOTUS ROOT TEA*, ½ cup of *WINTER SQUASH AND WALNUT TEA*, 1 tablespoon of *DAIKON JUICE WITH RICE SYRUP*, ½ cup of *BLACK SOYBEAN TEA*, or 1 tablespoon of *DAIKON SEED COUGH DRINK*.
To relieve severe cough	Try drinking ½ cup of *BROWN RICE TEA WITH LOTUS ROOT AND SHISO LEAVES* or *BROWN RICE TEA WITH KUMQUAT LEAVES* 2 to 3 times per day. *and* Use a GINGER SESAME OIL MASSAGE on the throat when coughing.
To relieve nursing babies	If a nursing baby gets whooping cough, the mother should drink the teas listed above.
To maintain energy and a more alkaline condition	Avoid hot baths; use sponge baths only.

Dietary Recommendations

Use the following dietary suggestions until your condition improves or up to two months. Then, widen your choices using a macrobiotic dietary approach (see page 11).

☐ Main foods: Brown Rice Balls with Gomashio, Azuki Rice, Brown Rice Gruel with Mochi, Fried Rice, Brown Rice Cream. Take one small bite at a time and chew well. Parents should teach their children to do this. If there is a lot of vomiting, try a diet of Brown Rice Balls served with Gomashio only until this condition improves.

☐ Side dishes (one-third of main foods): Tekka Miso, Hijiki Lotus Root Nitsuke, Burdock Carrot Nitsuke, Vegetable Tempura, Azuki Beans with Kombu.

☐ Miso soup ingredients: wakame, scallions, onions, dried daikon, Brown Rice Mochi.

☐ Beverages: Brown Rice Tea, Brown Rice Bancha Tea, Grain Milk, Kuzu Bancha Tea.

☐ Avoid especially: all fruit, sweet foods and drinks, tomatoes, eggplant, cocoa, tofu, potatoes, all beans (except azuki), salads, all dairy (including ice cream).

PART THREE

EXTERNAL REMEDIES

INTRODUCTION

Part Three—External Remedies—provides details about the major uses of the remedies that appear in SMALL CAPITAL LETTERS in Part Two. Some of the remedial techniques discussed here are based upon practices that are thousands of years old. Although these remedies use foods, herbs, and spices that Western medicine may not commonly use, the techniques and ingredients have been used for generations in both the East and West.

Heat therapy, for instance, is frequently used to control pain and is often applied through *compresses*. Moist heat relaxes tense areas, soothes inflamed areas, and draws toxins from infected areas. Hip (sitz) *baths* increase blood flow to the pelvic and abdominal areas and are, therefore, commonly used by health-care professionals to treat such ailments as cystitis, hemorhoids, and prostate problems. *Massage* is so well-recognized a technique that it is defined in the *Signet/Mosby Medical Encyclopedia* as the manipulation of soft tissue of the body to increase circulation, improve muscle tone, and relax the patient.

Still, people at our residential macrobiotic Vega Study Center frequently ask such questions as, "Why do we use ginger compresses to relieve pain? Why do we use albi plasters in cases of cancer? If foods have healing power, why do we need these external remedies? If these techniques are effective, do we still need a good diet? And if so, which is more important?" You also may have these questions and may be interested in learning the relationship between external remedies and diet.

According to our macrobiotic understanding, healing power originates in our body's homeostasis, our ability to maintain healthy internal conditions. This ability, improved and passed down through millions of years of mankind's evolution, is achieved by natural eating and drinking as described in Part One. The most natural healing, then, is returning to a natural diet and letting the body's healing power effect a cure.

Sickness will be cured by simply following a natural, healthy diet if the sickness is not too advanced and if the body's digestion, assimilation, elimination, and immunity are not damaged too much. In these cases, we often experience discomfort such as pain, swelling, itching, etc. This discomfort shows us that our healing power is not so strong. Thus, external remedies are used to relieve discomfort while the healing process is proceeding.

The external remedies in Part Three are all made of natural materials and can be prepared in your home without the danger of adverse side effects so often associated with synthetic drugs and over-the-counter preparations. It is important to understand and remember that these remedies do not cure diseases. However, they are helpful in the healing process.

APPLICATIONS

Topical applications of many different substances can be used for therapeutic reasons. These applications range from the juice of plant tissues to various food products. Actually, compresses, packs, plasters, and certain treatments may also be considered applications. (See these sections for more information.) Here, we refer to those substances that are applied directly to the skin, providing a covering over an affected area. Secure with a bandage if needed (see Figure 3.1).

BANCHA TEA LEAVES APPLICATION

These leaves are useful for insect stings or bites. Chew 1 teaspoon of leaves long enough to thoroughly mix the leaves with saliva. Cover the insect sting and surrounding area with the chewed leaves. Green tea leaves may be used if you can't find bancha tea leaves.

BURDOCK SEEDS APPLICATION

Burdock seeds are useful for skin infections such as boils. Chew a small amount of seeds so that they are thoroughly mixed with saliva. Place the chewed seeds directly on boils to help open the boils and allow them to drain.

CRAB WATER APPLICATION

Crab water is useful for poison oak or ivy rash. Boil a fresh crab in several cups of water. Remove the crab; dip a cotton cloth in the remaining water and use it to pat the skin of the affected areas.

GINGER SESAME OIL APPLICATION

This can be used in a variety of ways from putting one drop inside the ear for adult ear infections to covering insect bites. Ginger sesame oil is also used as a massage, spinal treatment, and special ear treatment. Grate 1 to 2 teaspoons of fresh ginger with a fine Japanese grater. Squeeze the juice into a small bowl and add an equal amount of sesame oil. Pure dark sesame oil is preferred.

GREEN LEAFY VEGETABLES APPLICATION

These are useful for arthritis pain or facial pain resulting from any skin infection. Take any kind of dark-green

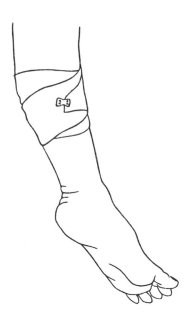

Figure 3.1 Securing the application with a bandage

leafy vegetable such as kale, collards, mustard greens, or any wild plant and chop fine. Place directly on the affected area and secure with a bandage if needed. Change to new greens after about 2 hours or when the old greens have become dry.

GREEN LEAVES APPLICATION

Applications of green leaves are used most often in conjunction with tofu plasters for fever or headache relief. They are also useful for persistent pain or swelling of a finger infection, in severe cases of frostbite, or for unconsciousness due to fainting. The leaves of any green leafy vegetable such as kale, collards, mustard greens, or any wild plant can be used directly on an affected area. For cooling relief from fever, the greens may be placed at the back of the neck while lying down. Secure with a bandage if needed.

LOTUS ROOT JUICE APPLICATION

This juice is useful to help clear nasal passages blocked by a sinus infection or nostrils obstructed by excess mucus. Finely grate fresh lotus root and squeeze out the juice (see Figure 3.2). Soak a small piece of cotton in this juice and insert the cotton into the nostrils for 30 minutes at a time or overnight.

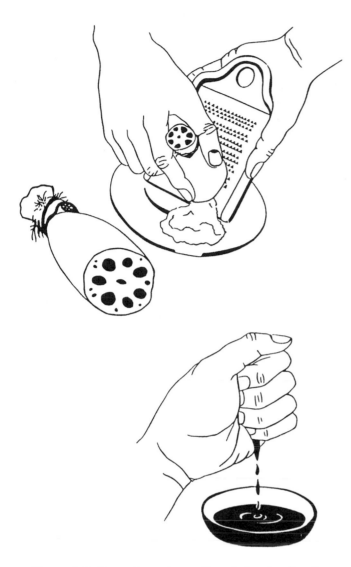

Figure 3.2 Preparing a Lotus Root Juice Application

MUSTARD POWDER APPLICATION

This is useful for pain resulting from dental caries. Mix ¼ teaspoon mustard powder with ½ teaspoon of warm water. Mix well to remove all the lumps and add 2 more teaspoons of warm water. Strain through a cotton cloth. Soak a cotton ball in this juice and place into the nostril on the side of the face where you are experiencing tooth pain.

TOFU APPLICATION

Applications of tofu are useful for skin abscesses, for pain from burns, and when acne flares up. Any kind of tofu will do for topical applications. Put tofu in a cotton cloth, fold up the corners, and squeeze (wring) out the water.

The tofu will become like mush. For burns, use immediately. For nonemergency skin problems, grind tofu in a suribachi until it becomes more firm again. Apply directly on the affected area and secure with bandages if needed.

BATHS

A bath refers to a medium in which the body is wholly or partly immersed or with which the body is cleansed. The medium may vary from water or liquid that is mostly water to vapor, sand, or mud. The hip bath, also called a sitz bath, is a special bath used for therapeutic purposes and is listed in its own section (see pages 181–182). The bath medium may also be used as a sponge bath. In this case, cleanse the body by dipping a washcloth in the medium and rubbing the body with it. Frequently rinse and redip the washcloth in the medium.

ARAME BATH

Arame Baths are useful to help increase circulation, remove excess salt, and afford relief from poison oak or ivy rash. They are also useful for controlling diarrhea resulting from enteritis. Arame Baths and Daikon Baths are interchangeable in all cases. Bring 20 cups of water to a boil and add 8 cups of arame. Simmer for 20 minutes and shut off the heat. Strain and place the arame water in a bathtub. Add enough warm to hot water to cover your belly when you are lying down in the tub.

With Grated Ginger

This is useful to help reduce fever resulting from malaria. After straining the arame water, add a small cotton bag containing ⅔ cup of freshly grated ginger. Let it sit for 5 to 10 minutes. Squeeze the bag with chopsticks or other utensils. Add arame water with ginger (including the bag) to your bath.

With Mustard Powder

This is useful to improve circulation, especially in cases of leprosy. After straining the arame water, add ⅓ cup of mustard powder to the bath.

With Salt

This is useful to improve circulation, especially in cases of leprosy. Add ⅓ cup of salt along with the 8 cups of arame.

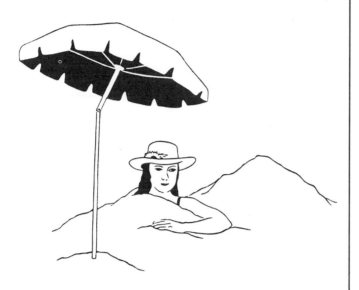

Figure 3.3 Sitting in a Sand Bath

BEACH SAND BATH

Sand Baths are useful for helping to remove toxins from the body, especially in cases of food or heavy metal poisoning, and to strengthen the kidneys. For this remedy, you bury yourself in the sand for several hours at a time. Do not eat or drink anything for several hours before burying yourself. Take a small amount of water, a shovel, and an umbrella or head-tent to a sandy beach (near saltwater is best). Dig a pit as long as the distance from your buttocks to your toes and as deep as the distance from your buttocks to your neck. Pile the removed sand within arm's reach. Line the pit with some of the warm surface sand. Position the umbrella so that your head will be shaded. Sit in the pit and cover all but your head, shoulder, and one arm with 4 inches of sand (see Figure 3.3). Stay in as long as you feel comfortable. Bathe in the ocean, lake, or river for at least 10 minutes after getting out of the sand. Then, take a hot bath to keep warm.

CEDAR LEAVES BATH

This remedy is useful for pain or swelling in the hands or feet. In these cases, immerse only your hands or feet in the cedar leaves water. Take about 2 cups of young cedar leaves and bring them to a boil in 7 cups of water. Simmer 20 minutes. Remove the leaves and let the water cool slightly so that you don't burn yourself.

CHESTNUT LEAVES BATH

A bath of chestnut leaves is useful for poison oak or ivy rashes, skin abscesses, itchy skin, or other skin disorders. Boil about 2 handfuls (5–6 cups) of chestnut leaves in 16 cups of water until the water turns brown (about 20 minutes). Place this water in a bathtub and add enough warm to hot water to cover your belly when you're lying down in the tub, or use as directed in Part Two under the appropriate disorder. You may use fresh leaves or dried ones; however, fresh leaves or those that have dried in the shade will be more effective than those that have dried in the sun. If you do not have chestnut leaves, use pine needles, oak leaves, or any strongly alkaline leaves that turn dark brown in color when boiled.

DAIKON BATH

Daikon Baths are useful to help increase circulation, remove excess salt, and relieve itchy skin, especially in cases of poison oak or ivy rash. They are also useful for controlling diarrhea resulting from enteritis. Daikon Baths and Arame Baths are interchangeable in all cases. First, dry daikon greens; cut the greens off the daikon and hang them outside in a shady place until they are dry (turn brown). (See Figure 3.4.) Drying takes about 1 week in a hot, dry climate. Bring about 10 cups of dried daikon greens to a boil in 20 cups of water. Simmer over low heat for 20 minutes. Turn off the heat; strain and place

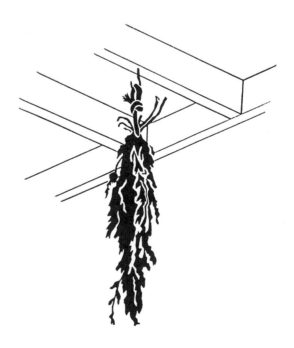

Figure 3.4 Drying daikon greens

this water in a bathtub. Add enough warm to hot water to cover your belly when you are lying down in the tub.

With Grated Ginger

This is useful for skin abscesses and to help reduce fever from malaria. After straining the daikon water, add a small cotton bag containing 1/2 cup of freshly grated ginger. Let sit for another 5 to 10 minutes. Squeeze the bag with chopsticks or other utensils. Add daikon water with ginger (including the bag) to your bath.

With Mustard Powder

This is useful to improve circulation, especially in cases of leprosy. After straining the daikon water, add 1/3 cup of mustard powder to the bath.

With Salt

This is useful to improve circulation, especially in cases of leprosy. Add 1/3 cup of salt along with the 10 cups of dried daikon greens.

GINGER BATH

Ginger Baths are useful for relieving itchiness and other skin disorders, improving circulation, helping to remove old salts from the body, relieving frostbite, and helping to remedy night sweating. Use Ginger Baths for adults only. Bring 20 cups of water to a boil and shut off the heat. Finely grate about 2/3 cup of ginger and tie it up in a cheesecloth bag. (Use more ginger if it is old or if you want a stronger bath.) Put the bag into the hot water. After a couple of minutes, squeeze the bag with chopsticks or other utensils so that all the ginger juice is expelled into the hot water. Place this water in a bathtub and add enough warm to hot water to cover your belly when you're lying down in the tub.

GINGER FOOT BATH

Ginger Foot Baths are good for blood circulation, kidney disorders, and insomnia. They are useful for cooling the head in cases of sunstroke because they pull circulation away from the head and toward the feet. Prepare water as for the Ginger Bath (above) and use it as a Water Foot Bath (see page 174).

MUSTARD POWDER BATH

Mustard Powder Baths are useful for improving circulation. Bring 24 cups of water to a boil and add 2/3 cup of mustard powder. Simmer for a few minutes and then

place this water in a bathtub. Add enough warm to hot water to cover your belly when you're lying down in the tub.

MUSTARD POWDER FOOT BATH

Mustard Powder Foot Baths are good for improving circulation, and in cases of sunstroke, they cool the head by pulling circulation away from the head and toward the feet. Prepare water as for the Mustard Powder Bath (see above) and use it as a Water Foot Bath (see page 174).

PEACH LEAVES BATH

Peach Leaves Baths are especially good for dandruff, prickly heat, and ringworm on the scalp or face. Put one handful of peach leaves into 8 cups of water. Bring to a boil and simmer for 20 minutes. Strain and use this water as a sponge bath.

PINE NEEDLES BATH

Pine Needles Baths are especially good for dandruff and for ringworm on the scalp or face. Put one handful of pine needles into 8 cups of water. Bring to a boil and simmer for 20 minutes. Strain and wash your hair with this water or use as a sponge bath.

RICE BRAN BAG

The Rice Bran Bag is very useful in the event of skin problems because the rice bran gives natural oil to the body whereas soap usually takes natural oil from the skin, leaving the body colder. Make or purchase a cotton bag 2 inches by 4 inches. Put 2 heaping tablespoons of rice bran in the bag. Tie the bag (see Figure 3.5) and soak it in hot water for a few minutes until white juice comes out. Scrub your skin with the bag. The bag may be reused if it is emptied and washed between uses.

RICE BRAN BATH

Rice Bran Baths are useful for itchy skin due to chicken pox and for other skin problems. Put 5 cups of rice bran in a cotton bag and place the bag in 20 cups of water. Bring to a boil and simmer for a few minutes. Squeeze the Rice Bran Bag with chopsticks or with other utensils so that all the juice is expelled into the hot water. Place this water in a bathtub and add enough warm to hot water to cover your belly when you're lying down in the tub. Use the Rice Bran Bag to gently rub your body.

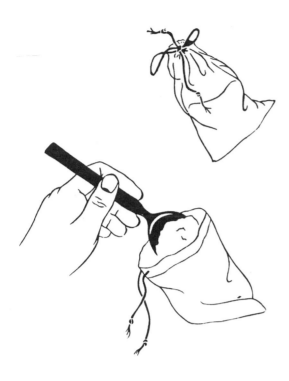

Figure 3.5 Preparing a Rice Bran Bag

SALT BANCHA EYE BATH

This bath is useful for improving the blood circulation in the eyes, reducing swelling and protruding eyes, and relieving eye inflammation. Add 1/3 teaspoon salt to 1 cup warm Bancha Tea (100° to 104°F). Take a large cotton ball and soak it in the warm tea. Use the ball to swab the eye from the inside corner to the outside corner of the eye (see Figure 3.6), wash the eyelid, and then hold the cotton on the eyelid and apply slight pressure for about 10 minutes.

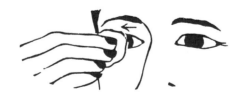

Figure 3.6 Placing a cotton ball on the eye for a Salt Bancha Eye Bath

SALT BANCHA NASAL BATH

This bath is useful for clearing nasal passages and stopping nosebleeds. Add 1/3 teaspoon salt to 1 cup of Bancha Tea. The tea can be room temperature or slightly warmer (100° to 104°F). Hold the left nostril shut and snort a handful of salted Bancha Tea into the right nostril. Pus and mucus will come out. Hold the right nostril shut and snort a handful of salted Bancha Tea into the left nostril. Continue until the nasal passages are clear or until all the tea is used.

This remedy can also be used for ear infections by soaking a small piece of cotton in the salted Bancha Tea and placing the cotton inside the ear.

SALT BATH

Salt Baths are very useful for improving the condition of the kidneys, correcting mineral imbalances in the body, removing excess toxins or poisons, and relieving pain, insomnia, worry, or other stressful conditions. Add 1 pound of any kind of salt (we use the least expensive available) to 12 gallons of bath water. (One pound of salt in 12 gallons of water makes a 1 percent salt bath. Salt baths can be varied by changing the amount of salt used. Do not use less than a 1 percent solution.) Any comfortable temperature of water may be used. Sit in the tub for 20 minutes or longer unless you have a weak heart. In this case, stay only a short time, and if your heart starts beating faster, get out of the bath immediately.

SALTWATER BATH

Cool Saltwater Baths are useful for burns. Mix salt and water in the proportion of 1/4 teaspoon of salt to 1 cup of boiling water. Let cool and then immerse the affected area in this water.

WATER FOOT BATH

Hot foot baths are good for blood circulation, kidney disorders, insomnia, and cold feet resulting from diarrhea. Boil enough water to cover your feet and put the water in a big pan. Being careful not to burn them, carefully place your feet in the pan for about 10 minutes, You might try putting one foot in at a time for a brief time until the water cools a bit or until you are accustomed to the hot water.

BREATHING EXERCISE

This Breathing Exercise is useful for anemia and insomnia. Extra oxygen in the lungs helps create more red blood cells and a better quality of blood. Sit on a chair or on the floor. Keep your backbone straight. Slowly exhale through the mouth, pushing in your abdomen. Then quickly inhale through the nose, pushing abdomen out. Repeat 5 or 6 times.

You can do this exercise before sleeping, while lying in bed. Inhale lots of oxygen to aid in sound sleep. Give appreciation for the air, the oxygen, and the end of the day. Give thanks for a lack of trouble during the day.

Sleeping is important because during sleep all diseases recover naturally. There is no aggression, no ego desire during sleep. Such sleep can create peace and health. A macrobiotic diet helps you to have a good sleep, short but deep.

CHARCOALED TREATMENTS

Charcoaled substances are prepared in a special manner for therapeutic reasons. They may be eaten, drunk, or used as applications. To make charcoaled foods, fill an unglazed ceramic flower pot (saucer needed) one-third full of the food you wish to charcoal. Cover the top edge of the pot with pie dough, then place the saucer on top to seal the pot (see Figure 3.7). Leave the pot in an oven set to a high temperature until the pot starts to smoke.

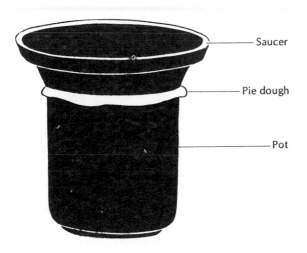

Figure 3.7 Sealing of ceramic pot with pie dough

Turn the oven to medium, about 350° to 400°F. Cook 1 hour and remove from the oven. Shake the pot and if the contents sound dry, they are done. If the contents sound wet, then bake them longer. Completely cool the pot before opening it or black ashes will form. Remove the contents and grind them into a fine powder. All charcoals are very yang, so make sure to grind them very finely.

CHARCOALED HAIR

Charcoaled Hair is useful to control bleeding. Men's hair is used for female bleeding, especially in childbirth. Women's hair is used to stop bleeding in men. Completely wash hair (don't use scented shampoo or conditioner) to remove dirt and excess oil. Cut hair and charcoal it as directed (see above). Swallow ½ teaspoon of charcoaled hair with a little water 2 to 3 times per day until bleeding stops.

CHARCOALED HAIR TEA

This tea is also useful for bleeding. Mix 1 teaspoon of charcoaled men's hair in ½ teaspoon of water and drink. In cases of bleeding, drink ¼ teaspoon several times per day until the bleeding stops.

CHARCOALED KOMBU

Charcoaled Kombu is useful for tooth pain. It can be added to Kuzu Bancha Tea and is good for tonsillitis or sore throat pain. Mix Charcoaled Kombu with roasted salt, 3 to 1, for tooth pain.

CHARCOALED KOMBU WITH LOTUS ROOT POWDER

This powder is useful to help control asthma. Mix 7 parts of lotus root powder with 3 parts Charcoaled Kombu and use as directed under the appropriate disorder.

CHARCOALED MULBERRY BARK

Charcoaled Mulberry Bark is useful to help promote hair growth. Charcoal a small amount of mulberry bark and/or roots and mix with an equal amount of sesame oil. Apply to the scalp.

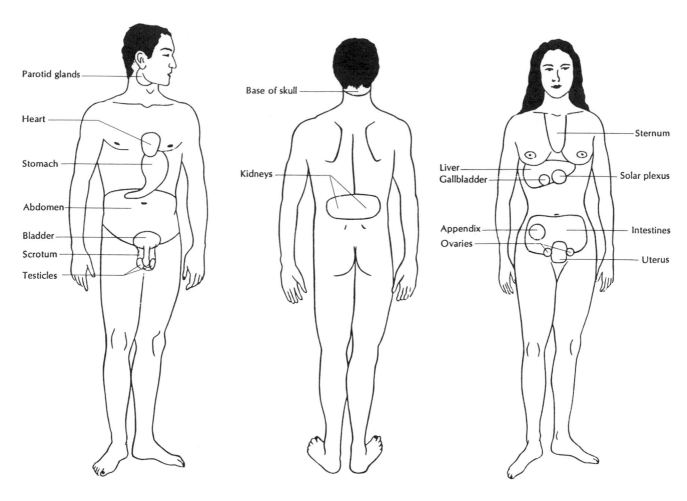

Figure 3.8 Parts of the human body: front view of male body on left, back view of male or female body, center; front view of female body, right

CHARCOALED UMEBOSHI

Charcoaled Umeboshi is useful for diarrhea and stomach cancer. Charcoal umeboshi plums and use as directed in Part Two under the appropriate disorder.

CHARCOALED UMEBOSHI TEA

This preparation is good for reducing fever due to a cold and swelling due to laryngitis. Mix ¼ teaspoon of charcoaled umeboshi with ½ to ¾ cups of boiling water. Drink as directed in Part Two under the appropriate disorder.

COMPRESSES

A compress refers to a pad of folded cloth (linen or cotton), moistened with hot or cold liquid, and applied to the skin to help relieve discomfort by providing heat, cold, pressure, etc. Compresses are used to help bring circulation to a particular area of the body (see Figure 3.8). The Ginger Compress is most helpful in relieving pain and is used for almost any painful condition except in cases of breast cancer where swelling may be a problem. (See the section on Breast Cancer for more information and alternatives.) Because the Ginger Compress is so useful, it is wise to purchase a fine Japanese grater and to always keep a good supply of fresh ginger or know where it can be found quickly.

To use a compress, first prepare the liquid to be used. Using an enamel pan will yield the best results; stainless steel is next best. Then, dip a hand towel (cotton or linen) or other cloth into the liquid and squeeze the excess back into the pan. If the liquid is hot, you will need to wear rubber gloves. Otherwise, you may try folding the towel in half several times lengthwise. Hold each end of the towel by the fingers of each hand and lower it into the pan so that the ends do not become wet. Squeeze out excess water by twisting the towel from the ends (see Figure 3.9). This takes some practice but is useful if rubber gloves are unavailable or are not desired. Cover the compress liquid if it has been heated so that it will maintain its heat.

Before applying the hot towel to the affected area, place a thin, dry cotton cloth (room temperature) over the area. If the hot towel is too hot, cool it by briefly swinging it back and forth before applying it over the thin, dry cloth. As the liquid is used, it becomes less hot and as succeeding towels are applied the skin becomes used to the heat so that eventually the towels are applied directly from the liquid to the affected area. Cover hot, soaked towels with dry towels to help keep the area warm.

Apply newly dipped towels, whether heated or not, every few minutes for about 20 minutes, until the area is red, until the pain is gone, or as directed in Part Two under the appropriate disorder. One method is to use two alternating towels, having one soaking in the pan of liquid while the other is applied to the skin. Or, you may use the same towel over and over by redipping it in the liquid every few minutes.

ARAME COMPRESS

Arame Compresses are useful for improving circulation and relieving rheumatism pain. Bring 10 cups of water to a boil and add 4 cups of arame. Simmer for 20 minutes and shut off the heat. Strain. Use this water as the compress liquid.

With Grated Ginger

This is useful as a substitute for the Daikon Ginger Compress. After straining the arame water, add a small cotton bag containing 1/3 cup of freshly grated ginger. Let sit for 5 to 10 minutes. Squeeze the bag with chopsticks or other utensils. Use this water as the compress liquid.

BANCHA TEA EYE COMPRESS

This compress is useful for relieving mild eye pain, especially in cases of corneal diseases. Add 1/3 teaspoon salt

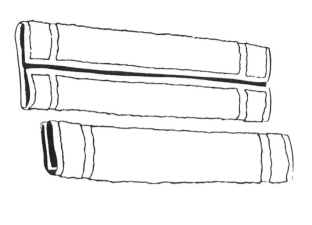

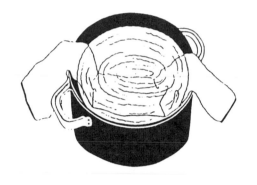

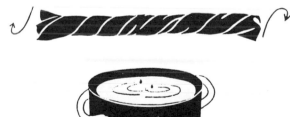

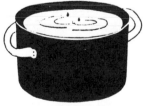

Figure 3.9 Preparing a Hot Towel Compress

to 1 cup warm to hot Bancha Tea (warmer than 98.6°F). Take a cotton ball and soak it in the tea. Place the wet cotton ball over the closed eyelid and swab the eye from the inside corner to the outside corner of the eye. Wash the eyelid and then use the cotton ball as a compress by holding it against the eye for 10 minutes. Soak a new cotton ball and treat the other eye if needed.

CASTOR OIL COMPRESS

Castor Oil Compresses are useful for diverticular pain and as a follow-up for body pain when Ginger Compresses aren't effective. Heat 2 to 4 cups (or the amount needed) of castor oil such that the oil is not too hot to touch. Saturate 2 to 4 layers of heavy flannel by dipping them in the oil. Wring out the flannel cloths and apply these directly on the affected area. Place oilpaper or a dry cloth over the layers of flannel and apply dry heat such as a Roasted Salt Pack (see page 187) on top. Leave the pack on the body for an hour or so. Then, cleanse the body with a weak baking soda solution. Castor Oil Compresses may be used daily for several hours at a time but should not be used during periods of menstruation.

DAIKON GINGER COMPRESS

Daikon Ginger Compresses are helpful in relieving itchiness, improving circulation, controlling skin abscesses, and reducing swelling or pain. If you have no daikon, try a Ginger Compress (see below) or an Arame Compress with Grated Ginger (see page 177). Add 3 to 4 bunches of dried daikon greens to 16 cups of water and bring to a boil. Simmer over low heat for 20 minutes. Shut off heat and strain the water. Put ⅓ cup grated ginger in a cheesecloth bag, tie it up, and put it in the hot water. Squeeze the bag with chopsticks or another utensil to get all the ginger juice out of the bag and into the water. Use this water as the compress liquid.

GINGER COMPRESS

The Ginger Compress is used for any kind of pain. The Ginger Compress works because the blood circulation is improved, bringing fresh oxygen to the painful area. If Ginger Compresses do not alleviate the pain and none of the other alternatives listed under the appropriate disorders is effective, try a Castor Oil Compress (see above). Ginger Compresses are also useful for strengthening the kidneys, reducing swollen organs, removing excesses and blockages, and relieving numbness and itchiness.

To prepare a Ginger Compress, bring 10 cups of water to a boil, then shut off the heat. Put ⅓ cup of grated ginger in a cheesecloth bag, tie it up, and put it in the hot, not boiling, water (see Figure 3.10). If the ginger is boiled, it loses its effectiveness. The amount of ginger used will vary slightly according to the size of the person's body—use more for a larger person and less for a smaller per-

son or child. Also, if the ginger is old, use a little bit more. Squeeze the bag with chopsticks or another utensil to get all the ginger juice out of the bag and into the water. Use this water for your compress. You may reheat the water and use it again for up to 24 hours. Be careful not to bring the ginger water to a boil.

When using a Ginger Compress on some areas (such as over the kidneys), it is best to lie down. In these cases, having a support person applying the towels so that you can relax fully is extremely helpful. If you don't have the luxury of a second person to apply the towels for you, position the pan and towels next to you so that you don't have to get up and run to the stove when changing towels. A heating pad is useful for this purpose.

With Saké or Rubbing Alcohol

This is useful for severe coughing. Add 1 cup of saké or rubbing alcohol to the Ginger Compress water and use as the compress liquid.

With Salt

This is useful for severe nerve pain. Use only on the body and not on the head. Add 1 tablespoon of salt to the Ginger Compress water at the same time you add the ginger and use as the compress liquid.

HOT TOWEL COMPRESS

This compress is useful for easing cramps, clearing blocked nasal passages, and temporarily relieving fainting, unconsciousness, or a concussion. Bring 10 cups of water to a boil. Soak a towel in this water and make a compress to apply over the affected area.

Alternating Hot Towel Compress

This compress is useful for relieving leg cramps. Soak a towel in cold water and apply to the affected area as a compress for 1 minute. Bring 10 cups of water to a boil. Soak a second towel in the hot water and apply as a compress for 2 minutes. Repeat, alternating a cold towel for 1 minute and a hot towel for 2 minutes as long as needed.

OIL COMPRESS

Oil Compresses are useful for burns. Take a cotton cloth, soak it in any kind of cooking or edible oil (unheated), and cover the affected area with this cloth as a compress.

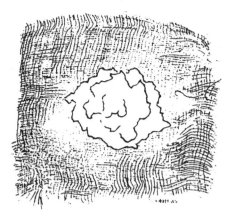

1. Put ⅓ cup of grated ginger in a cheesecloth bag.

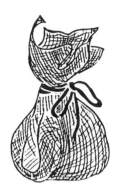

2. Tie the bag.

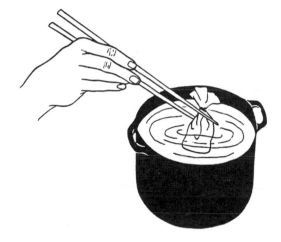

3. Place the bag in hot water.

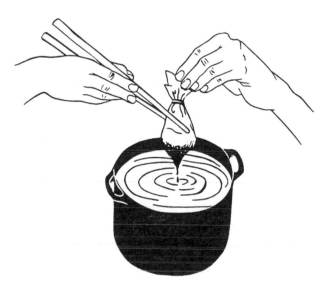

4. Squeeze the bag to get the ginger juice into the water.

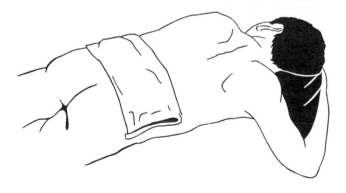

5. Use the water to prepare a compress that will be placed on the painful area.

Figure 3.10 Preparing a Ginger Compress

RICE BRAN COMPRESS

Rice Bran Compresses are useful for itchy skin and bed sores. Put 4 handfuls of rice bran in a cotton bag and place the bag in 3 quarts of water. Bring to a boil and simmer for 20 minutes. Shut off the heat and let cool slightly. Use the liquid for a compress. The bag may be used as a Rice Bran Bag (see page 173).

UME EXTRACT COMPRESS

This compress is useful for nonpoisonous snakebites. Mix 1 tablespoon Ume Extract and 1/4 teaspoon of salt with 1 cup of cold water. Soak a hand towel in this liquid and apply as a compress on the bite or affected area.

WARM TOWEL COMPRESS

This compress is useful for insomnia. Heat 12 cups of water to a warm (not hot) temperature. Soak a hand towel in this water and use it as a compress on the head and/or the back of the neck.

ENEMAS

Usually constipation is remedied with food such as Azuki Beans with Kombu or Green Leafy Vegetables with Homemade Agé. However, some conditions, such as emergency cases, require a faster method and in these cases, an enema of warm water may be used, but only once. To administer the enema, follow the directions on the enema syringe package.

PYRETHRUM TEA ENEMA

This enema is useful for ridding the body of pinworms. Add 1 cup of pyrethrum flowers and stems to 3 cups of water and bring to a boil. Simmer 20 minutes. Strain and let cool so that it's not too hot. Use 1 cup of this tea for an enema.

UME EXTRACT TEA

This enema is useful for pain due to colon cancer. Mix 1 teaspoon of Ume Extract with 1/2 cup of water. Administer it deeply with a syringe. Hold the Ume Extract water in for about 10 minutes by lying on your back with your knees on your chest. After 10 minutes, go to the bathroom and then lie down for a while longer.

FASTS OR FASTING

There are many variations on fasting. For complete fasting you need an experienced guide; otherwise, it can be very dangerous. Perhaps strong people can undertake complete fasting for a quick cleansing, but what does this do to a person's inner acid and alkaline balance? Sometimes fasting can make you weak; however, you sometimes need to cleanse your body by eliminating old stools or you want to improve your thinking. In such cases, we recommend the following macrobiotic fasts.

BROWN RICE BALL FAST

The Brown Rice Ball Fast is useful in cases of nervous system malfunction. Eat only Brown Rice Balls with Gomashio plus 3 slices of Takuan Pickle as a way of partial fasting. Eat 2 times a day, using a total of 1–1 1/2 cups of cooked rice per day. Do this for 2 weeks if your condition allows it.

MACROBIOTIC FASTING

This fast is useful for cleansing the body, improving thinking, and clearing up skin disorders. Use thin (watery) Brown Rice Cream, Brown Rice Gruel, Buckwheat Cream, or a cream made from any kind of grain. Eat only 2 to 3 bowls per day, chew well, and keep physically active. Try the fast for 7 days, if possible. The body still makes hemoglobin, which it does not do during complete fasting, and there is less fatigue. Old stools are eliminated.

Breaking the macrobiotic fast must be done carefully. The intestines will have become like those of a baby, and it is best to eat soft foods like baby food. Some people become so hungry after a fast that they are tempted to eat solid foods right away; this can tear the intestines. Eat progressively thicker rice (or other) cream. If you have trouble with the macrobiotic fast for 7 days, you can do shorter fasts more often, say once a month.

GARGLES

To gargle is to use a solution to rinse or medicate the mucous membranes of the throat by forcing air in an agitating manner through the solution while it is in the throat. Warm salt water is often used for general gargling purposes.

BANCHA TEA WITH SALT GARGLE

This gargle is useful for sore throats and throat swelling. Add ½ teaspoon of sea salt to 1 cup of hot Bancha Tea and gargle.

DENTIE WATER GARGLE

This gargle is useful for tonsillitis. Mix ¼ teaspoon of dentie powder with 1 cup of hot water and gargle.

LOTUS ROOT TEA GARGLE

Lotus Root Tea Gargle is useful for loss of voice. Use the adult proportion of Lotus Root Tea for gargling whether to be used by adults or children.

SHO-BAN TEA GARGLE

This gargle is useful for tonsillitis. Add ⅔ cups of boiling Bancha Tea to 1 teaspoon of soy sauce and gargle.

UME EXTRACT GARGLE

This gargle can be used to kill the bacteria on the tonsils. It is especially useful in the case of scarlet fever. Mix 1 part Ume Extract to 30 parts hot water.

HIP BATHS

A hip bath, also called a sitz bath, is a special therapeutic bath in which you soak your hip area in a tub of water with daikon, ginger, arame, mustard powder, and/or salt. The hip-bath water is placed in a big wash basin (big enough to sit in) that is usually placed in your bathtub or shower. Hip baths are especially good for bladder problems, skin diseases, and female disorders. Daikon hip baths are so popular with macrobiotic persons that many people grow their own daikon in order to have the best-quality organic greens to dry and later use for hip baths.

To take a hip bath, start by preparing the water using the desired ingredients. Put this liquid in a wash basin or tub and add enough hot water so that when you sit in the tub, the liquid covers your hip bones. Sit in this tub with your hands and feet outside the tub. If the room is cold, cover your upper body and legs with a large towel or blanket (see Figure 3.11). When you start to sweat or after 15 to 20 minutes, dry off and keep warm by going to bed. Hip baths are most effective taken immediately before going to sleep. If you take a hip bath during the

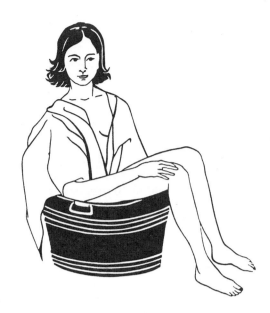

Figure 3.11 Sitting in a Hip Bath

day, rest for at least 30 minutes to an hour before becoming active.

ARAME HIP BATH

Arame Hip Baths are good for skin diseases such as itchiness and for anal pain, bladder inflammation, menstrual cramps, ovarian or uterine problems, and other female disorders. A Daikon Hip Bath may be used in place of an Arame Hip Bath if daikon is unavailable. Add 4 cups of arame to 10 cups of cold water. Bring to a boil and simmer for 20 minutes. Shut off heat and add ¼ cup salt. Strain and let sit for 5 to 10 minutes before using arame water as a hip bath.

With Grated Ginger

This is useful for relieving diarrhea, stomach and sciatica pain, and numb legs, and for balancing bodily hormones. After straining the arame water, add to the hip bath a small cotton bag containing 3 tablespoons of grated ginger. Let it sit for 5 to 10 minutes. Squeeze the bag with chopsticks or other utensils. Use the water (including the bag) for a hip bath.

With Mustard Powder

This is useful for severe diarrhea due to enteritis, and for tuberculosis of the intestines, and leg cramps from cholera. After straining the arame water, add ⅓ cup of mustard powder to the hip bath.

181

Daikon Hip Bath

Daikon Hip Baths are good for skin diseases such as itchiness, and for anal pain, bladder inflammation, menstrual cramps, ovarian or uterine problems, and other female disorders. If daikon is unavailable, an Arame Hip Bath may be used in place of a Daikon Hip Bath. The greens from 1 daikon are considered to be 1 bunch. Some grocery stores cut off the greens and throw them away, so perhaps you can purchase some inexpensively. Hang the greens to dry in the shade for 1 to several weeks.

To prepare the hip-bath liquid, bring 7 bunches of dried daikon greens (about 8 cups) to a boil in 15 cups of water and simmer for 30 to 60 minutes until the water is dark brown in color. Then, add 1/4 cup of salt and shut off the heat. Strain and let the water sit for 5 to 10 minutes before using as a hip bath.

With Grated Ginger

This is useful for relieving diarrhea, stomach and sciatica pain, and numb legs, and for balancing bodily hormones. After straining the daikon water, add to the hip bath a bag containing 3 tablespoons of freshly grated ginger. Let it sit for 5 to 10 minutes. Squeeze the bag with chopsticks or other utensils. Use the water (including the bag) for a hip bath.

With Mustard Powder

This is useful for severe diarrhea from enteritis, and for tuberculosis of the intestines, and leg cramps from cholera. After straining the daikon water, add 1/3 cup of mustard powder to the hip bath.

Ginger Water Hip Bath

This hip bath is useful for diarrhea, and for stomachaches from enteritis or children's dysentery. Bring 10 cups of water to a boil and shut off the heat. Finely grate about 1/3 cup of ginger and tie it up in a cheesecloth bag. Use more ginger if it is old or if you want a stronger bath. Put the bag into the hot water. After a couple of minutes, squeeze the bag with chopsticks or other utensils so that all the ginger juice is expelled into the hot water.

Mustard Powder Hip Bath

This hip bath is useful for diarrhea and stomachaches from children's dysentery. Bring 12 cups of water to a boil and add 1/3 cup of mustard powder. Turn off the heat and let the water sit several minutes.

Saltwater Hip Bath

This hip bath is useful for pain and other symptoms of vaginitis, endometriosis, or uterine tumors. Add any kind of salt to hot water in the proportion of 1/2 pound of salt to 6 gallons of hot water.

Juices

"Juice" refers to the fluid from plant tissue. Juice is often obtained by chopping various leaves finely, then grinding them in a suribachi, and finally squeezing out the liquid. It is quicker to use a blender, adding a little water before blending; however, the juice is not as strong (effective) as when you use the slower manual method. In this section, juice is used as a drink. Juices of plants can also be used as applications, massages, and special treatments.

Burdock Juice

Burdock Juice may be helpful for appendicitis, scabies or infestation with mites, phlegm in the throat, and meat poisoning. Finely grate burdock root with a Japanese grater and squeeze out the juice. Drink as directed in Part Two under the appropriate disorder.

Daikon Juice

Daikon Juice is useful for tension headaches and food poisoning from Udon Noodles. Finely grate daikon and squeeze out the juice. Drink as directed in Part Two under the appropriate disorder.

With Rice Syrup

This juice is good for relief of coughing (including whooping cough), and for asthma attack, headaches, and hoarseness. Add 1 to 2 tablespoons of rice syrup to 1/3 cup of Daikon Juice and drink.

With Rice Syrup and Ginger

This drink is good for improving circulation. Add 1 to 2 tablespoons of rice syrup and 1/2 teaspoon of ginger juice (obtained by finely grating and squeezing fresh ginger) to 1/3 cup of Daikon Juice and drink.

With Spring Water

This variation is good for children's swollen throat glands, especially in cases of esophageal stricture. Mix equal amounts of Daikon Juice and pure spring water and drink. If pure spring water is unavailable, use the best-quality water you can find.

LEEK JUICE

Leek Juice is useful for poisonous bites and food poisoning from crab meat. Chop and grind leeks in a suribachi or blender and squeeze out the juice. Drink as directed in Part Two under the appropriate disorder.

LOTUS ROOT JUICE

This juice is useful for asthma attacks, uterine bleeding, and coughing up of blood due to tuberculosis. Finely grate fresh lotus root and squeeze out the juice. Then add a pinch of salt. Drink as directed in Part Two under the appropriate disorder.

RICE SYRUP JUICE

This juice is useful for coughs, especially during cases of the measles. Use a 2-inch-thick piece of daikon that is about 1½ inches in diameter, quarter it vertically, and cut each quarter into eight ¼-inch-thick pieces (32 pieces in all). Put these pieces into ½ cup of rice syrup. About an hour after adding the daikon, a juice will appear on the top of the syrup. Skim off the juice and drink as directed in Part Two under the appropriate disorder.

SCALLION JUICE

This juice is useful for asthma attacks, uterine bleeding, and coughing up of blood due to tuberculosis. Chop and grind scallions (or wild scallions) in a suribachi or blender and squeeze out the juice. Drink as directed in Part Two under the appropriate disorder.

SOUR APPLE JUICE

Sour Apple Juice is useful for helping control diarrhea, slowing a pulse that is too strong, and reducing a high fever, especially a child's fever. Grate ½ of a sour apple and squeeze out the juice. Add 2 or 3 drops of lemon juice and drink as directed in Part Two under the appropriate disorder.

Sour Apple Juice can be used in place of Daikon Ginger Tea to reduce fever in children who don't like the tea. Grate ½ of a sour apple and give it to the child to eat. Grate the other half, squeeze out the juice, mix it with 2 or 3 drops of lemon juice and give this to the child to drink. If the fever is 102°F or more, the apple juice should be given raw. If the fever is below 102°F, lightly boil the apple juice before giving it to the child.

SWEET UMEBOSHI JUICE

This juice is helpful for children's diarrhea. Mix 1 teaspoon of ume zu, 2 drops of ginger juice (obtained by finely grating and squeezing fresh ginger), and ½ teaspoon of rice syrup with 2 tablespoons of boiling water. This juice should be drunk as directed in Part Two under the appropriate disorder.

MASSAGES

Massage refers to the systematic therapeutic manipulation of the body by friction, stroking, and kneading to help stimulate circulation and make muscles or joints supple. Massages in this book involve lightly rubbing an affected area with a therapeutic substance. (The substances that are worked into the skin or hair in massages are also sometimes used as applications.) To give a massage, put the substance on your fingers and rub the affected area with your fingers or palms for 3 to 5 minutes. Repeat as needed.

APPLE JUICE MASSAGE

Apple Juice Massages are useful for relieving headaches from any cause. Finely grate an apple and squeeze out the juice. Massage this juice into the scalp.

CHLOROPHYLL JUICE MASSAGE

Chlorophyll juice is especially useful for all yang skin diseases such as dry eczema. The juice can be derived from various greens and vegetables such as parsley, daikon greens, carrot leaves, endive, turnip greens, Swiss chard, spinach, scallion greens, spring chrysanthemum, mustard greens, pine needles, persimmon greens, mugwort, chickweed, plantain, goosefoot, or shepherd's purse. Use 4 to 5 different kinds of greens, always including parsley if possible. Chop fine and grind in a suribachi or use a blender. Squeeze out the juice and use as a massage on the affected area.

DAIKON JUICE MASSAGE

A Daikon Juice Massage is especially good for headaches. Finely grate daikon and squeeze out the juice. Massage this juice into the scalp.

EGGPLANT SULFUR MASSAGE

This massage is useful for removing red birthmarks. Put a small amount of sulfur in a shallow bowl and add enough rubbing alcohol to cover. Mix and let sit overnight. Mix again. Then, take an eggplant and cut off a section near the stem such that the surface area of the cut eggplant is about 2 inches in diameter. Dip the cut surface in the yellow sulfur water and rub the skin with it, using the stem to hold the eggplant. When the skin is dry, dip the eggplant in the sulfur water and rub the skin with it again. Repeat a third time.

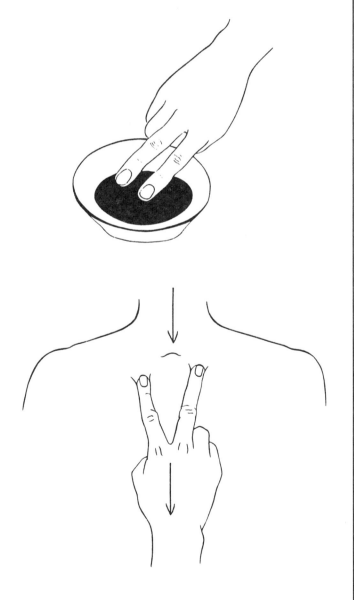

Figure 3.12 Giving a Ginger Sesame Oil Massage

GINGER SESAME OIL MASSAGE

A Ginger Sesame Oil Massage can be used for a variety of symptoms including hair loss, ear trouble, headaches, dandruff, rheumatism or other pain, skin diseases, numbness, and crooked spine. (For a crooked spine, see also Ginger Sesame Oil Spinal Massage.) Grate about ¼ cup fresh ginger with a fine Japanese grater. Squeeze the juice into a small bowl and add an equal amount of sesame oil. Pure dark sesame oil is preferred. Use as a massage on the affected area.

GINGER SESAME OIL SPINAL MASSAGE

This massage is useful for helping correct any curvature of the spine. Grate 1 to 2 teaspoons of fresh ginger with a fine Japanese grater. Squeeze the juice into a small bowl and add an equal amount of sesame oil. Pure dark sesame oil is preferred. Put ginger sesame oil on the index and second fingers. With one finger on each side of the spine, massage down the spine for about 30 minutes at a time (see Figure 3.12).

PINE NEEDLE SCALP MASSAGE

This treatment helps promote hair growth. Bundle pine needles together to form a brush 1 inch in diameter. Stimulate the scalp by lightly poking it with the pine needles (see Figure 3.13). Sometimes the scalp may bleed slightly at first, but the skin will become stronger as you continue for short periods each day. Use new pine needles daily.

RICE BRAN MASSAGE

This massage is used for very severe cases of frostbite. Put 4 handfuls of rice bran in a cotton bag and place it in 3 quarts of water. Bring to a boil and simmer for 20 minutes. Shut off the heat and let cool slightly.

In the case of frostbite, after the area has warmed gradually, the rice bran water is used to make a compress (see page 180) that is applied around the frostbitten area and not directly on it. Gently massage the surrounding area with the towel each time you change towels. After applying the last towel, leave the bran water on the skin until it has dried. (The soft rice bran from the cotton bag may be used as well.) Then, wash with plain, warm water and gently pat the skin dry.

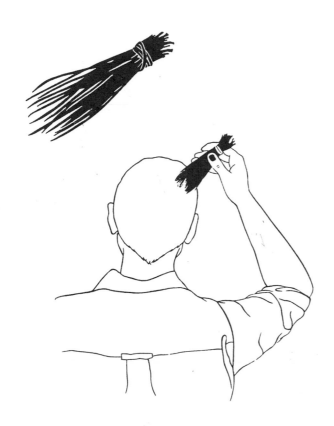

Figure 3.13 Massaging the scalp with pine needles

STOMACH MASSAGE

This massage (see Figure 3.14 on page 186) is effective in relieving constipation and diverticular pain, and in eliminating stagnant stools. Those interested in enhancing the effects of a change in dietary habits may do this massage every morning.

To start, lie on your back in a relaxed position with the soles of your feet flat on the ground about 18 inches from your buttocks. There are four parts to this exercise.

Step 1

1. Beginning at the solar plexus (the center of the stomach just under the rib cage) with the hands bent at a 90° angle to the body and the back of the fingers together, push in slowly as you exhale.
2. Then inhale, move the fingers one inch lower, and push in slowly as you exhale.
3. Continue in this manner moving down the body, skipping the belly button, until you reach the pelvic bone. There will be 5 to 6 places in which you push at one-inch intervals.

Step 2

1. Next, imagine a clock (circle) with the solar plexus as 12:00 and the pelvic bone as 6:00 with 3:00 and 9:00 just inside the rib cage on both sides.
2. Bend the left hand as in part I and hold the left wrist with the right hand. Beginning at 12:00, push in slowly until your little finger touches the skin.
3. Move in a clockwise direction down the left side of your body until you reach 6:00.
4. Then, reverse the hands so that the left hand holds the right hand and push down on the left side of the body in a counter-clockwise direction, moving from 12:00 to 6:00.
5. Repeat for a total of 3 times in each direction.

Step 3

1. Next, position the heel of the right hand just under the rib cage at about 10:30.
2. Push in while moving the heel of the right hand toward the lower left side of the circle (4:30).
3. Then, pull against the skin while pushing down with your fingers as you return to the original (10:30) position.
4. Repeat 10 times, pushing with the heel and pulling with the fingers.
5. Change to the left hand and push downward with the heel of the left hand and pull back with the fingers for a total of 10 repetitions going from 1:30 to 7:30 and back.

Step 4

1. Next, place the right hand flat on the stomach at 12:00 and put the left hand on top of the right hand.
2. Gently push in while rotating around the clock in a clockwise direction 30 times.

A good time to do this exercise is in the early morning before eating or at night before sleeping. It is best not to have eaten for at least 3 hours before doing this massage.

VINEGAR MASSAGE

This massage is useful for skin discolorations and for helping to remove red birthmarks. Take a good-quality vinegar, heat it slightly, and then rub it on the affected area with a cotton cloth.

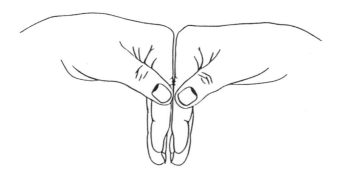

1. Bend your hands at a 90° angle to your body (Step 1).

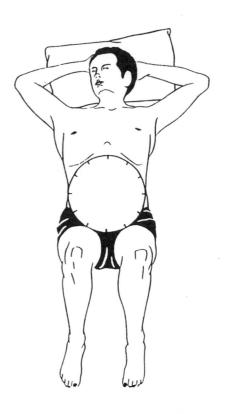

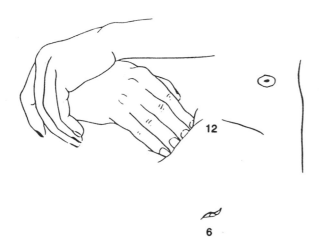

2. Imagine your body is a clock (Step 2).

3. Reverse the position of your hands and move them in a counter-clockwise direction (Step 2).

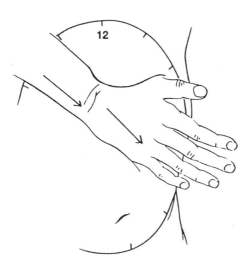

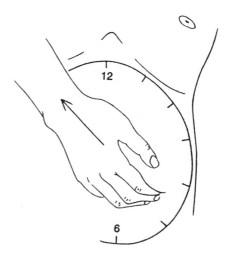

4. Push in, moving the heel of your right hand to the lower left (Step 3).

5. Pull against your skin while pushing down with your fingers (Step 3).

Figure 3.14 Giving a Stomach Massage

PACKS

Packs are similar to plasters but a more firm substance is used and is usually wrapped in cotton or put into a cotton bag and then applied.

ROASTED SALT PACK

Roasted Salt Packs are often used on top of plasters to help keep them warm during their use. They are also useful for warming the body—especially the stomach—increasing circulation, and relieving pain. Roast 1 cup of salt in a dry frying pan until it is very hot. Put it in a cotton bag with a tie (long, heavy cotton socks work very well) and let it cool a little so it does not burn the skin. Tie the bag or socks and place on the area being treated. Repeat as necessary.

PLASTERS

A plaster refers to a pastelike mixture spread on a cloth and applied to the body, or applied directly on the skin without a cloth, to provide relief or to help remove toxins from the body. Among macrobiotic followers, use of an Albi Plaster is the most popular way to help remove toxins from the body; the Tofu Plaster is most often used to help reduce fever and to alleviate headaches and other head problems.

ALBI PLASTER

Albi plasters are used to help remove excess toxins and alleviate pain. They are used mostly on the body but may be used on the head in special circumstances as directed in Part Two under the appropriate disorders. Albi Plasters are also useful for severe or persistent coughs, swelling, and sore throats. The Albi Plaster is usually applied after a Ginger Compress.

To prepare the plaster, use white, not red, albi. Peel the albi and discard the skin. Finely grate the albi; mix in freshly grated ginger to equal 10 percent of the albi. Grated albi is very wet so it needs to be mixed with flour until it is the consistency of an earlobe; use approximately the same amount of unbleached white flour as albi and ginger. Place this mixture about ½-inch thick on cotton flannel and apply to the affected area or apply the mixture directly onto the skin as directed under the appropriate disorder. Secure with a gauze bandage. Albi

absorbs toxins so an Albi Plaster can be used only once. If your condition is not so serious, you may leave the plaster on overnight. However, for a serious illness such as cancer, apply a new Ginger Compress followed by a new Albi Plaster every 4 hours.

If albi is out of season or if you cannot find it, any kind of dark green vegetable leaves such as spinach, chard, kale, or mustard greens along with potatoes will do. Chop the vegetable leaves very fine. Add a little grated potato (⅓ the amount of green vegetable). Mix the green vegetable and potato with a little ginger. If you do not have fresh ginger, use ginger powder, adding enough water to make it as close to the consistency of grated ginger as you can. Or use black or white pepper instead of the ginger powder. Add white flour until the mixture is earlobe consistency. Spread this mixture ½-inch thick on a piece of cotton flannel and apply as with albi. It takes longer for this plaster to remove toxins than it takes an Albi Plaster.

In order to have albi available all year, you may want to make dried albi-plaster-powder. Dry albi and ginger in the shade. Then, grind each separately to a fine powder and mix 9 parts albi with 1 part ginger. Keep this ready to make Albi Plasters by adding a green vegetable juice (see the directions for making juice on page 182) and flour to the powder to make a plaster of earlobe consistency and applying as above.

APPLE PLASTER

An Apple Plaster is useful for headaches, migraine headaches with low fever, and heart palpitations. Finely grate an apple and spread it ½-inch thick on a piece of cheesecloth. Apply to the head or to the affected area as directed in Part Two under the appropriate disorder.

BUCKWHEAT PLASTER

This plaster helps remove excess water and toxins from the body and is useful for reducing swelling and relieving pain. A Buckwheat Plaster is often used before an Albi Plaster because an Albi Plaster is ineffective if there is too much water in the body. Buckwheat Plasters are especially effective for conditions of the bladder and surrounding areas.

To make a Buckwheat Plaster, mix 4 cups of buckwheat flour with about 9 cups of hot water. Adjust the amount of water to make a pastelike consistency. Spread the buckwheat mixture about 1-inch thick on a cotton-flannel cloth. To apply the plaster, place the cloth so that the buckwheat touches the skin. If using the plaster over the belly button, place a piece of paper over the belly button so the plaster does not enter it. On top of the

Buckwheat Plaster, place a Roasted Salt Pack (see page 187). This will keep the Buckwheat Plaster warm for about an hour. Apply a new hot salt pack after 1 hour to keep the plaster warm for another hour (total of 2 hours).

With Salt

This plaster is useful for relieving arthritis pain. Add 2 teaspoons of sea salt to the Buckwheat Plaster, mixing thoroughly. Increase the recipe if necessary to produce enough plaster to cover all the painful places. Apply as you would a Buckwheat Plaster.

CARP PLASTER

The Carp Plaster is used mostly to reduce fever and is also effective to help relieve congestion in pneumonia. Use the meat from as fresh a carp as you can find. Grind the meat and add a bit of flour. Cover the carp mixture with aluminum foil, plastic wrap, or wax paper. Leave on the chest area (all the way around the front and back) until the body temperature returns to normal. If carp is unavailable, you may try hamburger or other fatty meat in the plaster.

DAIKON PLASTER

A Daikon Plaster is useful for heart diseases, flu, mumps, rectal prolapse, and syphilis. Finely grate daikon and spread it 1/2-inch thick on a piece of cheesecloth or wrap it in a cotton cloth. Apply to the affected area as directed under the appropriate disorder.

With Ginger

This is useful for ringworm on the body from the neck down. Mix 1 tablespoon of grated ginger with 2 cups of freshly grated daikon. Wrap in a cotton cloth and apply to the affected area.

GREEN PLASTER

This plaster is good for sprained ankles or similar accidents, eardrum pain, or inhibited breast-milk flow. Use any kind of dark-green vegetable. Chop and grind finely in a suribachi or blender. Mix 9 parts vegetable to 1 part dried and crushed peppermint leaves and a little unbleached white flour to make a pastelike consistency. Apply to the painful area.

MISO PLASTER

This plaster is useful for constipation. Spread barley, soybean, or rice miso 1/3-inch thick on a cotton-flannel cloth. Put 4 layers of wax paper or a piece of cardboard over the belly button so that the miso does not enter it. Apply the plaster to the abdomen with the miso side touching the skin for about 20 minutes at a time.

MUSTARD PLASTER

This plaster is useful for yin heart diseases, sore throats, chest colds, or other chest pain. It is a very quick and effective way to get the circulation going. The Mustard Plaster is also used to draw blood away from the head, to help one regain consciousness, and to relieve cramps or nausea. Mix equal amounts of dried mustard powder and white flour with warm water until a pastelike mixture forms. Put this mixture on a cheesecloth and roll up the cloth. Do not let the Mustard Plaster mixture touch the skin as it will burn. Apply to the area being treated until the skin becomes red. Do not leave the plaster on too long.

RICE PLASTER

This is a traditional Japanese remedy for twisted ankles and bruises since it helps remove stagnated blood. It is also useful for body odor. Cook either white or brown rice by any method. If you use brown rice, cook it until the skins are broken. Cool the rice to room temperature. Cover a cotton-flannel cloth with a 1–1 1/2-inch thick layer of rice. Apply to the affected area. When the rice becomes spoiled (turns yellow or smells funny), change the plaster. If the skin becomes itchy, remove the plaster and massage the area with sesame oil.

SALT PLASTER

This plaster is useful for those suffering from a sore throat or sore tonsils. Mix 2 cups of sea salt with 5 to 6 tablespoons of water (room temperature) so that the salt is only slightly damp, not wet. For children, use 1 cup of sea salt and 2 to 3 tablespoons of water. Put the salt in the center of a rectangular kitchen towel and roll the towel along the longer side. Wrap the towel around your neck and place a clean dry towel over it (see Figure 3.15). Apply before sleeping and leave on overnight. In the morning, all the salt will be dry.

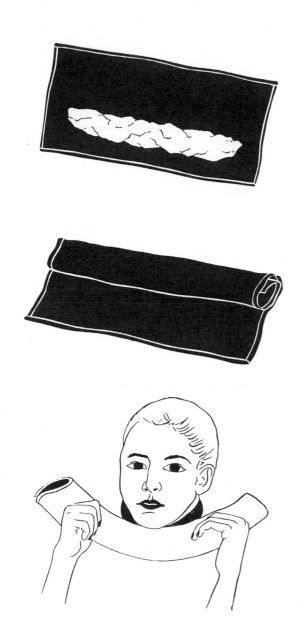

Figure 3.15 Preparing a Salt Plaster

TOFU PLASTER

Tofu Plasters are used to reduce fevers, to help a person regain consciousness, and to relieve pain, especially head pain. They provide cooling relief and are used anywhere there is too much heat on the body or head. Use any kind of commercial tofu. It is often sold in 1–pound blocks; if so, cut it into 3 or 4 pieces. Squeeze out water from the tofu blocks by applying weight; a block may, for instance, be squeezed between two cutting boards. Mash the tofu. Next, mix tofu with grated ginger in the

proportion of 1 tablespoon of ginger per 8 ounces of tofu and add a little unbleached white flour until the mixture becomes sticky. Then, put the tofu mixture in cheesecloth and apply about 3/4-inch thick to the affected area. For fevers, apply to the forehead. The tofu will become yellow after a while. Change the plaster every 2 to 3 hours, or when the tofu becomes hot or yellow in color. Change more often in cases of high fever or when used on the chest. For cerebral hemorrhage in cases where help is unavailable, shave the head and apply a 1 1/2-inch-thick Tofu Plaster to the entire head.

UMEBOSHI EYE PLASTER

This plaster is useful for glaucoma, corneal diseases, bloodshot eyes, and trachoma. Glaucoma can be improved in one month using this plaster every night. Grind umeboshi, including the pits, and add a little white flour to make a paste. For bloodshot eyes or eye infections, apply a thin layer of umeboshi paste on a piece of rice paper; cover the eyes with the paper so that the umeboshi paste does not touch the eyes. Cover the eye plaster with an eye bandage to hold it in place.

Rice paper is best to use; however, if you don't have any rice paper, put a double layer of paper towel over the eyes; spread the umeboshi paste on a paper towel. Place the paper towel with the umeboshi paste on it on top of the double layer of toweling. (There will be 3 layers of paper towel between the eye and the umeboshi paste.) Cover with a bandage.

UMEBOSHI PLASTER

This plaster is used for tension headaches, sprains, and arthritis or rheumatism. Grind umeboshi, including the pits, and add a little white flour to make a paste. Apply to the affected area.

- For headaches, put a thin layer of umeboshi paste on rice paper and apply to the temples.
- For sprains, apply umeboshi paste 1/4-inch thick over the area that is sprained. Cover with a cotton-flannel cloth. Leave the paste on until the pain has lessened.
- For arthritis or rheumatism, apply umeboshi paste to the painful area and cover with cheesecloth or rice paper. Secure with a bandage. The umeboshi helps take out excess heat so the pain will be lessened.

UMEBOSHI SAKÉ PLASTER

This plaster is useful for pain from bone marrow diseases. Open about 10 umeboshi pits, remove the kernels, and grind them in a suribachi. Cover with saké in the proportion of 2 to 3 tablespoons of saké per tablespoon of ground umeboshi kernels. Mix well. Then, add enough white flour so that the umeboshi-saké mixture will keep its shape when put on the body but not so much that the paste is hard. Spread this on a cotton-flannel cloth or rice paper and apply to the affected area. Change the plaster 3 to 4 times per day.

SAUNA (FAR-INFRARED)

The relationship between fat and degenerative disease is becoming more and more understood. In order to prevent or cure degenerative diseases, it is very important to reduce fat intake. The trouble is that most people living in modern civilized countries already have deposits of excess fat in their bodies. The question is, therefore, how can we eliminate these old deposits of fat in our tissues? This is where the sauna comes in.

Below 104°F, fat is insoluble in water. This means that at our normal body temperature, the fat deposits in our bodies cannot be dissolved in the blood or in the intercellular or intracellular fluids. This is a significant problem because we cannot eliminate fat deposits from our tissues, organs, and blood stream unless we can dissolve the fat.

The Scandinavian peoples invented the sauna, a very good way to reduce fat deposits caused by the overconsumption of cheeses and other fatty foods. The Scandinavian sauna, however, raises the temperature to 200°F, which is too high for people whose hearts are weak.

In answer to this problem, Tadashi Ishikawa, a ceramics manufacturer and inventor in Japan, invented a sauna that uses very long-wave far-infrared radiant heat. Since this sauna employs the very low end of the infrared spectrum, it causes the user to sweat at temperatures just under 150°F, a temperature that is much safer for the aged and for people with weak hearts. In addition, the heat of Mr. Ishikawa's sauna penetrates 2 to 4 inches beneath the skin and can melt fat deposits there because it is produced by the very long-wave portion of the far-infrared spectrum.

Another important benefit of this sauna is that it helps the body discharge heavy metals. When fat is discharged as sweat, the fat contains such metals as cadmium, mercury, nickel, lead, etc., which cannot be discharged by the kidneys or the lungs. These metals—which enter our bodies by way of chemical fertilizers, food processing, herbicides, and insecticides—are poisonous to us. The far-infrared sauna's ability to help us eliminate these substances is very advantageous to us.

After extra fat is eliminated, blood circulation will increase, leading to increased general health and particularly to improved heart conditions (including high blood pressure) and strengthened kidneys. For these reasons we recommend that you take saunas, especially saunas that use long-wave far-infrared heat.

TREATMENTS

Listed here are special therapeutic uses of foods (uses other than eating) for the ears, eyes, mouth, and skin.

DENTIE POWDER TREATMENT

This treatment is useful for relief from canker and cold sores. Mix dentie powder with enough saliva to form a pastelike material. Apply directly on cold sores or fever blisters in the mouth. For ongoing pain, use your index finger to gently rub dentie powder into the gums and teeth twice a day.

GINGER SESAME OIL EAR TREATMENT

This ear treatment is useful for ear infections, ringing in the ears, and pain from a ruptured eardrum. In cases of ruptured eardrum, the ginger may be omitted. In either case, use this treatment for adults only. Grate 1 to 2 teaspoons of fresh ginger with a fine Japanese grater. Squeeze the juice into a small bowl and add an equal amount of sesame oil as juice. Pure dark sesame oil is preferred. Bring to a boil. Filter through a sterilized cotton bandage and let cool. Apply only 1 drop into the ear using an eye-dropper.

MOXA TREATMENT

A Moxa Treatment is useful for removing warts and controlling bed-wetting. Roll a small piece of moxa 1/2 the size of a grain of rice for a child and the size of a whole grain for an adult. Place on the skin of the area to be treated. Take a stick of lit incense (see Figure 3.16) and heat the moxa with the burning end. Brush the moxa off before it burns the skin. Repeat using 5 pieces for a child and 10 for an adult or use as directed in Part Two under the appropriate disorder.

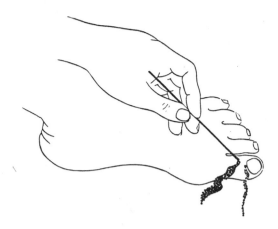

Figure 3.16 Administering a Moxa Treatment

SESAME OIL EYE TREATMENT

This treatment is useful for all eye problems such as swelling, pain, and infections. It helps improve the circulation around the eyes. Before sleep, put 1 drop of sterilized, organic sesame oil in the eyes in the following manner: Sterilize the oil by heating it up and staining it through a piece of sterile cotton. Dip the pad of your ring finger in the heated oil and rub gently around the edge of the eye allowing the oil to enter the eye slowly. (Putting a drop of heated oil directly in the eye may sting and cause temporary blindness.) Or, 1 to 2 drops of breast milk from a macrobiotic mother may be placed in your eyes before sleep.

WOOD ASH FACIAL TREATMENT

This treatment is useful for facial pain from a skin infection. Use 2/3 cup wood ashes, 1 egg white, and enough water to make a thick pancake-batter mixture. Apply a layer to the infected area on the head and face and leave on until dry. Rinse it off and pat the area dry. Reapply more of the mixture for up to a total of 3 times per treatment.

WOOD ASH WATER TREATMENT

This treatment is useful for itchy skin, swollen gums, and mouth pain from dental caries, canker sores, cold sores, or periodontal disease.

- For pain in the mouth, place 1/4 cup natural wood ashes in a bowl. Cover with 3/4 cup boiling water. Mix and let the ashes settle to the bottom. Pour the clear water on top into another bowl and add a teaspoon of salt. Hold this ash water in the mouth a few minutes and then rinse with plain water. Rest. Again hold the ash water in the mouth for a few minutes and rinse. Repeat several times for pain relief.

- For skin problems, put 2 tablespoons of wood ashes in a pan and mix with 8 cups of boiling water. Let this mixture settle. Take the clear water from the top and rub the affected area with this liquid. Let it dry on your body, then take a shower or wash the ash water off with a cloth. The treatment can be done at any time but is most effective before bedtime so that it works while you sleep.

191

PART FOUR

RECIPES

INTRODUCTION

The healing powers of certain foods have been recognized since ancient times. The ancient Romans thought that mushrooms gave warriors great strength. The reishi mushroom was first on the list of ancient Chinese medicines. Hippocrates, known as the Father of Modern Medicine, wrote, "Food should be our medicine and our medicine should be our food." He recognized and taught that foods and drinks have varying effects—some are laxative or binding, some are drying or moisturizing, some are astringent, some are diuretic.

Today, American health-care professionals acknowledge the benefits of fiber, fish oils, bran, and many other foods. However, just as these foods are partial foods, so is the modern dietary approach a partial one. On the other hand, the macrobiotic approach is a holistic one that begins with whole foods—namely, whole grains. Whole grains provide vitamins, minerals, and fiber, and are a slow-burning and long-lasting source of energy. They are ideal complex carbohydrates, which nutritionists today highly recommend as the basis of a healthful diet.

The macrobiotic recipes in Part Four are those used for therapeutic reasons and referred to in Part Two under "Dietary Recommendations." In Part Four, each recipe includes a listing of the main disorders for which it is useful. Still, knowing which foods and condiments to choose for healing is only the first step. How these recipes are prepared is of at least equal importance. Therefore, until you have learned macrobiotic cooking, follow the recipes in this section very carefully. Also, reread the section on the proper selection, preparation, and consumption of foods within a macrobiotic dietary approach (see pages 11–12). See the Suggested Readings on pages 249–250 for macrobiotic cookbooks that will provide more information on daily macrobiotic cooking.

We cannot emphasize enough that it is not specific foods that cure specific illnesses. Rather, it is the total effect of natural eating and drinking that corrects our homeostasis and allows our natural healing power to maintain a natural, healthy condition. However, eating and drinking these foods while eliminating the foods and drinks listed under "Avoid especially" in Part Two, does improve the body's healing power and makes the transition from sickness to health more smooth. Most of these preparations may also be used in a daily macrobiotic dietary approach.

MAIN FOODS

Whole grains and grain dishes are considered main foods by those following a macrobiotic dietary approach. The recipes listed here are used as main foods for therapeutic reasons. Pressure-cooked Brown Rice (or other grain) is recommended in most cases. Boiled grain is useful for very yang conditions, for those living in yang climates (hot and dry), and whenever a change is desired. See the Brown Rice (Boiled) recipe for instructions on boiling other grains.

AZUKI MILLET RICE

Preparation time: 15 minutes   *Yield:* 7–8 servings
Soaking time: 5 hours
Cooking time: 45 minutes
Standing time: 15 minutes

Azuki Millet Rice is useful specifically with excessive fatigue, hunchback, and the yin types of arthritis and rheumatism.

> 4 cups brown rice
> 2/3 cup azuki beans
> 1 cup millet
> 6 cups water
> 1/2 teaspoon sea salt

1. Wash rice, beans, and millet separately. Leave millet in a strainer to dry.
2. Soak rice and beans together in 6 cups water for 5 hours or overnight.
3. Put rice and beans, millet and salt in a pressure cooker. Slowly bring to pressure and pressure cook 45 minutes.
4. Remove from heat and let stand 15 minutes. Reduce pressure following the instructions for your cooker.
5. Remove cover and spoon rice into a serving bowl, mixing thoroughly.
6. Serve warm.

AZUKI RICE

Preparation time: 15 minutes   *Yield:* 4–5 servings
Soaking time: 5 hours
Cooking time: 45 minutes
Standing time: 15 minutes

This recipe is useful with all disorders. (The Japanese custom is to serve Azuki Rice on the first and fifteenth of every month.)

> 3 cups brown rice
> 2/3 cup azuki beans
> 5 cups cold water
> 1/4 teaspoon sea salt

1. Wash rice and azuki beans separately.
2. Soak together in cold water 5 hours or overnight.
3. Add salt. Slowly bring to pressure and pressure cook 45 minutes.
4. Remove from heat and let stand 15 minutes. Reduce pressure following the instructions for your cooker.
5. Remove cover and spoon rice into a serving bowl, mixing thoroughly.
6. Serve warm.

AZUKI RICE BALLS

Preparation time: 5 minutes   *Yield:* 1 rice ball

These rice balls are useful for kidney and intestinal problems, cancer, breast infections, and nerve pain.

> 1/2–1 cup of Bancha Tea (see page 232) or water
>   (use same tea for each ball)
> 1/2 cup cooked Azuki Rice (see above)
> 2–3 pieces of Shio Kombu (see page 224)
>   or 1 piece of umeboshi
> 2 pieces of toasted nori, 2 inches x 2 1/2 inches

1. Wash and rinse your hands thoroughly. Slightly moisten your hands in the tea.
2. Hold Azuki Rice in your left hand.
3. In the center of the Azuki Rice put Shio Kombu or Umeboshi for flavor and to keep the rice from spoiling.
4. Form Azuki Rice into a ball and shape the ball into a 1 1/2-inch-thick, flattened triangle.
5. Cover Azuki Rice Ball with 2 pieces of toasted nori.

Variation

With Gomashio

When eating, dip each Azuki Rice Ball in Gomashio (see page 202), if called for in Part Two or desired.

BAKED MOCHI WITH SOY SAUCE

Preparation time: 5 minutes   *Yield:* 3–4 servings
Cooking time: 20 minutes

This preparation is useful in cases of lung and intestinal disorders, bed-wetting, spinal cord inflammation, or nerve pain.

7–12 bite-sized pieces of mochi
soy sauce

1. Bake mochi on a cookie sheet at 325°F until pieces are tender and puffy, about 20 minutes.
2. Lightly baste the mochi with soy sauce (Baked Mochi may be covered with nori.)
3. Serve hot.

BROWN RICE

Preparation time: 5 minutes   *Yield:* 5–7 servings
Soaking time: 5 hours
Cooking time: 50–80 minutes
Standing time: 15 minutes

Pressure-cooked Brown Rice is useful with all diseases and conditions. If you have a very yang condition or live in a very hot and dry climate, use Brown Rice, Boiled, as needed. Soft Brown Rice, made by increasing the amount of water by 2 to 3 cups, is useful when you have no appetite, diarrhea, or persistent pain.

> 4 cups brown rice
> 4–5 cups water
> 1/4–1/2 teaspoon sea salt

1. Wash rice until rinse water runs clear.
2. Soak in 4 to 5 cups water for 5 hours or overnight.
3. Add salt. In pressure cooker, cook 20 minutes over low heat.
4. Turn heat to high and bring to full pressure.
5. Reduce heat to low. Place flame-spreader under pressure cooker. Cook 30 to 60 minutes.
6. Remove from heat and let stand 10 minutes.
7. Reduce pressure following the instructions for your cooker. Let stand 5 more minutes.
8. Remove cover. Mix rice from bottom to top.
9. Serve warm or hot.

Variation
Boiled

Preparation time: 5 minutes   *Yield:* 5–7 servings
Soaking time: 5 hours
Cooking time: 1 hour and 50 minutes

Brown Rice is useful with all diseases. This recipe is used for very yang disorders when a more yin preparation is appropriate. It is also useful in climates that are hot and dry. For other conditions use Brown Rice (pressure cooked as above).

> 4 cups brown rice
> 6–8 cups water
> 1/4–1/2 teaspoon sea salt

1. Wash rice and soak it in 6 to 8 cups water for 5 hours or overnight.
2. Add salt. Cover and cook in a heavy pot for 20 minutes over low heat.
3. Turn heat to high. When steam escapes, turn heat to low and cook for 1 hour. Don't lift the cover.
4. Turn heat to high for 10 seconds.
5. Remove from heat. Let stand 30 minutes.
6. Mix rice from top to bottom.
7. Serve hot or warm.

BROWN RICE WITH BARLEY

Preparation time: 10 minutes   *Yield:* 3–4 servings
Soaking time: 5 hours
Cooking time: 50–80 minutes
Standing time: 15 minutes

This preparation is used in all cases of yang disorders.

> 3 cups brown rice
> 2/3 cup barley
> 4 1/2 cups water
> 1/4 teaspoon sea salt

1. Rinse rice and barley separately.
2. Combine and soak rice and barley in 4 1/2 cups water for 5 hours or overnight.
3. Add salt. In pressure cooker, cook 20 minutes over low heat.
4. Turn heat to high and bring to full pressure.
5. Reduce heat to low. Place flame-spreader under pressure cooker. Cook 30 to 60 minutes.
6. Remove from heat and let stand 10 minutes.
7. Reduce pressure following the instructions for your cooker. Let stand 5 more minutes.
8. Remove cover. Mix barley rice from bottom to top.
9. Serve hot or warm.

BROWN RICE WITH HATOMUGI

Preparation time: 10 minutes   *Yield:* 5–7 servings
Soaking time: 5 hours
Cooking time: 50–80 minutes
Standing time: 15 minutes

This preparation is useful for dissolving corns and removing warts.

> 3 cups brown rice
> 2/3 cup hatomugi
> 4 1/2 cups water
> 1/4 teaspoon sea salt

1. Rinse rice and hatomugi separately.
2. Combine and soak rice and hatomugi in 4½ cups water for 5 hours or overnight.
3. Add salt. In pressure cooker, cook 20 minutes over low heat.
4. Turn heat to high and bring to full pressure.
5. Reduce heat to low. Place flame-spreader under pressure cooker. Cook 30 to 60 minutes.
6. Remove from heat and let stand 10 minutes.
7. Reduce pressure following the instructions for your cooker. Let stand 5 more minutes.
8. Remove cover. Mix hatomugi rice from bottom to top.
9. Serve hot.

BROWN RICE WITH SOYBEANS

Preparation time: 10 minutes   *Yield:* 6–7 servings
Soaking time: 5 hours
Cooking time: 45–60 minutes
Standing time: 15 minutes

This preparation is useful with itchy skin or excessive tears.

> 5 cups brown rice
> ½ cup soybeans
> 7½ cups water
> ½ teaspoon sea salt

1. Wash rice and beans separately.
2. Soak rice in 7½ cups of the water; soak soybeans in the remaining 1 cup of water for 5 hours or overnight.
3. Drain soybeans and add to rice the water it soaked in.
4. Add salt and pressure cook 45 to 60 minutes.
5. Remove from heat and let stand 10 minutes.
6. Reduce pressure following the instructions for your cooker. Let stand 5 more minutes.
7. Remove cover. Mix rice from bottom to top.
8. Serve hot or warm.

BROWN RICE BALLS

Preparation time: 5 minutes   *Yield:* 1 rice ball

Brown Rice Balls are useful in cases of stomach, intestinal, and lung disorders, especially the yin types. Brown Rice Balls are also used with cancer, infections, and kidney or sexual problems.

> ½–1 cup of Bancha Tea (see page 232) or water (use same tea for each ball)

> ½ cup Brown Rice (see page 197)
> 2–3 pieces of Shio Kombu (see page 224)
>   or 1 piece of umeboshi
> 2 pieces of toasted nori, 2 inches x 2½ inches

1. Wash and rinse your hands thoroughly. Slightly moisten your hands in the tea.
2. Hold rice in your left hand.
3. In the center of the rice, put Shio Kombu or Umeboshi for flavor and to keep the rice from spoiling.
4. Form rice into a ball and shape the rice ball into a 1½-inch-thick, flattened triangle.
5. Cover rice ball with 2 pieces of toasted nori.
6. Serve warm or at room temperature.

Variation

With Gomashio

This variation is useful with nausea. Dip rice balls in Gomashio (see page 202) when eating.

BROWN RICE CREAM

Preparation time: 5 minutes   *Yield:* 2 servings
Cooking time: 50–60 minutes

Brown Rice Cream is useful when you have no appetite, difficulty swallowing, or persistent pain, or when breaking a fast. It is used in many disorders and may be made thick or thin as needed by adjusting the proportion of powder to water. To make thick rice cream, use 2½ to 3 cups water per cup of powder. To make thin rice cream, use 4½ to 5 cups water per cup of powder. Brown Rice Cream may even be used as a beverage by using 9 to 10 cups of water per cup of powder. Prepared rice cream powder can be purchased, but it is fresher when made at home: Wash 1 cup brown rice and dry-roast in a heavy skillet until it is golden in color and begins to pop. Grind it into powder in a grain mill or in an electric blender.

> 1 cup brown rice cream powder
> 3½–4 cups boiling water
> ¼ teaspoon sea salt

1. Dry-roast rice cream powder in a heavy pan or skillet over medium heat until it gives off a nut-like fragrance.
2. Place the pan in the sink and add boiling water and salt. Mix thoroughly to remove lumps.
3. Cook, covered, over low heat for 40 to 50 minutes, stirring occasionally to prevent burning.
4. Mix thoroughly before serving hot.

Variations

With Grated Daikon

This variation is useful with diarrhea, chills, scarlet fever, tetanus, or uremia. To serve Brown Rice Cream with Grated Daikon, add 1 tablespoon grated daikon for each cup of rice cream. Grated daikon may be mixed with soy sauce in the proportion of 1 teaspoon soy sauce to 1 tablespoon grated daikon before adding to rice cream.

With Umeboshi

This variation is useful when there is loss of appetite, especially when accompanied by diarrhea. Add 1/3 to 1/2 umeboshi per cup of Brown Rice Cream. Mix and serve.

BROWN RICE CREAM, SPECIAL

Preparation time: 5 minutes *Yield:* 2 servings
Cooking time: 1 hour, approximately

This thin cream is good for people who have swollen feet resulting from a weak heart, trouble digesting food because of a weak stomach, gastric pain, a fever with no appetite, and fatigue or low energy. It is good in the summer as a tonic and a health promoter.

    1 cup brown rice, roasted
    10 cups water
    1 pinch sea salt

1. Cook ingredients together until the volume is reduced to 7 cups.
2. Strain through a very fine colander or squeeze through a piece of cotton cloth. Eat only the creamy liquid.
3. Serve warm.

BROWN RICE CREAM WITH OIL

Preparation time: 10 minutes *Yield:* 2 servings
Cooking time: 30–60 minutes

Brown Rice Cream with Oil is good for arthritis, rheumatism, and heart conditions.

    1 cup brown rice
    1 teaspoon sesame oil
    7 cups water
    1 pinch sea salt

1. Roast brown rice in oil until it is golden brown.
2. Add water and salt. Bring to a boil and simmer, covered, until the rice is soft. Do not stir. It will resemble a thick soup when done.

3. Place 1 cup at a time in a triangular cotton bag or a very fine strainer. Push a rice paddle down onto the bag so that the cream (juice) comes out.
4. Eat this cream hot or warm. (The remaining rice may be used in bread or other dishes.)

BROWN RICE GRUEL

Preparation time: 5 minutes *Yield:* 2 servings
Cooking time: 30 minutes

Brown Rice Gruel is useful in cases of malaria, blood poisoning, or spinal-cord inflammation. It is also used to help induce a measles rash.

    3 cups water, stock, or soup
    1 cup cooked brown rice
    1 pinch sea salt

1. Bring water to a boil and add rice and salt.
2. Cover and simmer slowly for 30 minutes.
3. Serve hot.

Variations

With Grated Daikon

This variation is useful mostly with lung or intestinal disorders. Add 1 tablespoon grated daikon to gruel after removing from heat.

With Homemade Agé

This variation is useful mostly with lung problems. Cut 1 piece of agé into match-stick shapes. Add to the water along with rice and salt. Simmer as above.

With Miso

This variation is useful mostly with intestinal disorders. Add 1 teaspoon miso to gruel after removing from heat.

With Miso and Scallions

This variation is useful mostly with diarrhea, throat problems, or menstrual irregularities. Add 1/3 cup scallions to gruel and bring to a boil. Remove from heat. Dissolve 1 teaspoon miso in a little water and mix in.

With Mochi

This variation is useful mostly with lung, intestinal, or sexual organ problems. Bake or pan-fry mochi. Place on top of Brown Rice Gruel, Brown Rice Gruel with Miso, or Brown Rice Gruel with Miso and Scallions.

With Umeboshi

This variation is useful mostly with diarrhea. Add 1 to 1½ umeboshi plums when adding rice to water.

BROWN RICE GRUEL WITH SHIITAKE MUSHROOMS

Preparation time: 20 minutes
Cooking time: 40 minutes   *Yield:* 2 servings

This preparation is useful in cases of appendicitis or scarlet fever.

> 2 or 3 shiitake mushrooms
> 1 cup cooked brown rice
> 3 cups water
> 1–2 teaspoons soy sauce

1. Soak shiitake mushrooms until soft, about 15 minutes.
2. Slice mushrooms. Discard hard part of stem or reserve for use in soup stock.
3. Place mushrooms then rice in pot. Add water.
4. Cover and cook over low heat for about 40 minutes.
5. Add soy sauce and mix from top to bottom.
6. Serve hot.

Variation

With Miso and Mochi

This variation is useful for strong persons who have the flu. Replace soy sauce with 1 teaspoon miso and a pinch of sea salt. Top with baked or pan-fried mochi.

BROWN RICE KAYU

Preparation time: 5 minutes   *Yield:* 2 servings
Soaking time: 5 hours
Cooking time: 1 hour

This soft rice is very easy to digest and is useful with respiratory or intestinal problems.

> 1 cup brown rice
> 5 cups water
> 1 pinch sea salt

1. Wash rice and soak it in 5 cups water for 5 hours or overnight.
2. Add salt and pressure cook 60 minutes.
3. Serve hot.

BROWN RICE MOCHI, PAN-FRIED WITH OIL

Preparation time: 3 minutes   *Yield:* 5 servings
Cooking time: 7 to 12 minutes

Brown Rice Mochi is useful with most disorders. Prepare with or without oil depending on your condition and need for oil. Mugwort mochi is useful for parasites. Either variety may be baked (see Baked Mochi with Soy Sauce) or pan-fried, and eaten plain or with soy sauce sprinkled on top, or added to soup.

> 1 tablespoon sesame oil
> 7–12 bite-sized pieces of mochi
> oil for frying

1. Put oil in a heavy skillet and heat it over medium heat.
2. Pan-fry mochi 7 minutes, covered.
3. Turn mochi, cover, and cook over low heat 5 minutes more, or until soft.
4. Serve hot.

Variation

Without Oil

Heat the heavy skillet over medium-low heat. When skillet is hot, pan-fry mochi, covered, 7 to 10 minutes or until soft. Serve hot.

BROWN RICE MOCHI WITH AZUKI BEANS

Preparation time: 10 minutes   *Yield:* 2–3 servings
Soaking time: 5 hours
Cooking time: 1½ hours

This preparation is used specifically for helping to induce urination in cases of kidney failure.

> 1 cup azuki beans
> 1½ cups water for soaking
> 1½ cups cold water
> 3 cups winter squash, sliced
> 1 teaspoon sea salt
> Brown Rice Mochi, baked or pan-fried
>   without oil

1. Soak azuki beans in water for at least 5 hours or overnight.
2. Bring beans to a boil over high heat and add ½ cup of cold water.
3. Repeat this procedure 2 more times.
4. Cover the beans and cook over medium heat until they are tender; about 1 hour.

5. Add the squash and salt. Cook until the squash is tender.
6. Gently stir the mixture.
7. Cover pieces of mochi with the mixture and cook slightly to make mochi soft or warm as desired.
8. Serve warm in the winter or at room temperature in the summer.

BUCKWHEAT CREAM

Preparation time: 5 minutes   *Yield:* 1 serving
Cooking time: 30 minutes

Thick Buckwheat Cream helps build a strong constitution and is useful in all cases of cancer (except skin cancer), as well as in kidney or lung diseases. Increase or decrease the amount of flour to make thicker or thinner Buckwheat Cream.

sesame oil
2 tablespoons buckwheat flour
1 cup warm water or Kombu Stock (see
    page 216)
1 pinch sea salt
chopped raw scallions or parsley

1. Brush a pan with oil and heat it.
2. Roast the flour. (If Kombu Stock is used in place of water, it is not necessary to roast the flour.) Slowly add water or stock, stirring constantly.
3. Add salt. Cover, bring to a boil, and simmer for 20 minutes.
4. Serve hot with a pinch of raw scallions or parsley.

BUCKWHEAT GROATS

Preparation time: 5 minutes   *Yield:* 2–3 servings
Cooking time: 30 minutes

Sometimes used as a substitute for brown rice, buckwheat groats are good for people with cancer, parasites, or weak stomachs, but should be avoided by those with skin diseases.

1 cup whole buckwheat groats
2 cups boiling water
1/4 teaspoon sea salt

1. Wash then dry-roast buckwheat groats in a heavy skillet for 10 minutes or until groats are golden brown.
2. Add water and salt. Cover and simmer over low heat for 20 minutes.
3. Mix thoroughly before serving warm or hot.

BUCKWHEAT NOODLES

Preparation time: 5 minutes   *Yield:* 4–5 servings
Cooking time: 30 minutes

These noodles are sometimes used as a substitute for brown rice and are especially good for those with cancer of the esophagus, and for parasites, leprosy, or anal itch.

8 cups water
1–2 teaspoons sea salt
1 pound buckwheat noodles
3 cups cold water

1. Bring 8 cups water to a boil.
2. Add salt. Sprinkle the noodles into the boiling water. Stir and bring to a boil.
3. Add 1 cup cold water and bring to a boil again. Repeat 2 times.
4. Remove from heat. Cover and let stand for a few minutes. When noodles are the same color inside as out, they are done.
5. Drain noodles, reserving the water for making soup or cooking grain.
6. Quickly wash noodles in cold water. Continue washing them until they are completely cold. Drain.
7. Serve noodles in Kombu Stock Clear Soup (see page 216) or as directed in Part Two under the appropriate disorder.

BUCKWHEAT NOODLES WITH TEMPURA

Preparation time: 15 minutes   *Yield:* 4–5 servings
Cooking time: 10 minutes

Buckwheat Noodles with Tempura are useful in cases of nerve pain or extreme pain from a breast infection.

8 cups Kombu Stock (see page 216)
4–5 tablespoons soy sauce
1 lb. buckwheat noodles (soba),
    cooked and cooled (see above)
10 small pieces vegetable tempura
3 scallions, thinly sliced
2 sheets nori, roasted and crushed
grated daikon

1. Bring soup stock to a boil and add soy sauce.
2. Heat noodles in boiling water and drain before serving.
3. Pour soup stock over noodles in bowls. Arrange two pieces of tempura on top of each bowl of noodles.
4. Garnish with scallions, nori, and grated daikon.
5. Serve hot.

BUCKWHEAT PANCAKES

Preparation time: 5 minutes   *Yield:* 2–3 servings
Cooking time: 7 minutes per batch

Buckwheat Pancakes are useful in cases of esophageal problems, including cancer of the esophagus.

> 1 cup buckwheat flour
> 1–1½ cups water
> ½ teaspoon sea salt
> oil for frying

1. Mix flour, water, and salt to form a thin batter. (You may need to experiment to get the right consistency; if batter is too thick, the pancakes will not cook through and will taste raw.)
2. Spoon batter onto a hot, oiled skillet.
3. Cook about 5 minutes until bubbles appear and the pancakes turn slightly lighter in color.
4. Turn and cook the other side for about 2 minutes.
5. Serve hot.

FRIED NOODLES

Preparation time: 5 minutes   *Yield:* 1 serving
Cooking time: 40–50 minutes

Fried Noodles are useful in cases of esophageal problems, including cancer of the esophagus.

> 1 tablespoon sesame oil
> 1–2 cups cooked whole-wheat spaghetti or noodles
> 1–2 teaspoons soy sauce

1. Heat a cast iron skillet and add oil.
2. When the oil is heated, add a layer of noodles and press down. Cover and cook over medium-high heat for 7 minutes or until noodles are lightly browned.
3. Turn and cook another 7 minutes, covered.
4. Turn once more and remove from heat. Add soy sauce by sprinkling it around the edges of the cooked noodles.
5. Cover skillet and let stand for a few minutes, then stir. Remove noodles from pan and keep warm.
6. Repeat until all noodles have been fried.
7. Serve warm.

FRIED RICE

Preparation time: 10 minutes   *Yield:* 3–4 servings
Cooking time: 50–60 minutes

Fried Rice is used mostly in cases of head and brain prob-
lems, asthma, troubles in the rectal and sexual areas, or nervous system malfunction.

> 3-inch piece burdock
> 1 large onion
> 1½-inch-piece carrot
> 2 teaspoons sesame oil
> 1 teaspoon sea salt
> 5 cups cooked brown rice

1. Chop the burdock finely. Mince the onion and the carrot.
2. Heat oil in a heavy cast iron skillet. Add burdock with a pinch of salt; stir, cover, and cook 5 minutes.
3. Repeat salting and cooking burdock 2 times.
4. Add onion. Cover and cook until onion is translucent.
5. Add carrots. When burdock is completely tender, put rice on top of vegetables.
6. Cover and cook over low heat for about 20 minutes or until rice is hot.
7. Stir. Add Gomashio (see below) or soy sauce to taste if desired.
8. Serve hot.

GOMASHIO

Preparation time: 5 minutes   *Yield:* 1 cup
Drying time: 10 minutes to overnight
Cooking time: 5 minutes
Grinding time: 5–10 minutes

Gomashio is good for those who have morning or motion sickness, food poisoning, heartburn, epilepsy, hiccups, menstrual cramps, loss of blood, or insomnia with fever. Do not use Gomashio in cases of stomach ulcer or intestinal hemorrhaging.

Gomashio is a mixture of sea salt and sesame seeds that have been roasted and ground. The proportion of seeds to salt can range from 15 to 1 for children, up to 4 to 1 for hard-working adults. Brown, black, or white sesame seeds may be used. White sesame seeds grow in warm climates and have fewer minerals and more oil. They are usually used for salad dressings and baking rather than for Gomashio. Black sesame seeds grow in a cold climate and contain less oil and more minerals than the other sesame seeds. Buy black sesame seeds from a reputable source to be sure they have not been dyed. Avoid over-roasting the black seeds as they can become bitter. Brown sesame seeds are not as flavorful as the black, so they need to be roasted well for more flavor.

Fresh Gomashio is best so prepare a small amount and keep it tightly covered. Use as a general condiment; however, be careful not to feed young children too much Gomashio as the body and organs may become too contracted and not grow properly. If you do give Gomashio to your children, use brown rather than black sesame seeds. If the children don't want any, don't give it to them.

> 10 tablespoons sesame seeds
> 1 tablespoon sea salt

1. Wash the seeds and allow to dry overnight. Or dry over medium heat, stirring occasionally for about 10 minutes
2. Roast the salt until the acid, chlorine smell is gone.
3. Grind the salt in a suribachi until it becomes a fine powder.
4. Roast the seeds, a few tablespoons at a time, in a small frying pan over medium-high heat. When the seeds start to pop, cover and shake the pan. Roast each batch about 20 seconds to 1 minute maximum. (The seeds are done when you can crush them between your fourth finger and thumb.)
5. Add the roasted seeds to the suribachi on top of the powdered salt.
6. Grind them gently until 80 percent of the seeds are broken.
7. Serve at room temperature over grains or vegetables.

GRAIN MILK OR KOKKOH

See BEVERAGES.

HATOMUGI, BOILED

Preparation time: 5 minutes   *Yield:* 5–7 servings
Soaking time: 5 hours
Cooking time: 1 hour and 20 minutes
Standing time: 10–15 minutes

Hatomugi is used specifically to help dissolve corns or remove warts. Use this preparation in hot weather or if you have a very yang condition; in other cases, use Hatomugi, Pressure Cooked (see below).

> 4 cups hatomugi
> 8 cups water
> 1/4–1/2 teaspoon sea salt

1. Wash hatomugi. Soak it in 8 cups water for 5 hours or overnight.
2. Add salt. Cook in a heavy, covered pot for 20 minutes over low heat.
3. Turn heat to high. When steam escapes, turn heat to low and cook for 1 hour. Don't lift the cover.
4. Turn heat to high for 10 seconds. Remove from heat.
5. Let stand 10 to 15 minutes.
6. Mix hatomugi from top to bottom.
7. Serve hot, warm, or at room temperature.

HATOMUGI, PRESSURE COOKED

Preparation time: 5 minutes   *Yield:* 5–7 servings
Soaking time: 5 hours
Cooking time: 50–80 minutes
Standing time: 15 minutes

Hatomugi is used specifically to help dissolve corns or remove warts. Use this preparation in cold or warm weather or if you have a more yin condition.

> 4 cups hatomugi
> 4–5 cups water
> 1/4–1/2 teaspoon sea salt

1. Wash hatomugi until rinse water runs clear.
2. Soak in 4 to 5 cups of water for 5 hours or overnight.
3. Add salt. In pressure cooker, cook 20 minutes over low heat.
4. Turn heat to high and bring to full pressure.
5. Reduce heat to low. Place flame-spreader under pressure cooker. Cook 30 to 60 minutes.
6. Remove from heat and let stand 10 minutes.
7. Reduce pressure following the instructions for your cooker. Let stand 5 more minutes.
8. Remove cover. Mix hatomugi from top to bottom.
9. Serve hot, warm, or at room temperature.

MILLET RICE

Preparation time: 10 minutes   *Yield:* 5 servings
Soaking time: 5 hours
Cooking time: 1 1/4–1 1/2 hours

Millet Rice is useful with more yin types of disorders, especially sexual organ problems, spinal-cord inflammation, or pneumonia.

> 3 cups brown rice
> 6 cups water
> 1 cup millet
> 1 teaspoon sea salt

1. Rinse rice and soak 5 hours or overnight in the 6 cups of water. (Reduce water to 5 cups if using a pressure cooker.)
2. Wash millet.
3. Add millet and salt to rice and water. Cover and cook over low heat for 30 minutes.
4. Bring to a boil over high heat and simmer for 1 hour or pressure cook for 45 minutes.
5. Mix thoroughly from top to bottom.
6. Serve hot or warm.

MOCHI SOUP

Preparation time: 10 minutes   *Yield:* 5–7 servings
Cooking time: 1 hour

This soup is useful with several disorders including children's dysentery, tonsillitis, spinal-cord inflammation, and impotence.

> 1 medium burdock root
> 1 carrot
> 1 piece daikon, 7 inches long
> 5 albi
> 2 teaspoons sesame oil
> 1/3 teaspoon sea salt
> 7 cups boiling water
> 2 scallions
> 2–3 tablespoons soy sauce
> plain or mugwort mochi

1. Cut burdock and carrot into shavings. Cut daikon in sections 1½ inches long, then slice in vertical pieces; slice vertical pieces lengthwise, thinly. Scrub albi and scrape off hairy skin. Cut albi in ¼-inch rounds. Cut scallions in ¼-inch diagonals.
2. Heat the oil and sauté the burdock in a pot covered with an otoshibuta or lid that drops inside the pot, and with the pot lid. After 5 minutes, dip chopsticks in salt and stir the salt into the burdock.
3. Re-cover with both covers and cook for 5 minutes more.
4. Repeat the salting and cooking process 2 times. The burdock will begin to smell sweet.
5. Add the daikon, albi, and carrot in that order, sautéing each before adding the next.
6. Sprinkle with a few pinches of salt. Add boiling water. Cover and cook 30 minutes.
7. Add scallions and soy sauce.
8. Bake mochi on a cookie sheet at 325°F until tender and puffy, about 20 minutes, or pan-fry in a dry, covered skillet over medium-low heat for 7 to 10 minutes or until soft. Place a piece of mochi in a soup bowl, cover it with hot soup, and serve immediately.

Variations

With Homemade Agé

This variation is useful for the yang type of leprosy. Cut 2 pieces of Homemade Agé (see page 215) into matchstick shapes. Add agé, then the boiling water. Cook 30 minutes and continue as directed above.

With Miso

This variation is useful for appendicitis, diphtheria, and tuberculosis of the intestines. Eliminate soy sauce. Soften 1 heaping tablespoon of miso in a small amount of soup stock and add to soup along with the scallions.

RAW BROWN RICE

Preparation time: 5 minutes   *Yield:* 1 serving

Eating Raw Brown Rice is good for eliminating parasites, especially hookworms, and helpful for cleansing the system in those who have jaundice.

> 1 handful of brown rice

1. Wash and drain rice.
2. This can be eaten every morning before breakfast. Chew very well.

SWEET BROWN RICE

Preparation time: 5 minutes   *Yield:* 1 serving
Soaking time: 5 hours
Cooking time: 40 minutes
Standing time: 1 hour

This preparation is useful in cases of breast cancer, stomach ulcer, peritonitis, or tuberculosis of the intestines. Chew very well, especially in the case of stomach ulcer.

> 1 cup sweet brown rice
> 1 cup water

1. Wash and soak rice for 5 hours or overnight in 1 cup water.
2. Place in a pressure cooker over medium-high heat until cooker comes to pressure (about 20 minutes).
3. Turn heat to low and cook 20 minutes more.
4. Remove from heat and let stand 1 hour.
5. Serve warm.

UDON NOODLES

Preparation time: 2 minutes   *Yield:* 2–3 servings
Cooking time: 30–40 minutes

Udon Noodles are useful with more yang types of disorders, including leprosy, non-insulin-dependent diabetes, or skin infections on the body.

> 8 cups water
> 2 teaspoons sea salt
> 8 ounces udon
> 3 cups cold water

1. Bring 8 cups salted water to a boil.
2. Sprinkle the udon into the pot, stir, and bring to a boil.
3. Add 1 cup cold water and bring to a boil again. Repeat 2 times.
4. Remove from heat. Cover and let stand 20 minutes.
5. Drain udon, rinse in cold water, and drain again.
6. Use udon in clear soup or vegetable soup.

VEGETABLE BROTH

See BEVERAGES.

VEGETABLE FRIED RICE

Preparation time: 15 minutes   *Yield:* 5–7 servings
Cooking time: 30–40 minutes

This preparation is useful in cases of excessive fatigue or the yin types of arthritis and rheumatism.

> 1 medium onion
> 5 cabbage leaves
> 1 stalk celery
> 1 tablespoon sesame oil
> 1/2 teaspoon sea salt
> 7 cups cooked Brown Rice (see page 197)
> 1 tablespoon soy sauce
> 1 tablespoon minced parsley

1. Cut the onion in thin crescents. Cut the cabbage leaves into match-stick shapes. Cut the celery stalk in diagonals.
2. Heat the oil in a heavy pan and sauté the onions with a pinch of salt until they are translucent.
3. Add the cabbage and celery with the remaining salt and sauté for 10 minutes.
4. Spread the rice over the vegetables. (If the rice is very dry, add 1/2 cup water.) Cover and cook over low heat until steam rises from the rice.
5. Mix the rice and vegetables. Cover and cook for 5 minutes more or until the rice is hot.
6. Remove from heat and sprinkle with soy sauce. Garnish with parsley.
7. Serve hot or warm.

SIDE DISHES

Side dishes are usually vegetables, or grain and vegetable combinations and commonly comprise one-third to one-fourth of the main foods depending on an individual's condition. Side dishes are used to provide variety. Presented here are recipes for those dishes called for in Part Two; see Suggested Reading (page 249–250) for cookbooks that offer additional side-dish recipes.

AMASAKE

See BEVERAGES.

ARAME NITSUKE

Preparation time: 10 minutes   *Yield:* 5–7 servings
Cooking time: 25–35 minutes

Arame nitsuke is useful in cases of itchy skin, grey hair, or leprosy.

> 2 cups arame
> 3–5 cups cold water
> 1 tablespoon sesame oil
> 1 tablespoon soy sauce

1. Rinse arame in the 3 to 5 cups cold water and reserve the rinsing water.
2. Place arame in a strainer or basket. Let the arame remain in the basket for 7 minutes. (Arame may be cut in 1-inch lengths if desired.)
3. Heat the oil and sauté the arame about 5 minutes. (Thinly-cut vegetables such as carrot, onion, or burdock may be cooked with the arame. Sauté the vegetable in the oil until slightly soft, then add the rinsed arame and continue as directed.)
4. Add 1 cup of the reserved rinsing water (the rest may be saved for use in soup). Cook mixture uncovered over high heat 20 to 30 minutes until tender.
5. Add soy sauce and cook 5 more minutes.
6. Serve warm or at room temperature.

AZUKI BEANS WITH KOMBU

Preparation time: 10 minutes   *Yield:* 2–3 servings
Soaking time: 5 hours
Cooking time: 1 hour

This preparation is useful in cases of urination troubles, constipation, or intestinal problems. It is also beneficial for the sexual organs or strengthening the kidneys.

> 1 cup azuki beans
> 8 pieces kombu, 2 inches by 2 inches
> 3 cups water
> 3 cups cold water
> 1/4–1/2 teaspoon sea salt

1. Sort and wash azuki beans.
2. Soak beans and kombu in 3 cups water for 5 hours or overnight.

3. Bring to a boil.
4. Add 1 cup cold water and bring to a boil again. Repeat 2 times.
5. Cover and simmer until the beans are soft, adding more water if necessary.
6. Add salt and simmer for 20 minutes more.
7. Serve hot or warm.

AZUKI BEANS WITH KOMBU AND WINTER SQUASH

Preparation time: 10 minutes   *Yield:* 2–3 servings
Soaking time: 5 hours
Cooking time: 1 hour

This dish is useful with many illnesses including eye problems, heart and circulatory disorders, diabetes, kidney diseases, beriberi, and nervous system malfunction.

    1 cup azuki beans
    1 piece kombu, 2 inches by 2 inches
    1½ cups water
    1½ cups cold water
    4 cups winter squash, cut in ½-inch squares
    ½ teaspoon sea salt

1. Sort azuki beans, picking out debris, discolored beans, and empty shells.
2. Wash the beans and soak with kombu in 1½ cups water for 5 hours or overnight.
3. Bring to a boil over high heat.
4. Add ½ cup cold water and bring to a boil again. Repeat 2 times.
5. Cover and cook over low heat for about 1 hour.
6. When the beans are tender, add squash and salt. Continue cooking until the squash is tender.
7. Stir the mixture until it becomes partly mashed.
8. Serve hot or warm.

BAKED WHITE FISH

Preparation time: 15 minutes   *Yield:* 5 servings
Standing time: 1 hour
Cooking time: 45–60 minutes

Baked white fish is useful specifically with insulin-dependent diabetes.

    3 pounds whole fish (sea bass, rex sole, or cod)
    1 tablespoon fresh ginger juice
    2 tablespoons sea salt

1. Preheat oven to 450°F.
2. Clean the fish and remove the scales. Make 2 deep, diagonal cuts to the bone on both sides of the fish.
3. Cover the entire fish with ginger juice and 1 tablespoon salt, and let it stand 1 hour.
4. Wipe the salt off the fish with a paper towel, and place the fish in a baking pan or on a cookie sheet.
5. From a height of about 1 foot, sprinkle the remaining 1 tablespoon of salt on the sides of the fish. This will give the fish a white glaze when it is baked.
6. Place the fish in the preheated oven and bake it for 45 to 60 minutes.
7. Serve warm.

BAKED YAMS OR SWEET POTATOES

Preparation time: 2 minutes   *Yield:* 1–2 servings
Cooking time: 2 hours

This dish is used with yang disorders such as appendicitis, itchy skin, or hypoglycemia. Do not use it if you have a yin disorder, a bladder infection, or hemorrhoids.

    1–2 yams or sweet potatoes

1. Place whole yams or sweet potatoes on a cookie sheet. Don't make any holes in the potatoes.
2. Bake at 350°F for about 2 hours.
3. Serve warm or hot.

BOILED DAIKON

Preparation time: 10 minutes   *Yield:* 5–7 servings
Cooking time: 30 minutes

Boiled daikon is useful with yang types of disorders, including eye and skin problems, sexual organ disorders, and measles.

    1 large daikon
    1 tablespoon sweet brown rice
    4 cups water

1. Cut the daikon in 1-inch rounds.
2. Place the sweet brown rice in a cotton bag and tie it securely. Place the bag of rice in the water with the daikon.
3. Cover and boil for about 30 minutes or until the daikon is tender.
4. Remove the daikon from the water and serve immediately with Lemon Miso (see page 217) or Oily Miso (see page 219).

BURDOCK CARROT NITSUKE

Preparation time: 10 minutes   *Yield:* 7–10 servings
Cooking time: 1 hour and 5 minutes

This preparation is useful with almost all disorders.

> 3 or 4 burdock roots, about ½-inch diameter
> and 12 inches long
> 1 carrot, about ¾-inch diameter and
> 8–10 inches long
> 1–2 tablespoons sesame oil
> sea salt
> cold water
> 3–5 tablespoons soy sauce

1. Gently wash burdock without removing the skin.
2. Cut burdock and carrot into match-stick shapes, 1½ inches long.
3. Heat oil and add burdock. Add a pinch of salt and stir.
4. Cover with both an otoshibuta or a lid that fits inside the pot, and with the pot lid. Cook for 5 minutes.
5. Repeat salting and cooking 2 more times (total 15 minutes) until the burdock smells sweet.
6. Add the carrot and sauté for 5 minutes without a cover.
7. Add water to just cover the vegetables and add the soy sauce. Stir and cook uncovered for 30 minutes over high heat.
8. When the water is almost gone, turn the heat to low and continue to cook 15 more minutes, stirring often.
9. Serve 1 to 2 tablespoons per meal, warm or at room temperature.

Variation

With Umeboshi

This variation is useful for children's dysentery. Sauté the burdock in umeboshi vinegar instead of sesame oil.

BURDOCK CARROT DAIKON NITSUKE

Preparation time: 15 minutes   *Yield:* 5 servings
Cooking time: 1 hour and 10 minutes

This preparation is useful in cases of peritonitis or infertility problems.

> 1½ medium burdock roots
> daikon, 2-inch section
> 1 carrot
> 1–2 tablespoons sesame oil
> sea salt
> cold water
> 3–5 tablespoons soy sauce

1. Gently wash burdock without removing the skin.
2. Cut each of the vegetables in match-stick shapes, 1½ inches long.
3. Heat oil and add burdock. Add a pinch of salt and stir.
4. Cover with both an otoshibuta or a lid that fits inside the pot, and with the pot lid. Cook for 5 minutes.
5. Repeat salting and cooking 2 more times (total 15 minutes) until the burdock smells sweet.
6. Add the daikon and sauté for 5 minutes without a cover.
7. Add the carrot and sauté for 5 minutes without a cover.
8. Add enough water to just cover the vegetables and add the soy sauce. Stir and cook uncovered for 30 minutes over high heat.
9. When the water is almost gone, turn the heat to low and continue to cook 15 more minutes, stirring often.
10. Serve 1 to 2 tablespoons per meal, warm or at room temperature.

BURDOCK CARROT LOTUS ROOT NITSUKE

Preparation time: 15 minutes   *Yield:* 5 servings
Cooking time: 1 hour and 10 minutes

This preparation is useful for people with hysteria, stroke, or a cough from tuberculosis.

> 1½ medium burdock roots
> lotus root, 2-inch section
> 1 carrot
> 1–2 tablespoons sesame oil
> sea salt
> cold water
> 3–5 tablespoons soy sauce

1. Gently wash burdock without removing the skin.
2. Cut each of the vegetables in match-stick shapes, 1½ inches long.
3. Heat oil and add burdock. Add a pinch of salt and stir.
4. Cover with both an otoshibuta or a lid that fits inside the pot, and with the pot lid. Cook for 5 minutes.
5. Repeat salting and cooking 2 more times (total 15 minutes) until the burdock smells sweet.
6. Add the lotus root and sauté for 5 minutes without a cover.
7. Add the carrot and sauté for 5 minutes without a cover.
8. Add water to just cover the vegetables and add the soy sauce. Stir and cook uncovered for 30 minutes over high heat.

9. When the water is almost gone, turn the heat to low and continue to cook 15 more minutes, stirring often.
10. Serve 1 to 2 tablespoons per meal, warm or at room temperature.

BURDOCK LOTUS ROOT NITSUKE

Preparation time: 10 minutes   *Yield:* 3–4 servings
Cooking time: 1 hour and 5 minutes

This preparation is useful in cases of pleurisy, ruptured eardrum, or breast cancer.

> 1½ medium burdock roots
> lotus root, 2-inch section
> 1–2 tablespoons sesame oil
> sea salt
> cold water
> 3–5 tablespoons soy sauce

1. Gently wash burdock without removing the skin.
2. Cut each of the vegetables in match-stick shapes, 1½ inches long.
3. Heat oil and add burdock. Add a pinch of salt and stir.
4. Cover with both an otoshibuta or a lid that fits inside the pot, and with the pot lid. Cook for 5 minutes.
5. Repeat salting and cooking 2 more times (total 15 minutes) until the burdock smells sweet.
6. Add the lotus root and sauté for 5 minutes without a cover.
7. Add water to just cover the vegetables and add the soy sauce. Stir and cook uncovered for 30 minutes over high heat.
8. When the water is almost gone, turn the heat to low and continue to cook 15 more minutes, stirring often.
9. Serve 1 to 2 tablespoons per meal, warm or at room temperature.

BURDOCK NITSUKE

Preparation time: 5 minutes   *Yield:* 7–10 servings
Cooking time: 1 hour

Burdock Nitsuke is useful with many disorders including appendicitis, mumps, stroke, and uremia.

> 3 or 4 burdock roots, about ½-inch diameter
>   and 12 inches long
> 1 tablespoon sesame oil
> sea salt
> cold water
> 3 tablespoons soy sauce

1. Gently wash burdock without removing the skin.
2. Cut in match-stick shapes, 1½ inches long.
3. Heat oil and add burdock. Add a pinch of salt and stir.
4. Cover with both an otoshibuta or a lid that fits inside the pot, and with the pot lid. Cook for 5 minutes.
5. Repeat salting and cooking 2 more times (total 15 minutes) until the burdock smells sweet.
6. Add water to just cover the burdock and add the soy sauce. Stir and cook uncovered for 30 minutes over high heat.
7. When the water is almost gone, turn the heat to low and continue to cook 15 more minutes, stirring often.
8. Serve 1 to 2 tablespoons per meal, warm or at room temperature.

CARP SOUP

Preparation time: 40 minutes   *Yield:* 10 servings
Cooking time: 2 hours (using pressure cooker);
   7–8 hours (boiling)

Carp Soup is good for mothers who need to produce more milk; people with weak bones; and those with periostitis, tuberculosis, yin cancer, polio, thyroiditis, swollen glands in armpit or groin, lymph problems, skin infections, mumps, or general weakness.

The carp is a fish that lives at the bottom of a river or lake. It moves very slowly and carries a lot of oxygen. Eating carp helps make one strong to fight diseases, especially more yin type diseases. Use as fresh a carp as you can find. If you can't find carp, use plain river fish of any kind. If you can't find river fish, try small ocean fish that have pink or white meat, not red meat.

> 1 whole carp, about 1 pound, or substitute
>   (see above)
> burdock root, 3 times the volume, after cutting,
>   as carp
> 1 tablespoon sesame oil
> ⅓ cup bancha tea twigs (previously used
>   twigs are okay), tied in a cotton bag
> water, 3 times the volume of carp and
>   burdock combined
> 3 tablespoons hatcho or barley miso
> ginger, grated

1. Clean carp and cut whole fish into 1-inch slices. Cut burdock into shavings.
2. Sauté burdock in sesame oil until it smells sweet.
3. Add the carp on top of the burdock, then the bag of tea twigs.
4. Add the water and bring to a boil. Simmer 6 to 7 hours or until the bones are completely soft. If using a pressure cooker, add only enough water to cover and

pressure cook for about 1 hour. Remove from heat and allow the pressure to come down.

5. Remove the bag of tea. If using a pressure cooker, add the remaining water.
6. Soften miso in soup stock and add to soup. Simmer 30 to 40 minutes longer.
7. Serve hot with a pinch of grated ginger in each bowl. Eat just 1 small bowl per day, but eat everything, including the bones.

CHINESE CABBAGE PICKLES

Preparation time: 10 minutes   *Yield:* 10–15 servings
Pickling time: 1–2 days

These pickles are useful in cases of uremia or kidney failure.

    1 whole Chinese cabbage
    1–2 tablespoons sea salt

1. Cut cabbage in 1-inch crosswise slices.
2. Mix the cabbage with the salt.
3. Press in a salad press, or place in a bowl, cover with a plate, and weight the plate with a rock. Press for several days.
4. It is ready to serve when it is covered with liquid and tastes pickled, usually 1 to 2 days.

CHUBA IRIKO NITSUKE

Preparation time: 5 minutes   *Yield:* 7 servings
Cooking time: 10 minutes

This nitsuke is useful for people with osteomyelitis, the yin types of leprosy, periostitis, or peritonitis.

    1 cup chuba iriko (small dried fish)
    1 teaspoon sesame oil
    1 tablespoon soy sauce
    1/4 teaspoon ginger juice

1. Roast chuba iriko in a dry pan over medium heat for about 7 minutes or until crisp.
2. Add sesame oil and put cover on pan. Heat for another 3 minutes.
3. Mix well and remove from heat.
4. Sprinkle with soy sauce and ginger juice.
5. Serve warm or at room temperature.

CUCUMBER WITH KUZU SAUCE

Preparation time: 5 minutes   *Yield:* 3–5 servings
Cooking time: 35 minutes

This preparation is useful for those who have yang disorders such as appendicitis, kidney failure, leprosy, and itchy skin.

    1 cucumber
    1/2 cup water or stock
    1 pinch sea salt
    1–2 teaspoons soy sauce
    1 tablespoon kuzu mixed with
        3 tablespoons water

1. Peel the cucumber if it is not organic. Cut into 1-inch slices.
2. Add pinch of sea salt and cucumber to water or stock; cook until cucumber is tender.
3. Add soy sauce, then the kuzu mixture.
4. Stir and cook until thick.
5. Serve warm or at room temperature.

Variation

And Tofu

This variation is useful for a very yang condition. Add 1/2 pound of tofu, cut in cubes, after cooking cucumber. Add 1 additional tablespoon soy sauce and proceed as above.

CUCUMBER PRESSED SALAD

Preparation time: 10 minutes   *Yield:* 7–10 servings
Pressing time: 20–30 minutes
Standing time: 5 minutes

This pressed salad is useful in cases of insomnia, stroke, non-insulin-dependent diabetes, or skin discoloration.

    3 cucumbers
    2 teaspoons sea salt
    3 tablespoons lemon juice or rice vinegar

1. Peel the cucumbers if they are not organic. Cut 1/2 inch from the stem end of each cucumber.
2. Dip the cut-off piece of the cucumber in salt and replace it on the cucumber.
3. Rub the cut surfaces together to eliminate any bitterness.
4. Cut the cucumbers in very thin slices.
5. Sprinkle with salt, mix well, and press in a salad press for 20 to 30 minutes or until water comes out of the cucumbers.

6. Drain cucumbers and squeeze out excess water.
7. Mix with lemon juice and serve after 5 minutes.

CUCUMBER SALAD WITH RICE VINEGAR

Preparation time: 10 minutes   *Yield:* 7–10 servings
Standing time: 15 minutes

This preparation is useful with cases of tetanus or beriberi.

>   3 cucumbers
>   2 teaspoons sea salt
>   3 tablespoons rice vinegar

1. Peel the cucumbers if not organic. Cut ½ inch from the stem end of each cucumber.
2. Dip the cut-off piece of each cucumber in salt and replace it on the cucumber.
3. Rub cut surfaces together to eliminate any bitterness.
4. Cut the cucumbers in very thin slices.
5. Sprinkle with salt and let stand for 10 minutes.
6. Squeeze out any excess water.
7. Mix with rice vinegar and let stand 5 minutes before serving.

DAIKON NITSUKE

Preparation time: 5 minutes   *Yield:* 7–10 servings
Cooking time: 35–50 minutes

Daikon Nitsuke is useful mostly in cases of yang disorders, including sexual organ and intestinal problems. It is also used in cases of the yin type of bladder infection.

>   1 medium daikon
>   2 teaspoons sesame oil
>   ¼ teaspoon sea salt
>   2 tablespoons soy sauce

1. Cut daikon in match-stick shapes.
2. Sauté daikon in oil until translucent.
3. Add salt and 1 tablespoon soy sauce. Cook over low heat, covered, for 10 minutes or until daikon releases its juice.
4. Raise heat to medium and continue to cook daikon for 20 minutes or until it is tender, stirring occasionally.
5. If much juice remains, remove the cover and simmer until juice evaporates.
6. Sprinkle 1 tablespoon soy sauce on top and mix.
7. Serve hot.

Variation

With Homemade Agé

This variation is useful with respiratory or kidney problems. Cut 2 or 3 pieces of Homemade Agé (see page 215) in match-stick shapes. Add along with salt and soy sauce. Cook as above.

DEEP-FRIED CHUBA IRIKO

Preparation time: 2–3 minutes   *Yield:* 10–15 servings
Cooking time: 5–7 minutes

This preparation in useful with more yin disorders, including arthritis, rheumatism, impotence, and leukemia.

>   oil for deep-frying
>   1 package chuba iriko (small dried fish),
>   about 3 ounces
>   2–4 tablespoons soy sauce
>   1 teaspoon ginger juice

1. Heat oil over medium-high heat to approximately 350°F.
2. Add chuba iriko and fry until they become slightly brown in color. Drain.
3. Heat soy sauce in a pan and add hot fish and ginger juice. Cook, shaking pan or stirring, over medium heat until dry.
4. Serve at room temperature. Any leftover will keep well in a tightly closed jar.

Variation

Pan-Fried Chuba Iriko

If you wish to use less oil, fish may be pan-fried in 2 tablespoons oil. Sauté fish and cook with soy sauce as above.

DEEP-FRIED KOMBU

Preparation time: 5 minutes   *Yield:* 5 servings
Cooking time: 3–5 minutes

Deep-Fried Kombu is useful with many disorders, mostly those of the yin type; however, it is useful for the yang type of arthritis or rheumatism.

>   1 or 2 pieces kombu
>   sesame oil for deep-frying
>   5 teaspoons grated daikon
>   soy sauce

1. Clean the kombu with a damp towel to remove any sand.

2. Cut kombu in 10 pieces, 1½ inches square.
3. Heat oil to about 350°F. Fry kombu on both sides until crispy. Let cool.
4. Drain in a colander and place on a paper towel to remove excess oil.
5. Add a few drops of soy sauce to the daikon.
6. Serve each person 2 pieces of kombu at room temperature with 1 teaspoon daikon.

DRIED DAIKON NITSUKE

Preparation time: 3–5 minutes   *Yield:* 7–10 servings
Soaking time: 20 minutes
Cooking time: 50–65 minutes

This nitsuke is useful for those who have the yang type of diarrhea or enteritis.

> 1 package dried daikon, about 3 ounces
> 2–3 cups water
> ¼ teaspoon sea salt
> 2 teaspoons soy sauce

1. Cover daikon with water and soak for 20 minutes. Drain and reserve the water used for soaking.
2. Cut daikon in pieces 1½ inches long.
3. Place the soaking water and the daikon in a pot and bring to a boil. Cook, covered, for 30 to 45 minutes or until tender.
4. Add salt and soy sauce. Cook over high heat, uncovered, until water is evaporated, about 20 minutes.
5. Serve warm.

Variation

With Homemade Agé

This option is useful for variety. Cut 3 or 4 pieces of Homemade Agé (see page 215) into match-stick shapes. Add agé to the cooking pot with the daikon and cook as above.

DRIED DAIKON PICKLES

Preparation time: 15 minutes   *Yield:* 5–7 servings
Standing time: 24 hours

These pickles are useful in cases of asthma or breast cancer.

> 1 package dried daikon, about 3 ounces
> 1 piece kombu, 3 inches square

Sauce
> ⅔ cup soy sauce
> ⅔ cup water or stock
> ¼ cup brown rice vinegar or umeboshi vinegar

1. Wash dried daikon quickly in a strainer. Squeeze out the water.
2. Cut kombu in ⅛-inch match-stick shapes.
3. Mix sauce ingredients together in a porcelain or glass container and add daikon and kombu.
4. Let stand for 24 hours in a cool place, mixing 2 or 3 times.
5. Serve with brown rice.

EGG OIL

Preparation time: 2–3 minutes   *Yield:* ⅓–½ cup
Cooking time: 1 hour

Egg oil is good with a yin heart condition or any time the heart needs to be strengthened. It is also used topically to help hair growth and to relieve pain from a rectal prolapse.

> 12 egg yolks (use fertile chicken eggs only)

1. Beat the egg yolks and cook in a heavy iron frying pan over high heat.
2. Eventually, the yolks will turn dark brown, and begin to smoke. The eggs will become black, like coal tar. In this process, smoke will be produced, so be sure to open windows and use a fan, or cook outdoors.
3. Slowly, a black-colored oil will appear.
4. Skim off the oil. (About ⅓ to ½ cup egg oil is produced from 12 egg yolks.) The oil will stay fresh for many years in a jar kept at room temperature.

EGGPLANT MUSTARD PICKLES

Preparation time: 50–60 minutes   *Yield:* 3–4 cups
Pressing time: 2–3 days
Cooking time: 20 minutes
Standing time: 14 minutes
Pickling time: 1–4 weeks

These pickles are useful for those who have yang intestinal problems, scarlet fever, or typhoid fever.

> 2 pounds small, young eggplant
> 2 tablespoons sea salt
> ½ cup water
> ⅔ cup soy sauce
> 4 tablespoons rice syrup
> 1 tablespoon sea salt
> 1 cup mustard powder

½ cup boiling Bancha Tea (see page 232)
1 cup rice koji
½ cup water or stock

1. Wash the eggplant and cut each in half lengthwise.
2. Mix with 2 tablespoons salt and place in a salad press with ½ cup water. Press hard for 2 or 3 days.
3. Remove eggplant and cut in strips ½ inch wide. Squeeze the strips firmly to remove water.
4. Mix soy sauce, rice syrup, and 1 tablespoon salt. Bring to a boil and allow to cool.
5. Marinate the eggplant in this mixture for 7 minutes.
6. In a small oven-safe bowl, combine mustard powder with enough of the boiling Bancha Tea to make a thick, creamy paste that will stick to the bowl when turned upside down.
7. Turn the bowl upside-down and let it stand 7 minutes.
8. Place the bowl upside-down on a burner turned to very low heat for 7 minutes, or until the mustard paste is dried out.
9. Combine the mustard paste with rice koji and ½ cup water or stock and mix well.
10. Spread a thin layer of this mustard mixture on the bottom of a clean crock.
11. Place a layer of eggplant strips on the mustard mixture and press down.
12. Continue making layers of eggplant and mustard mixture, ending with mustard on top.
13. Cover with a clean cotton cloth. Place the crock lid on top and seal it with tape.
14. Keep in a cool place. The pickles will be ready to eat in 1 to 4 weeks.
15. Serve at room temperature.

Eggplant Nishime

Preparation time: 5 minutes   *Yield:* 3 servings
Cooking time: 2–3 hours

Eggplant nishime is useful in cases of itchy skin or nocturnal emission.

    3 small eggplants
    1 tablespoon sesame oil
    ¼ cup water
    1 tablespoon soy sauce

1. Cut each eggplant in half and slash each half lengthwise into 3 or 4 slices, leaving the eggplant connected at the stem end.
2. Sauté eggplant in oil for 3 to 5 minutes.
3. Add water and soy sauce.
4. Cover and simmer over very low heat for 2 to 3 hours.

Eggplant Nitsuke with Miso

Preparation time: 10 minutes   *Yield:* 5 servings
Cooking time: 35 minutes
Standing time: 30 minutes

This nitsuke is useful with many yang disorders, especially kidney, blood, and nerve problems, or breast and lung cancer.

    1 large or 5 small eggplants
    2 teaspoons sea salt
    2–3 tablespoons sesame oil
    1 tablespoon sesame oil
    3 tablespoons barley miso
    5 tablespoons boiling water
    1 tablespoon grated ginger
    2 teaspoons grated orange rind

1. Remove the stem end of the eggplant. Cut eggplant in ½-inch lengthwise slices. Score each slice diagonally in a basketweave design.
2. Sprinkle with salt and let stand for 30 minutes. Remove the surface moisture with a paper towel.
3. Heat 1 tablespoon oil in a cast iron skillet over medium-high heat.
4. Place a layer of eggplant slices in the pan and cover. Cook 1 minute.
5. Turn the slices and press them slightly with a spatula. Cover and cook 5 minutes.
6. Turn the slices again. Cover and cook until tender. Eggplant will be translucent.
7. Repeat steps 3 through 6, adding oil each time as needed (approximately 2 to 3 tablespoons will be needed), until all eggplant slices have been cooked.
8. In another pan, heat the 1 tablespoon of oil. Combine with miso and cook until fragrant, about 5 minutes.
9. Add boiling water, stir until creamy, and bring to a boil.
10. Add the grated ginger and orange rind.
11. Pour miso sauce over eggplant and serve immediately.

Variation

And Lemon

This variation is useful in cases of insomnia. For step 10, add grated ginger, 2 tablespoons lemon juice, and 2 teaspoons grated lemon rind.

212

EGGPLANT PRESSED SALAD

Preparation time: 10 minutes   *Yield:* 5 servings
Pressing time: 30–60 minutes

This pressed salad is useful with more yang disorders, including constipation, facial skin infections, beriberi, and anal fissure.

> 3 small eggplants
> 2 teaspoons sea salt
> soy sauce

1. Cut the eggplant in match-stick shapes, 2 inches long.
2. Mix with salt.
3. Place in a salad press for 30 to 60 minutes, or until liquid appears.
4. Rinse the eggplant and squeeze out the water.
5. Serve with a small amount of soy sauce.

GINGER MISO

Preparation time: 5 minutes   *Yield:* 3–5 servings

This condiment is useful with many yang disorders. It is especially useful to help improve circulation.

> 1 teaspoon freshly grated ginger
> 1 tablespoon barley miso

1. Mix ginger and miso together.
2. If desired, 1 tablespoon boiling water may be added.
3. Serve at room temperature a little bit at a time on grains or side dishes.

GRATED DAIKON

Preparation time: 5 minutes   *Yield:* 1 serving

This condiment is used with many recipes and is appropriate for most disorders. It is used mostly with tempura to help digest oil, and with natto, Brown Rice Gruel, mochi, and vegetables. It may also be added (without soy sauce) to miso soup.

> 1 tablespoon freshly grated daikon
> 1/4–1/2 teaspoon soy sauce

1. Mix grated daikon with soy sauce.
2. Serve as a condiment.

Variations

With Soy Sauce

This variation is used as a side dish for many yang disorders and is helpful in removing excess poor-quality salt. Mix 1 tablespoon of grated daikon with 1/2 to 1 teaspoon of soy sauce.

With Sesame Oil and Soy Sauce

This variation is an easy way to digest oil and is useful for excessive fatigue, nerve pain, or peritonitis. Mix 1 tablespoon grated daikon with 1 tablespoon soy sauce and 1 tablespoon boiled sesame oil. Eat with Brown Rice or other grain.

GREEN LEAFY VEGETABLES

Preparation time: 10 minutes   *Yield:* 5–7 servings
Cooking time: 15–25 minutes

Green Leafy Vegetables are good in any healing diet, but especially with yang disorders of the lungs, intestines, or sexual organs.

> 1 bunch collard greens or other dark-green
>   leafy vegetables
> 2 teaspoons sesame oil
> 1/4 teaspoon sea salt
> 1 tablespoon soy sauce

1. Wash greens and cut in 1-inch strips.
2. Sauté the greens in sesame oil until they are bright green in color.
3. Add salt and soy sauce. Cover the pan and cook over low heat for 5 minutes. Water will come out of the vegetables.
4. Cover and cook over medium heat 5 to 10 minutes or until tender.
5. Serve hot, warm, or at room temperature.

Variations

With Homemade Agé

This variation is useful for many disorders, specifically bladder infections, diphtheria, and peritonitis. Cut 3 pieces of Homemade Agé (see page 215) into match-stick shapes. After greens have been cooked over low heat for 5 minutes, add agé on top of the greens. Cover and cook over medium heat 5 minutes. Mix agé into the vegetables and cook until they are tender, about 5 or 10 minutes.

With Mock Goose

This variation is useful for diphtheria. Place pieces of Mock Goose (see page 218) on top of the greens after they have been cooked for 5 minutes. Cover and cook over medium heat 5 minutes. Mix Mock Goose into the vegetables and cook until they are tender, about 5 or 10 minutes.

GREEN SALAD

Preparation time: 10–15 minutes   *Yield:* 7–10 servings

Green Salad is useful specifically for those experiencing headache, including migraines, or hair loss.

> 1 head of lettuce
> 1 medium cucumber
> sea salt

Dressing

> 2 tablespoons sesame or olive oil
> 1 tablespoon lemon juice
> 3 tablespoons orange juice
> 1 tablespoon minced onion
> 2 teaspoons sea salt

1. Wash lettuce leaves and tear in 1-inch squares.
2. Cut ½ inch from the stem end of the cucumber.
3. Dip the cut-off piece of the cucumber in salt and replace it on the cucumber. Rub the cut surfaces together to eliminate any bitterness.
4. Cut the cucumber in half lengthwise and slice thinly.
5. Place dressing ingredients in a jar; cover securely and shake until blended.
6. Toss salad with dressing.
7. Serve immediately.

HIJIKI BURDOCK NITSUKE

Preparation time: 10 minutes   *Yield:* 7–10 servings
Soaking time: 10 minutes
Cooking time: 1–1¼ hours

This side dish is useful with many yin or yang types of disorders.

> 1 package hijiki, about 2.5 ounces
> 3–4 cups water
> burdock, 3-inch piece or about 1 cup
>   after cutting
> 1–2 tablespoons sesame oil
> 3–4 tablespoons soy sauce

1. Rinse hijiki quickly in a bowl of water and drain.
2. Soak hijiki in 3 to 4 cups water for 10 minutes. (Water should rise 2 inches above hijiki.)
3. Cut burdock in match-stick shapes.
4. Drain hijiki. Strain soaking water through a cotton cloth and reserve.

5. Place hijiki in a bowl and hold it under running water. Hold a strainer in the other hand and allow ⅓ of the hijiki at a time to float from the bowl into the strainer. Any sand will remain in the bottom of the bowl. Repeat washing if necessary.
6. Heat oil and sauté burdock for a few minutes.
7. Add hijiki and sauté until it is almost dry.
8. Add strained soaking water and soy sauce. Cook, uncovered, over medium-high heat for about 40 minutes, stirring occasionally.
9. When water is almost evaporated, turn heat to low and continue to cook for about 15 minutes, stirring occasionally. Hijiki will appear very shiny.
10. Serve warm or at room temperature.

HIJIKI CARROT NITSUKE

Preparation time: 10 minutes   *Yield:* 7 to 10 servings
Soaking time: 10 minutes
Cooking time: 1–1¼ hours

This nitsuke is useful for those who have problems of the upper body, especially the head.

> 1 package hijiki, about 2.5 ounces
> 3–4 cups water
> carrot, 3-inch piece or about 1 cup after cutting
> 1–2 tablespoons sesame oil
> 3–4 tablespoons soy sauce

1. Rinse hijiki quickly in a bowl of water and drain.
2. Soak hijiki in 3 to 4 cups water for 10 minutes. (Water should rise 2 inches above hijiki.)
3. Cut carrot in match-stick shapes.
4. Drain hijiki. Strain soaking water through a cotton cloth and reserve.
5. Place hijiki in a bowl and hold it under running water. Hold a strainer in the other hand and allow ⅓ of the hijiki at a time to float from the bowl into the strainer. Any sand will remain in the bottom of the bowl. Repeat washing if necessary.
6. Heat oil and sauté carrot for a few minutes.
7. Add hijiki and sauté until almost dry.
8. Add strained soaking water and soy sauce. Cook, uncovered, over medium-high heat for about 40 minutes, stirring occasionally.
9. When water is almost evaporated, turn heat to low and continue to cook for about 15 minutes, stirring occasionally. Hijiki will appear very shiny.
10. Serve warm or at room temperature.

214

Hijiki Lotus Root Nitsuke

Preparation time: 10 minutes   *Yield:* 7–10 servings
Soaking time: 10 minutes
Cooking time: 1–1¼ hours

Hijiki Lotus Root Nitsuke is useful for yin people whose body condition is expanded and loose. It helps contract the body and is good for the lungs. It is also helpful for those with nearsightedness, hemorrhoids, arthritis, and many other disorders; eat 2 to 3 tablespoons of this dish every day. Don't use bleached lotus root; its color should be tan, not white. Choose smaller, more yang roots.

> 1 package hijiki, about 2.5 ounces
> 3–4 cups water
> lotus root, 3-inch piece or about 1 cup
>   after cutting
> 1–2 tablespoons sesame oil
> 3–4 tablespoons soy sauce

1. Rinse hijiki quickly in a bowl of water and drain.
2. Soak hijiki in 3 to 4 cups water for 10 minutes. (Water should rise 2 inches above hijiki.)
3. Cut lotus root in quarter moons or match-stick shapes.
4. Drain hijiki. Strain soaking water through a cotton cloth and reserve.
5. Place hijiki in a bowl and hold it under running water. Hold a strainer in the other hand and allow ⅓ of the hijiki at a time to float from the bowl into the strainer. Any sand will remain in the bottom of the bowl. Repeat washing if necessary.
6. Heat oil and sauté lotus root for a few minutes.
7. Add hijiki and sauté until almost dry.
8. Add strained soaking water and soy sauce. Cook, uncovered, over medium-high heat for about 40 minutes, stirring occasionally.
9. When water is almost evaporated, turn heat to low and continue to cook for about 15 minutes, stirring occasionally. Hijiki will appear very shiny.
10. Serve warm or at room temperature.

Hijiki Nitsuke

Preparation time: 5 minutes   *Yield:* 5–7 servings
Soaking time: 10 minutes
Cooking time: 1–1¼ hours

Hijiki Nitsuke is useful with almost all disorders.

> 1 package hijiki, about 2.5 ounces
> 3–4 cups water
> 1–2 tablespoons sesame oil
> 3–4 tablespoons soy sauce

1. Rinse hijiki quickly in a bowl of water and drain.
2. Soak hijiki in 3 to 4 cups of water for 10 minutes. (Water should rise 2 inches above hijiki.)
3. Drain hijiki. Strain soaking water through a cotton cloth and reserve.
4. Place hijiki in a bowl and hold it under running water. Hold a strainer in the other hand and allow ⅓ of the hijiki at a time to float from the bowl into the strainer. Any sand will remain in the bottom of the bowl. Repeat washing if necessary.
5. Heat oil and sauté hijiki until it is almost dry.
6. Add strained soaking water and soy sauce. Cook, uncovered, over medium-high heat for about 40 minutes, stirring occasionally.
7. When water is almost evaporated, turn heat to low and continue to cook for about 15 minutes, stirring occasionally. Hijiki will appear very shiny.
8. Serve warm or at room temperature.

Homemade Agé

Preparation time: 10 minutes   *Yield:* 10 servings
Cooking time: 15 minutes

Agé is used with grain and vegetable dishes and in soup. It is useful in cases of adult dysentery, insomnia, or hemorrhoids.

> 1 pound soft tofu
> sesame oil, for deep frying
> 1 cup grated daikon
> 5 teaspoons soy sauce

1. Cut the tofu in slices 1½ inches by 1 inch by ⅜ inches, or about 16 pieces per pound.
2. Place a clean cotton towel on a cutting board. Arrange the slices of tofu on the towel and cover with another towel. Place another cutting board on top. Set the cutting boards near the sink and tilt them slightly so excess water will drain into the sink. Place a heavy pot or weight on top of the cutting boards and allow tofu to drain for about 20 minutes. As an alternate method, you may gently squeeze the tofu with your hands by placing one slice at a time between 2 paper towels.
3. Heat the oil to about 350°F.
4. Deep-fry tofu slices until both sides are golden brown. Or, to use less oil, dust tofu slices with buckwheat flour or whole-wheat pastry flour and pan-fry.
5. Serve warm with 1 heaping tablespoon grated daikon, and ½ teaspoon soy sauce per person, or use agé in soup or vegetable dishes.

KOMBU ROLLS

Preparation time: 20 minutes   *Yield:* 7–10 servings
Soaking time: 10–15 minutes
Cooking time: 1¼ hours

Kombu rolls are useful with sexual organ disorders, especially ovarian inflammation.

> 1 piece kombu, 3 inches by 15 inches
> 3 cups water
> 1 carrot
> 1 burdock
> corn husk, or toothpicks
> 2 tablespoons soy sauce

1. Soak the kombu in 3 cups of water for 3 to 5 minutes. Reserve the soaking water.
2. Allow kombu to dry for 10 minutes.
3. Quarter the carrot and the burdock lengthwise. Cut the carrot and burdock in lengths equal to the width of the kombu, about 3 inches.
4. Cover the corn husk with water and soak until it is soft, about 10 minutes. Cut the corn husk in strips.
5. Place the kombu on a flat surface and arrange 2 pieces each of carrot and burdock across one end of the kombu.
6. Roll up the kombu with the carrot and burdock inside and roll once more so that there are 2 layers of kombu.
7. Trim the Kombu Roll at each end of the roll if necessary to produce even ends.
8. Tie the roll in 2 places with corn-husk strips or fasten with toothpicks.
9. Continue making rolls with the rest of the kombu and vegetables.
10. Cook the rolls in the soaking water for about 1 hour or until tender. (Or pressure cook for 7 minutes.)
11. Add soy sauce and cook a few minutes more. (If using a pressure cooker, add soy sauce, and cook over high heat until water evaporates.)
12. Cut each roll in 2 pieces.
13. Serve at room temperature or warm.

Variation

With Chuba Iriko

This variation is useful for sexual organ problems. It is also useful for bone, stomach, and spinal cord disorders. Substitute 20 chuba iriko (small dried fish) for the burdock.

KOMBU STOCK

Preparation time: 5 minutes   *Yield:* 7 cups
Soaking time: 10–20 minutes
Cooking time: 20 minutes

This stock is used for making soup or as a substitute for water in grain or vegetable dishes.

> 2 pieces kombu, 3 inches by 12 inches
> 7 cups water

1. Soak the kombu in the water until it softens, 10 to 20 minutes.
2. Slice into 1-inch strips and put back in the water. Cook over medium heat for 20 minutes. Do not boil.
3. When kombu comes to the surface, remove it. The kombu may be used in bean or vegetable dishes or to make Shio Kombu with Oil (see page 224).

KOMBU STOCK CLEAR SOUP

Preparation time: 5 minutes   *Yield:* 5–7 servings
Cooking time: 3–5 minutes
Standing time: 3–5 minutes

This clear soup is used for noodle dishes.

> 5 cups Kombu Stock (see above)
> 2–3 tablespoons soy sauce
> 1 sheet nori, roasted and crumbled
> several scallions, cut in thin rounds

1. Bring Kombu Stock to a boil and shut off the heat.
2. Add soy sauce and let stand for a few minutes.
3. Serve garnished with nori and scallions.

KUZU SOUP

Preparation time: 10–15 minutes   *Yield:* 5–7 servings
Cooking time: 45 minutes

Kuzu has a contracting quality and helps make the digestive organs strong. Kuzu Soup is especially useful for those experiencing sharp intestinal pains, diarrhea, dysentery, or cholera.

> 1 cauliflower
> 3 onions
> 1 carrot
> 2 stalks celery
> 1 tablespoon sesame oil
> ½ teaspoon sea salt

5 cups boiling water
1 heaping tablespoon kuzu
½ cup cold water
2–3 tablespoons soy sauce

1. Separate the cauliflower flowerets from the stems and heart. Cut the stems in diagonals and the heart in match-stick shapes. Cut the onions in ¼-inch crescents. Cut the carrot in large diagonal wedges. Cut the celery in ¼-inch diagonals.
2. Heat the oil and sauté the onions, carrot, cauliflower heart and stems, cauliflower flowerets, and celery, in that order.
3. Sprinkle salt over the vegetables and sauté them a few minutes more.
4. Add boiling water and cook over medium heat for 15 minutes.
5. Dissolve kuzu in ½ cup of cold water and add it to the soup. Stir the soup until it thickens.
6. When it begins to boil, add soy sauce.
7. Bring to a boil again and serve immediately.

LEMON DRESSING

Preparation time: 5 minutes   *Yield:* 5–7 servings

This dressing is used with many recipes.

2 tablespoons lemon juice
1 teaspoon soy sauce
1 tablespoon olive oil
¼ teaspoon sea salt

1. Place ingredients in a jar.
2. Cover securely and shake until creamy.
3. Serve at room temperature.

LEMON MISO

Preparation time: 10 minutes   *Yield:* 10–15 servings

This preparation is useful in cases of eye or skin problems, or infertility.

1 tablespoon rice miso
1 tablespoon barley miso
⅔ cup stock or water
2 teaspoons lemon rind, grated
1 tablespoon lemon juice

1. Combine miso and stock. Bring to a boil.
2. Remove from heat and add lemon rind and juice.
3. Serve at room temperature over boiled daikon or other cooked vegetables.

LOTUS ROOT NISHIME

Preparation time: 5 minutes   *Yield:* 3 servings
Cooking time: 55 minutes

Lotus Root Nishime is useful with coughs and in cases of tuberculosis.

1 cup lotus root (approximately)
1 teaspoon sesame oil
½ teaspoon sea salt
½ cup water
1 tablespoon soy sauce

1. Cut the lotus root in large rounds.
2. Heat the oil and sauté the lotus root for 5 minutes.
3. Add salt and water and cook over medium heat for 30 minutes.
4. Add soy sauce and cook 20 minutes more. Add more water if necessary. The lotus root should be slightly crisp when done.
5. Serve warm or at room temperature.

LOTUS ROOT NITSUKE

Preparation time: 5 minutes   *Yield:* 3 to 5 servings
Cooking time: 55 minutes

Lotus Root Nitsuke is useful for those who have respiratory, heart, or bladder disorders.

1 cup lotus root
1 teaspoon sesame oil
¼ teaspoon sea salt
½ cup water
1 tablespoon soy sauce

1. Dice lotus root.
2. Heat sesame oil and sauté the lotus root for 5 minutes.
3. Add salt and water. Cover and cook over medium to low heat for 30 minutes.
4. Add soy sauce and cook 20 minutes more. Add more water if necessary. The lotus root should be tender and slightly crisp when done.
5. Serve warm or at room temperature.

MISO PICKLES

Preparation time: 15–20 minutes   *Yield:* 30–50 servings
Pressing time: 24 hours
Pickling time: 3 months

These pickles are useful with all yin disorders.

vegetables (use any of the following: 7 or 8
small whole cucumbers, 1 daikon 2½ inches
in diameter and 12 inches long cut in lengths
to fit the crock and quartered, 6 or 7 small
whole eggplant, 3 burdock cut to fit the crock,
or peeled fresh ginger)
sea salt*
miso, about 3 pounds
crock or pickle press

1. Wash and clean vegetables.
2. Mix the vegetables with 10 percent of their weight
   in salt and place them in the crock.
3. Place a plate on the vegetables and weight it with a
   clean rock (see Figure 4.1), or press the vegetables in
   a pickle press.
4. When liquid comes to the top, in about 24 hours,
   remove the vegetables and discard the liquid.
5. Place a ¼-inch layer of miso on the bottom of the
   crock or pickle press.
6. Add a layer of vegetables then a 1-inch layer of miso.
   Continue layering miso and vegetables, ending with
   miso.
7. Place a board on the miso and weight it with a rock,
   or apply pressure with the pickle press.
8. Pickle at room temperature for about 3 months.
   Remove the pickled vegetables and discard the miso.
9. Serve 2 or 3 slices per meal at room temperature.

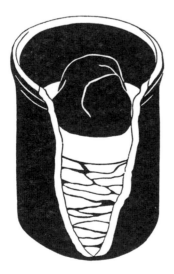

Figure 4.1 Cut-away view of plate weighted with a rock

* Kombu may be pickled dry (without salt). Cut kombu to fit the
crock and layer it with miso. Press as described above in steps 5
through 8.

MOCK GOOSE

Preparation time: 20 minutes   *Yield:* 10–15 servings
Standing time: 1 hour
Cooking time: 8–10 minutes

Mock goose is useful in cases of diphtheria.

> 1 pound soft tofu
> 5 shiitake mushrooms, soaked; or
>   10 fresh mushrooms
> 1 medium carrot
> 1 cup minced onions
> ½ cup scallions, cut in thin rounds
> 1 egg or 1 heaping tablespoon whole-wheat
>   pastry flour
> 1 teaspoon sea salt
> sesame oil for frying

1. Drain tofu. Wrap in a cotton cloth.
2. Place wrapped tofu between 2 cutting boards and
   weight with a rock. Raise at an angle so the water
   drains off.
3. Let stand for 1 hour. (Occasional pressing with your
   hands helps to drain off more water.)
4. Cut mushrooms in ½-inch pieces. Mince carrot.
5. Break pieces of tofu into a bowl. Knead by hand until
   tofu is well broken.
6. Add mushrooms, carrot, onions, scallions, egg or flour,
   and salt. Mix thoroughly and make into 10 rectangular shapes similar to slices of goose.
7. Deep fry one side of each slice for about 5 minutes at
   350°F. Turn over and deep fry the second side for
   about 3 minutes until golden yellow.
8. Drain excess oil and place on paper towels.
9. Serve warm or hot with mustard or soy sauce, or Grated Daikon with Soy Sauce (see page 213), or grated
   ginger with soy sauce.

MUGWORT BREAD

Preparation time: 20–30 minutes   *Yield:* 7–10 servings
Cooking time: 35 minutes

This bread is useful for helping to eliminate parasites.

> ½ cup fresh mugwort
> 1½ cups water
> ¼ teaspoon sea salt
> 1 cup sweet brown rice flour
> 1 cup brown rice flour
> 1 cup boiling water
> Azuki Beans with Kombu (see page 205)

1. Add ¼ teaspoon salt to 1½ cups water.

2. Boil mugwort, uncovered, in the salted water for a few minutes.
3. Drain and cool mugwort. Squeeze out water. Set aside.
4. Combine flours and add 1 cup boiling water. Mix and knead.
5. Add mugwort and knead until evenly mixed.
6. Place a damp towel inside a steamer. Make small balls of the dough and place them in the towel.
7. Cover the balls of dough with the towel and steam over high heat for 30 minutes.
8. Remove the balls of dough and pound them with a wooden pestle until they are sticky.
9. Form dough into tiny balls and serve them with a covering of Azuki Beans with Kombu.

MUSTARD GREEN PICKLES

Preparation time: 10 minutes   *Yield:* 10 servings
Drying time: 4 hours
Pickling time: 2 days

These pickles are useful for those who have kidney failure or uremia.

         1 bunch mustard greens
         2 teaspoons sea salt

1. Wash greens and let them drain and dry for 4 hours.
2. Cut greens in 1-inch slices and mix with the salt.
3. Press in a salad press in a cool place for 2 days. Greens may also be eaten as a pressed salad after about 5 hours of pressing.
4. Rinse and drain pickles before serving.

NATTO WITH SOY SAUCE AND SCALLIONS

Preparation time: 10 minutes   *Yield:* 10 servings

Natto with Soy Sauce and Scallions is useful with many yang disorders such as constipation, ovarian inflammation, and kidney troubles.

         1 cup natto
         1/8 teaspoon sea salt
         1 tablespoon soy sauce
         2 heaping tablespoons sliced scallions

1. Mix natto, salt, and soy sauce. Blend the mixture well.
2. Add scallions and mix again.
3. Serve at room temperature with Brown Rice (see page 195).

NORI NITSUKE

Preparation time: 5 minutes   *Yield:* 10–12 servings
Standing time: 5 minutes
Cooking time: 20–30 minutes

Nori Nitsuke is useful with nerve, joint, and bone problems as well as sexual organ or heart and circulatory disorders.

         1 1/2 cups water
         1 teaspoon sea salt
         10 sheets nori
         3–4 tablespoons soy sauce

1. Add salt to water.
2. Tear the nori in 1-inch squares and mix with salt water. Let stand 5 minutes or until nori becomes moist.
3. Add soy sauce. Cover and bring to a boil.
4. Cook over low heat for 20 to 30 minutes. Nori Nitsuke will keep for 1 week without refrigeration, in a cool place.
5. Serve at room temperature, 1 heaping teaspoon per person.

NORI ROASTED WITH OIL

Cooking time: 5 minutes   *Yield:* 3–4 servings

This preparation is useful for people who need to add oil to their diet but have trouble digesting it. It is useful for eye problems, for relieving thirst, and for many yin disorders.

         2 sheets nori
         sesame oil

1. Place 2 sheets of nori together and roast 1 side of each sheet by briefly passing over a flame.
2. Brush the heated side of each sheet with oil while the nori is still hot.
3. Serve at room temperature or warm.

OILY MISO

Cooking time: 3–5 minutes   *Yield:* 7–10 servings

This condiment is useful with many yin disorders, especially lung, heart, and circulatory diseases. It is also specifically useful for arthritis, near-sightedness, glaucoma, and rheumatism.

         3 tablespoons hatcho or barley miso
         1 tablespoon sesame oil
         5 tablespoons soup stock or water

1. Sauté miso in oil until it produces a rich aroma, about 3 to 5 minutes.
2. Add enough stock to make a very thick sauce.
3. Serve as a condiment.

OKARA NITSUKE

Preparation time: 20 minutes   *Yield:* 5–7 servings
Cooking time: 1–1¼ hours

Okara Nitsuke is useful with many yang disorders, especially eye, skin, kidney, and sexual organ problems.

⅓ cup burdock
⅓ cup carrot
⅓ cup onion
1 tablespoon sesame oil (approximately)
½ teaspoon sea salt
1 tablespoon soy sauce
1 cup okara
¼ cup chopped scallions

1. Cut burdock and carrot into shavings. Cut onion in thin crescents.
2. Heat the oil, add a pinch of salt to the burdock, and sauté, covered with an otoshibuta or lid that drops inside the pot, and with the pot lid.
3. After 5 minutes, add a pinch of salt and mix. Cover with both covers and cook for 5 minutes more.
4. Repeat the salting and cooking process 1 more time.
5. Add onion with a pinch of salt and sauté, covered, until translucent.
6. Add carrot and sauté for a few minutes, covered.
7. Add remaining salt and soy sauce. Cover and cook until vegetables are tender.
8. Spread okara over the vegetables and press it down. Cook over low heat, covered, for 30 minutes to steam the okara.
9. Gently mix the okara with the vegetables. Sprinkle with scallions and mix.
10. Serve hot or warm.

ORGANIC PHEASANT

Preparation time: 15–20 minutes   *Yield:* 10 servings
Cooking time: 20–30 minutes

This dish is useful in cases of leukemia or bedwetting.

1 organic pheasant
1 thumb-sized piece of ginger
2 tablespoons sesame oil
½ cup soy sauce

1. Cut up pheasant and remove bones.
2. Mince ginger and sauté in oil briefly, for about 1 minute.
3. Sauté pheasant for a few minutes until the color changes.
4. Add soy sauce. Cover and cook until soy sauce is absorbed and pheasant is somewhat dry.
5. Serve warm or at room temperature.

OYSTER TEMPURA

Preparation time: 15–20 minutes   *Yield:* 3–4 servings
Standing time: 5–7 minutes
Cooking time: 5–7 minutes

This tempura is useful for those who have tuberculosis, goiter, anal itch, or breast infection.

10–12 fresh oysters
saltwater
oil for deep-frying

Batter

whole-wheat pastry flour, enough to coat
    oysters
1½ cups whole-wheat pastry flour
1 heaping teaspoon arrowroot starch
¼ teaspoon sea salt
1 cup water

1. Wash oysters gently in salted water. Drain.
2. Coat oysters with whole-wheat pastry flour and let them stand for 5 minutes.
3. Mix 1½ cups whole-wheat pastry flour, arrowroot starch, salt, and water to make a batter.
4. Pour 2½ inches of oil in a heavy pan. Heat to 350°F.
5. Dip oysters in batter. If desired, oysters may be coated with bread crumbs or rice cake crumbs after dipping in batter.
6. Fry in oil until golden on both sides, about 3 minutes on one side and 2 minutes on the other.
7. Drain oysters in a colander and place them on a paper towel to absorb excess oil.
8. Serve hot.

OYSTERS AND TOFU WITH MISO

Preparation time: 10 minutes   *Yield:* 7–10 servings
Cooking time: 20 minutes

16 ounces tofu
1 bunch watercress
½ pound Chinese cabbage
1 bunch scallions

¼–½ cup soup stock
½–1 pound oysters
½–2 tablespoons barley miso
2 teaspoons grated orange peel

1. Cut tofu in 1-inch squares.
2. Separate the top leaves from the watercress stems. Cut the cabbage in 1-inch diagonals. Cut the scallions in long diagonals.
3. Put the soup stock in a pan. Place the tofu, Chinese cabbage, scallions, and oysters in the soup stock with the watercress and miso on top. *Do not mix them together.* Put the orange peel on the very top.
4. Cook, uncovered, over medium heat until the Chinese cabbage is tender, about 20 minutes. Do not overcook. Add more stock or water if necessary.
5. Mix all ingredients together and serve immediately.

OYSTERS COOKED WITH MISO

Preparation time: 5 minutes   *Yield:* 2–3 servings
Cooking time: 15 minutes

This preparation is useful with many yin disorders, especially respiratory illnesses.

5 or 6 fresh oysters
saltwater
1 teaspoon sesame oil
1–2 teaspoons barley miso
1 tablespoon water

1. Wash the oysters gently in salted water. Drain.
2. Heat oil and sauté oysters.
3. Dilute miso with water and add to oysters. Cook for 5 minutes.
4. Serve warm.

POACHED FISH

Preparation time: 5 minutes   *Yield:* 3–5 servings
Marinating time: 30 minutes
Cooking time: 30–40 minutes

This preparation is useful in cases of leukemia, pneumonia, or insulin-dependent diabetes.

water
sea salt
1 whole fish (flounder or other fresh fish), about 2 pounds
soy sauce

1. Prepare a marinade in the proportion of 1 cup water to 2 tablespoons sea salt, enough to cover the fish.
2. Marinate whole fish for 30 minutes.
3. Prepare poaching stock in the proportion of 1 cup water to 2 tablespoons soy sauce, enough to cover the fish.
4. Bring stock to a boil in a pan large enough to hold the fish.
5. Carefully place the fish in the poaching stock and bring to a boil. Simmer, uncovered, for 30 to 40 minutes.
6. Serve hot or warm.

POTATO CONCENTRATE

Preparation time: 30 minutes   *Yield:* 1 cup

This condiment is useful for those who have stomach or duodenal ulcers because it helps alkalize the body.

10 medium-sized potatoes

1. Wash potatoes very well. Remove and discard the eyes.
2. Finely grate the potatoes.
3. Extract the potato juice by squeezing the grated potatoes through a cotton cloth. Discard the pulp.
4. Using an uncovered ceramic or enamel pot, cook the juice over low heat for a long time, until it becomes thick and black. (The substance will be similar in texture and color to umeboshi extract.)
5. Serve at room temperature.

PRESSED SALAD

Preparation time: 10 minutes   *Yield:* 5–7 servings
Pressing time: 2–3 hours

Pressed salad is useful for yang disorders and avoided for yin disorders. For variety you may also use Cucumber Pressed Salad (see page 209) or Eggplant Pressed Salad (see page 213).

1 whole Chinese cabbage, or other salad greens
1–2 teaspoons sea salt

1. Cut the cabbage in 1-inch slices.
2. Mix the cabbage and salt together.
3. Press in a salad press for 2 or 3 hours.
4. Serve at room temperature.

RICE BRAN PICKLES

Preparation time: 6 days   *Yield:* 20 servings
Pickling time: varies with
    vegetable from hours to days

Rice Bran Pickles are useful with many yang disorders and avoided for certain disorders, especially yin ones. Rice Bran Pickles are very important to the digestion of whole grains and vegetables. You can make them yourself or purchase them from a number of natural food stores and mail-order suppliers (see pages 253–254).

> 10 cups rice bran (nuka)
> 2 cups sea salt
> vegetables (outer leaves of cabbage or
>   cauliflower, or carrot or daikon tops, and
>   vegetable to be pickled, such as celery,
>   peeled cucumbers, peeled watermelon rind,
>   whole cabbage*)

1. Mix bran and salt. Dry-roast over medium heat about 10 minutes, stirring constantly. The color will change slightly and the mixture will smell fragrant.
2. Remove from heat, cover, and let stand 1 hour.
3. Spread on a cookie sheet until completely cooled.
4. Place a 2-inch layer of bran in an 8-inch or 10-inch diameter crock or a pickle press and press it down. (You must use this size crock with a cover, or a pickle press.) Add a layer of vegetable leaves and/or tops and cover with the rest of the bran. Press down firmly. Cover the crock with a towel and the crock lid. Keep in a cool place.
5. After 2 days, remove the leaves or tops and discard them. Mix the rice bran thoroughly. Pickle 2 more batches of leaves or tops in the same way and discard them. (The bran will now be ready to use.)
6. Place a 2-inch layer of bran in the crock or pickle press and press it down firmly. Add a layer of vegetables to be pickled. Cover with the rest of the bran. If you wish, you can make 2 or 3 layers of vegetables, always pressing the bran firmly. Cover with a cotton towel, then the crock lid. Keep the crock in a cool place.
7. Celery will be ready in about 8 hours. Daikon takes 1 or 2 days. Peeled cucumbers take 6 to 8 hours. Peeled watermelon rind takes 2 to 3 hours. It will take from 3 to 5 days to pickle a whole cabbage.

* *Note:* For small whole cabbage, remove the core and pickle whole with the cored end up to contain the juice. Dis-card the excess liquid and remove 4 or 5 cabbage leaves every day as they pickle.

8. To speed up the pickling process, or in cold weather, place a board on the bran and weight it with a rock or apply pressure with the pickle press.
9. Remove pickled vegetables and store in the refrigerator. Wash the bran paste off pickles before slicing and serving.
10. After the vegetables have been pickled, mix the bran to keep it evenly moist.
11. After about a month of being used for pickling, the bran will become a wet paste. Roast 2 cups fresh rice bran with 1/3 cup sea salt. Cool and mix with the bran paste in order to keep the paste from spoiling.
12. If you cannot attend to the pickling for 1 month or longer, remove all the vegetables from the crock. Press the bran down and cover it with a board weighted with a rock. Cover the crock with a cotton towel and the crock lid and store in a cool place. Or put the bran in a pickle press, apply pressure, and store in a cool place.

RICE VINEGAR DRESSING

Preparation time: 5 minutes   *Yield:* 2–3 servings

This dressing is particularly useful for those experiencing hair loss or headaches, including migraines.

> 1 tablespoon rice vinegar
> 1/4 teaspoon sea salt
> 1 teaspoon soy sauce
> 1 tablespoon olive oil

1. Place ingredients in a jar.
2. Cover jar securely and shake until ingredients are blended.
3. Serve at room temperature.

ROASTED KOMBU

Preparation time: 2 minutes   *Yield:* 3–5 servings
Cooking time: 7–10 minutes

Roasted Kombu is useful with nausea or heartburn.

> several 2-inch squares of kombu

1. Roast kombu in a dry (no oil) skillet for 7 to 10 minutes. Let cool.
2. Eat a handful or so at a time.

Roasted Pumpkin Seeds

Preparation time: 30 minutes   *Yield:* 1–2 cups
Soaking time: 24 hours
Cooking time: 10 minutes

These seeds are useful in cases of parasites.

> 1 pumpkin
> cold water

1. After removing seeds from the pumpkin, soak them for 24 hours in cold water.
2. Wash seeds to remove the fibers. Drain.
3. Roast seeds in a dry pan until slightly brown, about 10 minutes. They will begin to pop. Let cool.
4. Eat 1 or 2 handfuls at a time or serve on grains.

Roasted Squash Seeds

Preparation time: 30 minutes   *Yield:* 1–2 cups
Soaking time: 24 hours
Cooking time: 10 minutes

These seeds are useful in cases of tapeworms.

> 1 winter squash, remove seeds
> cold water

1. After removing seeds from winter squash, soak them for 24 hours in cold water.
2. Wash seeds to remove the fibers. Drain.
3. Roast seeds in a dry pan until slightly brown, about 10 minutes. Let cool.
4. Eat 1 or 2 handfuls at a time.

Roasted Wakame

Preparation time: 2 minutes   *Yield:* 3–5 servings
Cooking time: 7–10 minutes

Roasted wakame is useful with nervous system malfunction, miscarriage, or premature birth.

> several 2-inch squares of wakame

1. Roast wakame in a dry (no oil) skillet for 7 to 10 minutes. Let cool.
2. Eat a handful or so at a time.

Roasted Watermelon Seeds

Preparation time: 5 minutes   *Yield:* 1 cup
Soaking time: 24 hours
Cooking time: 7–10 minutes

These seeds are useful in cases of parasites.

> 1 watermelon, remove seeds
> cold water

1. After removing seeds from the watermelon, soak them for 24 hours in cold water.
2. Wash seeds to remove the fibers. Drain.
3. Roast seeds in a dry pan until slightly brown, about 7 to 10 minutes. Let cool.
4. Eat 1 or 2 handfuls at a time.

Scallion Miso

Preparation time: 5 minutes   *Yield:* 5–7 servings
Cooking time: 15–20 minutes

Scallion Miso is useful with many disorders, especially yin respiratory or sexual organ problems, heart diseases, rheumatism, brain disorders, or insomnia.

> 1 bunch scallions
> 1 tablespoon sesame oil
> 1 heaping tablespoon barley miso

1. Mince scallion roots. Thinly slice the rest of the scallions, separating the green parts from the white parts.
2. Heat the oil and sauté the roots about 2 minutes until they are slightly brown.
3. Sauté the green parts about 2 minutes until the color changes slightly.
4. Sauté the white parts about 3 minutes.
5. Spread the miso on top of the scallions. Cook, covered, for 5 minutes or until the miso softens.
6. Stir gently and cook uncovered for 3 to 5 minutes more.
7. Serve warm or at room temperature as a condiment with Brown Rice (see page 197), Brown Rice Cream (see page 198), Brown Rice Kayu (see page 200), or cooked cereal.

Scallions Seasoned with Miso

Preparation time: 5 minutes   *Yield:* 3–5 servings

This condiment is useful for insomnia, parasites, or ulcers as it makes the stomach strong.

> 3 tablespoons scallions, chopped
> 1 tablespoon miso

1. Mix chopped scallions with miso. Do not cook.
2. Serve as a condiment or side dish.

SESAME MISO

Preparation time: 5 minutes   *Yield:* 10 servings
Drying time: 10 minutes to overnight
Cooking time: 25–30 minutes
Grinding time: 10 minutes

Sesame Miso is useful with constipation and many yang disorders, including arthritis, pneumonia, and insomnia.

  1/3 cup sesame seeds
  1–2 tablespoons barley miso
  2 teaspoons boiling water

1. Wash sesame seeds and allow to dry overnight. Or, dry over medium heat, stirring occasionally, for about 10 minutes.
2. Over medium heat, dry-roast 4 separate batches of seeds, 5 to 7 minutes per batch, until they crush easily between the thumb and fourth or little finger.
3. Grind seeds in a suribachi until all the seeds are crushed.
4. Add miso and boiling water and grind until smooth.
5. Serve at room temperature.

SESAME MISO DRESSING

Preparation time: 5 minutes   *Yield:* 7 servings
Drying time: 10 minutes to overnight
Cooking time: 25–30 minutes
Grinding time: 10 minutes

This all-purpose dressing is particularly useful for people who have bladder infections.

  1/4 cup sesame seeds
  1–2 tablespoons miso
  1 tablespoon rice vinegar, or
   1 tablespoon ume vinegar mixed with
   1 tablespoon water

1. Wash sesame seeds and allow to dry overnight, or dry over medium heat, stirring occasionally, for about 10 minutes.
2. Dry-roast sesame seeds in 4 batches, about 5 to 7 minutes per batch, and grind in a suribachi until 80 percent of the seeds are crushed.
3. Add miso and vinegar and grind with the sesame seeds.
4. Serve at room temperature.

SHIITAKE NITSUKE

Preparation time: 5 minutes   *Yield:* 2–3 servings
Soaking time: 20 minutes
Cooking time: 25–30 minutes

This nitsuke is useful with cases of appendicitis, skin infection, tetanus, diabetes, or nocturnal emission.

  5 shiitake mushrooms
  2 cups warm water
  1 teaspoon sesame oil
  1/4 teaspoon sea salt
  1–2 teaspoons soy sauce

1. Soak the shiitake mushrooms in the warm water for 20 minutes. Drain and reserve soaking water.
2. Remove and discard the hard parts of the stems and cut mushrooms in thin slices.
3. Heat the oil and sauté the mushrooms briefly.
4. Sprinkle with salt and add soaking water. Cover and cook for 10 minutes.
5. Add soy sauce and cook 10 minutes more. If liquid remains, remove cover and cook until liquid evaporates.
6. Serve warm or at room temperature.

SHIO KOMBU

Preparation time: 30 minutes   *Yield:* 50–70 servings
Drying time: 2 hours
Soaking time: overnight
Cooking time: 4 hours

This condiment is useful with all conditions, especially yin ones, as it is very strengthening. Shio Kombu is extremely salty and only 2 or 3 pieces should be eaten at a meal. It may be stored in a covered glass container for many years.

  8 ounces kombu
  3–4 cups soy sauce

1. Clean kombu with a damp cotton towel to remove sand.
2. Cut in 1/2-inch squares using a kitchen scissors. Allow the kombu to dry completely.
3. Put the kombu in a large bowl and add the soy sauce. Let kombu soak overnight.
4. Transfer the kombu and soy sauce to a pot. Cover with an otoshibuta and the pot lid. (To make Shio Kombu without an otoshibuta, use 4 cups soy sauce.)
5. Bring to a boil. Simmer for about 3 hours, stirring occasionally.

6. Continue cooking over low heat and stirring for about 1 hour, until all the liquid evaporates.
7. Serve at room temperature.

SHIO KOMBU WITH OIL

Preparation time: 10 minutes   *Yield:* 20 servings
Cooking time: 30–45 minutes

Shio Kombu with Oil is very effective in cases of arterial diseases, especially arteriosclerosis; varicose veins; grey hair; or hemorrhoids.

> 3–5 pieces of kombu (3 inches by 8 inches), left over from preparing Kombu Stock (see page 216)
> 1 teaspoon sesame oil
> 1/4–1/3 cup soy sauce

1. Cut kombu in match-stick shapes or 1/2-inch squares.
2. Briefly sauté kombu in oil.
3. Add soy sauce. Cover and cook over low heat until kombu is tender.
4. Shio Kombu can be kept for 2 to 3 weeks if refrigerated, or for 1 week if kept in a cool place.
5. Serve at room temperature.

SMALL FISH TEMPURA

Preparation time: 25 minutes   *Yield:* 5 servings
Standing time: 5 minutes
Cooking time: 7–8 minutes

Small Fish Tempura is useful for people who have tuberculsis, goiter, or anal itch.

> 10 smelt or other small whole fish
> 2 teaspoons ginger juice
> 1 teaspoon sea salt
> whole-wheat pastry flour
> sesame oil for deep-frying
>
> **Batter**
> 1 1/2 cups whole-wheat pastry flour
> 1 heaping teaspoon arrowroot starch
> 1/4 teaspoon sea salt
> 1 cup water

1. Clean fish and remove head and bones. (Head and bones can be coated with flour, but not batter, and deep-fried if desired.)
2. Sprinkle fish with ginger juice and salt. Let stand for 5 minutes.
3. Coat with a small amount of pastry flour.

4. Combine the batter ingredients.
5. Heat oil to 350°F.
6. Dip fish in batter and drop into hot oil. Deep-fry until golden on both sides, about 5 minutes on one side and 2–3 minutes on the other side.
7. Serve hot.

SOUR CABBAGE

Preparation time: 30 minutes   *Yield:* 20 servings

Sour Cabbage is useful with yang disorders, especially intestinal problems.

> 2 medium heads of cabbage, organic if available
> 2 tablespoons sea salt
> 5 bay leaves

1. Quarter the cabbage. Wash the quarters and let them drain for half a day.
2. Core quarters and save the cores for soup. Slice the cabbage as thinly as possible.
3. Place 2 handfuls of cabbage in a suribachi or bowl. Add 1 teaspoon salt and knead the cabbage gently until it begins to soften.
4. Place cabbage in a salad press with 1 or 2 bay leaves. Repeat steps 3 and 4 until all the cabhage is layered in the salad press.
5. Press the cabbage strongly for a few days, or until a white, bubbly fermentation appears.
6. Pressed cabbage can be packed tightly in a glass jar, or it can be kept in the salad press under very light pressure. It can be stored in the refrigerator for up to 5 weeks.
7. Serve at room temperature

SOY SAUCE WITH SESAME OIL

Cooking time: 7–8 minutes   *Yield:* 18 servings

This preparation helps disperse the yin quality of the oil and helps you avoid getting diarrhea from eating raw oil.

> 1 tablespoon sesame oil
> pinch of sea salt
> 2–3 tablespoons soy sauce

1. Heat oil until it sizzles when a pinch of salt is added.
2. Mix heated oil with soy sauce to taste and serve warm, 1/2 teaspoon per person, over grains and vegetables.

Variation

And Ginger Juice

This variation is useful for anemia or tuberculosis as it helps strengthen the whole body. Decrease sesame oil to 2 teaspoons. Mix the heated sesame oil, 4 teaspoons soy sauce, and 1 teaspoon juice squeezed from freshly grated ginger. Eat as is or serve on top of grains and/or vegetables.

SOYBEAN SOUP

Preparation time: 10 minutes   *Yield:* 5–7 servings
Soaking time: overnight
Cooking time: 50–60 minutes

This is useful with skin infections of the face or non-insulin-dependent diabetes.

> ¼ cup soybeans
> 2 cups water
> 1 small onion
> 2 small turnips
> 1 burdock
> 1 carrot
> ½ teaspoon sea salt
> 1 teaspoon sesame oil
> 1 tablespoon chirimen iriko (small dried fish), optional
> 5 cups water
> 1–2 tablespoons soy sauce

1. Soak the soybeans overnight in 1 cup water.
2. Drain and purée the beans in a blender with 1 cup fresh water.
3. Dice the onion into large pieces. Cut the turnips into bite-sized pieces. Cut the burdock and carrot into shavings.
4. Heat the oil and sauté the onion with a pinch of salt until onion is translucent.
5. Add dried fish, if desired, and burdock and sauté for a few minutes.
6. Add turnips, then carrots, and sauté for a few minutes.
7. Add the water. Cover, bring to a boil, and cook for 20 minutes or until vegetables are tender.
8. Add remaining salt and the puréed soybeans. Bring to a boil, being careful that the foam doesn't boil over.
9. Cook for 20 minutes more.
10. Season with soy sauce.
11. Serve hot.

SOYBEANS WITH KOMBU

Preparation time: 10 minutes   *Yield:* 7–10 servings
Soaking time: 7 minutes
Cooking time: 40–50 minutes

This dish is useful for people who have breast or skin cancer.

> 1 piece kombu, 3 inches by 12 inches
> 3 cups water
> 1 teaspoon sesame oil
> 1 cup soybeans
> 1–2 tablespoons soy sauce

1. Soak kombu in water for 7 minutes. Wash kombu in the soaking water and remove.
2. Strain the water through a cotton cloth and reserve.
3. Cut kombu in 1-inch squares.
4. Heat the oil in a pressure cooker.
5. Add the soybeans and roast until they become slightly brown.
6. Add the soaking water and the kombu. Bring to pressure and cook for 10 minutes.
7. Remove from heat and allow pressure to drop according to directions for your cooker.
8. Add soy sauce. Cook, uncovered, for 20 minutes more, stirring occasionally, to allow liquid to evaporate.
9. Serve warm or at room temperature.

TEKKA MISO

Preparation time: 10 minutes   *Yield:* 30 servings
Cooking time: 2½ hours
Standing time: 2 hours and 20 minutes

This condiment is useful with all disorders, especially arthritis, chronic constipation, gastritis, a weak pulse, and all yin diseases.

> 1 medium burdock root
> 1½-inch piece lotus root
> 3-inch piece carrot
> ½ cup sesame oil
> 1½ cups hatcho or barley miso
> 1 tablespoon minced ginger

1. Mince all the vegetables very finely.
2. Heat ¼ cup oil in a heavy pot. Sauté vegetables for 20 minutes or until they are tender.
3. Add remaining oil and miso and mix well. Remove from heat and allow pot to cool.
4. Return to heat and cook over very low heat for 20 minutes, stirring constantly. Remove from heat for

20 minutes. Repeat this process 5 times, being careful not to burn the tekka, which should become dry and crumbly.

5. Add ginger and cook for 10 minutes.
6. Tekka Miso will keep for about 6 months. It is not necessary to refrigerate it.
7. Serve at room temperature, 1 level teaspoon per meal.

TOFU WITH KUZU SAUCE

Preparation time: 5 minutes   *Yield:* 5 servings
Cooking time: 15–20 minutes

This dish is useful for those who have eye or kidney problems.

    1 pound tofu
    1 teaspoon sea salt
    6 cups water

Sauce

    1 cup stock or water
    1 tablespoon kuzu
    3 tablespoons cold water
    2 tablespoons soy sauce
    parsley for garnish

1. Cut tofu in 2-inch squares.
2. Bring the 6 cups water and salt to a boil.
3. Add tofu and simmer about 2 to 3 minutes, until it becomes puffy.
4. Remove tofu to a heated plate.
5. Bring the 1 cup stock to a boil.
6. Dissolve kuzu in the cold water and add to stock.
7. Add soy sauce. Bring to a boil and cook until clear.
8. Pour sauce over cooked tofu and garnish with parsley.
9. Serve hot.

TORORO KOMBU SOUP

Preparation time: 10 minutess   *Yield:* 1 serving

This soup is useful with insomnia, colds, or flu.

    1 teaspoon tororo kombu (shredded kombu)
    1 teaspoon sliced scallions
    1 teaspoon bonita flakes (optional)
    2/3 cup boiling water
    1/4 teaspoon soy sauce

1. In a bowl, layer the tororo kombu, scallions, bonita flakes (if desired), and soy sauce.
2. Cover with boiling water.
3. Serve hot or warm.

TURNIP ALBI BURDOCK COOKED WITH HOMEMADE AGÉ

Preparation time: 20 minutes   *Yield:* 5 servings
Soaking time: 10 minutes
Cooking time: 50–60 minutes

This preparation is useful for those who have the yang type of bladder infection.

    1 piece kombu, 6 inches long
    5 cups water (approximately)
    2 burdock roots
    10 albi (taro potato)
    3 turnips
    2 or 3 pieces Homemade Agé (see page 215)
    2 tablespoons soy sauce

1. Soak kombu in water for 10 minutes. Drain and reserve water.
2. Cut burdock in 2-inch lengths. Scrape albi and leave whole. Cut turnips in wedges. Cut agé in 1-inch slices.
3. Place kombu on the bottom of a heavy pot. Add burdock, albi, and turnips. Add the kombu soaking water and enough fresh water to cover. Add 1 tablespoon soy sauce.
4. Cover and bring to a boil. Simmer 30 to 40 minutes until nearly tender.
5. Add agé and cook 20 minutes more.
6. Add 1 tablespoon soy sauce or to taste.
7. Serve hot or warm.

UME EXTRACT

Preparation time: 20–30 minutes   *Yield:* ½–1 cup
Cooking time: several days

Ume extract is useful for alkalizing the system, controlling diarrhea and dysentery, and eliminating hookworms. Ume extract or concentrate can be purchased at natural food stores or made at home. In either case, mix ⅛ teaspoon of the extract with ⅓ cup warm water before eating.

    7 cups hard green ume plums

1. Grate the plums using a Japanese-style porcelain grater.
2. Squeeze the juice from the grated plums.
3. Cook the juice in a porcelain or glass pot over low heat for several days, stirring once in a while. The plum juice will become sticky and black.
4. After the extract cools, put it in a bottle. Ume Extract will keep for at least 5 years.

Umeboshi

Preparation time: 1–2 minutes   *Yield:* 2–3 servings

Umeboshi, a preparation of salted, preserved Japanese plums, contains citric acid and is a very powerful alkalizing agent. Citrus fruits are also alkalizing, but because they are yin, tend to further weaken a body that is already in a weakened condition. Umeboshi is more yang than citrus fruit and helps expanded (weakened) organs to contract (strengthen), so we recommend it instead of citrus fruit. Also, the citric acid from the Umeboshi helps the body's immune system clean up harmful bacteria. Umeboshi is very good with all cases of anemia, fatigue, or heartburn. If you are concerned about salt content, use Ume Extract (see page 227) or soak a whole umeboshi plum in warm water for 20 minutes.

1 umeboshi plum*

1. Remove pit.
2. Break umeboshi plum into small pieces and serve over grain or vegetable dishes.

Variation

With Soy Sauce

This variation is useful for those who have stomach cramps, morning sickness, or nausea. Proceed as above, mix with 1 to 2 teaspoons soy sauce and eat.

Vegetable Stew

Preparation time: 20 minutes   *Yield:* 5 servings
Cooking time: 50–55 minutes

Vegetable stew is useful with many disorders, whether yin or yang.

3 scallions
6-inch piece burdock (onion may be substituted)
1½ inch piece carrot
1-inch piece daikon (turnip may be substituted)

---

* Some umeboshi plums are colored with artificial dye. Use the following method to determine if plums have been dyed: Place 3 plums in an open basket and hang the basket outside, sheltered from rain, for 3 or 4 nights. Take the basket in during the day. If the plums turn brown, they were colored naturally with shiso (beefsteak) leaves. If the plums remain bright red, they were artificially colored. Umeboshi plums that are naturally colored and that have a round seed are the best quality. Artificially-dyed plums may be used but are less effective than natural ones.

---

2 or 3 albi (Jerusalem artichoke may be substituted)
⅓ pound tofu
2 teaspoons sesame oil
4 cups Kombu Stock (see page 216) or water
½ teaspoon sea salt
1 tablespoon miso or soy sauce

1. Slice scallions in thin rounds. Cut burdock and carrot in thin rounds. Cut daikon in quarter moons. Cut the albi and the tofu in ¼-inch bite-sized pieces.
2. Heat ½ teaspoon oil and sauté scallions for 3 to 5 minutes, until the color changes. Remove to a bowl.
3. Heat the remaining oil. Sauté burdock with a pinch of salt until it is fragrant, about 5 minutes.
4. Add carrot, albi, and daikon, sautéing each for 2 minutes with a pinch of salt.
5. Sauté tofu for 2 to 3 minutes.
6. Add Kombu Stock or water. Cover and cook about 30 minutes until vegetables are tender.
7. Add soy sauce or miso. Cook 5 minutes more.
8. Serve hot or warm in bowls garnished with sautéed scallions.

Vegetable Stew with Fish

Preparation time: 20 minutes   *Yield:* 5 servings
Cooking time: 35–45 minutes

This stew is useful with many disorders, the yin type of most diseases and the yang type of some.

2 small onions
3 small turnips
6-inch carrot
¼ Chinese cabbage or 5 cabbage leaves
½ pound white-meat fish
½ teaspoon sea salt
1 tablespoon sesame oil
water
2–3 tablespoons barley miso
3 tablespoons water

1. Cut onion in ⅓-inch crescents. Cut turnips in ½-inch pieces. Cut carrot in half moons. Cut cabbage in 1-inch squares. Cut fish in 5 pieces.
2. Heat oil and sauté onions with a pinch of salt until they are translucent.
3. Sauté fish for a short time.
4. Add turnips, carrots, and cabbage in layers. Add water to just cover.
5. Cover pan and cook 20 minutes or until ingredients are tender.

6. Add miso diluted in water and cook for 5 minutes more.
7. Serve hot or warm.

VEGETABLE TEMPURA

Preparation time: 20 minutes   *Yield:* 10 servings
Cooking time: 7–10 minutes per batch

Vegetable Tempura is useful with almost all disorders. Tempura may appear to be too oily for those who have eaten large amounts of fat in the past; however, the macrobiotic approach is relatively low in fat and some good-quality oil is needed daily. Adjust the amount of tempura eaten if you need to control your oil intake.

     4-inch piece burdock
     1-inch piece lotus root
     3-inch piece carrot
     1/2 small onion
     4–6 cups sesame oil for deep-frying
     1 tablespoon daikon or red radish, grated
     1/4–1/2 teaspoon soy sauce

Batter

     1 1/2 cups whole-wheat flour
     1/4 teaspoon sea salt
     1 1/2–1 3/4 cups water

1. Cut burdock, lotus root, and carrot in match-stick shapes. Cut onion in thin crescents.
2. Mix flour, salt, and water to make batter.
3. Add vegetables to batter and mix to coat.
4. In a heavy pot, heat oil to 350°F.
5. Drop tempura vegetables into the hot oil, a tablespoon at a time, until a layer of Vegetable Tempura pieces is floating on the oil.
6. When the vegetables are golden brown (about 5 minutes), turn them over. Fry until they are golden brown on the second side, about 2 minutes more.
7. Drain in a strainer and place on a paper towel to absorb excess oil.
8. Serve hot or warm with grated daikon or grated red radish and soy sauce to aid digestion of the oil.

VEGETABLES COOKED WITH MISO

Preparation time: 5 minutes   *Yield:* 5 servings
Cooking time: 30–35 minutes

This preparation is useful in cases of menstrual irregularities.

     2 onions
     12 cabbage leaves
     1 carrot
     1 tablespoon sesame oil
     1/2 teaspoon sea salt
     1 1/2 cups water
     2 tablespoons miso

1. Cut onions in large crescents. Cut cabbage leaves in 1-inch slices. Cut carrot in rounds.
2. Heat oil and sauté onions with a pinch of salt for a few minutes. Repeat with cabbage, then carrot.
3. Add water and remaining salt. Cover and cook 10 minutes, or until the vegetables are tender.
4. Add miso and cook 10 to 15 minutes more.
5. Serve vegetables hot or warm. Any liquid remaining in the pan may be served as a sauce over Brown Rice (see page 197).

WAKAME NITSUKE

Preparation time: 5 minutes   *Yield:* 10–15 servings
Soaking time: 7 minutes
Cooking time: 10 minutes

Wakame Nitsuke is useful for those who have leprosy or bone marrow disorders.

     1/2 ounce wakame
     3 cups cold water
     2–3 tablespoons soy sauce

1. Soak wakame in cold water until it is tender; about 7 minutes.
2. Remove wakame. Strain soaking water through a cotton cloth and reserve for use in cooking.
3. Cut wakame in 1-inch slices.
4. Cook in 1/4 cup of soaking water for 10 minutes.
5. Add soy sauce to taste.
6. Serve warm or at room temperature.

WATERLESS COOKED VEGETABLES

Preparation time: 15–20 minutes   *Yield:* 3–5 servings
Cooking time: 40–45 minutes

This preparation is useful with skin problems or trachoma. (Other vegetables and combinations may be cooked in this style for variety.)

     2 onions
     1/2 small cabbage
     1/2 carrot
     1 teaspoon sesame oil
     1 teaspoon sea salt

1. Cut onions in thin crescents. Cut cabbage in 1-inch squares. Cut carrot in half moons.
2. Heat oil and sauté onions with a pinch of salt until they become translucent, 5 to 7 minutes.
3. Sauté cabbage 3 to 5 minutes until it is bright green.
4. Sauté carrot for 2 to 3 minutes.
5. Add remaining salt. Cover and cook over low heat until vegetables are tender, about 30 minutes.
6. Remove cover and continue to cook to evaporate excess liquid.
7. Serve warm.

WATERMELON SYRUP

Preparation time: 20–30 minutes   *Yield:* ½–1 cup
Cooking time: 2–3 hours

Watermelon syrup is useful in cases of kidney failure or uremia. This concentrate keeps well. An average melon will yield about 1 pint of concentrate.

> 1 watermelon

1. Cut the red part of the watermelon in cubes.
2. Press through a colander or a food mill to extract the juice.
3. Boil the juice uncovered 2 to 3 hours until it becomes a thick syrup.
4. Serve at room temperature.

WINTER SQUASH AND ONION

Preparation time: 10 minutes   *Yield:* 5–7 servings
Cooking time: 50–60 minutes

This dish is useful for those who have hunchback or hypoglycemia, especially if they are craving sweets.

> 1 small Hokkaido squash or any winter squash
> 3 medium onions
> 1 tablespoon sesame oil
> ½ teaspoon sea salt
> 1 tablespoon soy sauce
> ⅓ cup boiling water as needed

1. Cut squash in 1½-inch squares. Cut onions in crescents.
2. Heat oil and sauté onions with a pinch of salt until they become translucent.
3. Add squash and sauté 5 minutes.
4. Add remaining salt and soy sauce. Cover and cook over low heat for 10 minutes.
5. If squash is dry, add boiling water around edge of pan. Cover and cook 25 minutes or until squash is tender.
6. Serve hot or warm.

MISO SOUPS

Miso Soup is recommended daily for those following a macrobiotic dietary approach for therapeutic reasons. In a sense, any soup can be made into Miso Soup by adding miso at the end of cooking. Where Miso Soup ingredients are suggested in Part Two, combine one or two of these ingredients with Wakame Miso Soup (see page 231) for your daily Miso Soup. Onions may be added to any combination of ingredients. For variety, use any combination of the listed ingredients and prepare as Miso Soup.

MISO SOUP

Preparation time: 10 minutes   *Yield:* 5–7 servings
Cooking time: 1 hour

> 1 medium onion
> 2 medium turnips
> ½ carrot
> 1 teaspoon sesame oil
> 6 cups boiling water
> 1 heaping tablespoon barley miso

1. Cut onion in thin crescents, turnips in bite-sized pieces ¼-inch thick, and carrot in match-stick shapes.
2. Heat oil and sauté onions until they become translucent.
3. Add turnips and sauté until their color changes.
4. Add carrots and sauté a few minutes more.
5. Add boiling water and turn heat to high. Cook uncovered for a few minutes to remove strong flavors of vegetables.
6. Lower heat to medium, cover, and simmer for 45 minutes or until vegetables are tender.
7. Remove pot from heat.
8. Put miso in a strainer and use a wooden spoon to mash miso through strainer into soup.
9. Bring soup to boiling point, but do not boil it.
10. Serve hot.

Variations

With Mochi

This variation is useful for diarrhea and helping to cool the body by removing excess perspiration. Cut Brown Rice Mochi (see page 200) in 2-inch squares. Bake mochi at 325°F for 20 minutes or until it is tender. Add 1 or 2 squares to each bowl of soup when serving.

With Dried Seitan

This variation is useful with many disorders. Soak dried seitan for 10 minutes. Cut into ½-inch-thick pieces, about 5 per serving, and cook with the other vegetables for at least 20 minutes before adding miso.

WAKAME MISO SOUP

Preparation time: 5 minutes   *Yield:* 5–7 servings
Soaking time: 5–10 minutes
Cooking time: 30–35 minutes

This soup may be used as the basis for your daily miso soup. It is especially good in cases of anemia or tuberculosis and is a good blood purifier.

    4 strips wakame
    1 medium onion
    1 teaspoon sesame oil
    5 cups water and wakame stock
    1 tablespoon barley miso

1. Cover wakame with cold water and soak it for 5 to 10 minutes.
2. Remove wakame. Strain soaking water through a cotton cloth and reserve as stock.
3. Remove hard stem sections of wakame and chop stems finely. Cut softer leafy sections into ½-inch pieces. Cut onion in thin crescents.
4. Heat sesame oil and sauté onion until it becomes translucent.
5. Add wakame soaking water and enough additional water to equal 5 cups.
6. Add chopped wakame stems and bring to a boil over high heat. Simmer ingredients, covered, for 20 minutes or until tender.
7. Add soft parts of the wakame and simmer 5 minutes more.
8. Remove pot from heat.
9. Place miso in a strainer and use a wooden spoon to mash miso through strainer into soup. Bring soup to boiling point, but do not boil it.
10. Wait a few minutes before serving hot.

BEVERAGES

Drinking the proper amount of liquid is very important for healing purposes. However, when eating a diet of whole grains and fresh vegetables that contain a lot of liquid, there is less need for concern about getting enough fluid.

For preparing teas, use an enamel, glass, ceramic, or clay pot; avoid iron, aluminum, and stainless steel. In most cases, teas should be simmered only since rapid boiling lessens the effectiveness of the tea.

AMASAKE DRINK

Cooking time: 10–15 minutes   *Yield:* 5 servings

Amasake Drink is useful with colds, flu, mumps, measles, and other ailments. If you buy an Amasake Drink, make sure it is unsweetened.

    3–4 cups water
    1 cup amasake, blended
    ½ teaspoon sea salt
    1 teaspoon lemon or orange rind

1. Bring water to a boil.
2. Add amasake and cook over medium heat, stirring, until mixture comes to a boil.
3. Add salt and cook 5 minutes.
4. Serve Amasake Drink hot with a pinch of lemon or orange rind in each cup.

AZUKI BEAN DRINK

Preparation time: 5 minutes   *Yield:* 1 cup

This drink is used to protect the intestines and kidneys from toxins, especially in cases of nonrabid dog bites.

    ½ cup azuki beans
    1 cup water

1. Grind raw azuki beans to powder in a blender.
2. Mix 2 tablespoons of powder with 1 cup of water. Retain extra powder for future use.
3. Drink as directed in Part Two under the appropriate disorder.

AZUKI BEAN TEA

Preparation time: 2–3 minutes   *Yield:* 1 serving
Cooking time: 2 hours

This tea is good for all kidney diseases. The cooked azuki beans can be used in other dishes.

    ⅓ cup azuki beans
    6 cups water
    pinch sea salt

1. Clean and rinse beans.

2. In a porcelain pot, bring beans and water to a boil and simmer for 30 minutes, uncovered.
3. Add salt and simmer about 1½ hours until 2 cups of liquid remain.
4. Strain and drink only the juice.

AZUKI KOMBU DRINK

Preparation time: 2–3 minutes   *Yield:* 3–4 servings
Cooking time: 50–60 minutes

This juice is useful with kidney problems, gonorrhea, or penis pain.

> 1 cup azuki beans
> 1 piece kombu, 3 inches by 6 inches
> 3 cups water
> 4½ cups cold water
> 1 pinch sea salt

1. Wash azuki beans.
2. Add kombu and the 3 cups of water. Bring to a boil.
3. Add 1½ cups cold water to stop the boiling. Repeat the process 2 times.
4. Cook until azuki beans are completely soft.
5. Add salt and cook 20 minutes more.
6. Strain.
7. Serve hot or warm.

BANCHA TEA

Cooking time: 25–30 minutes   *Yield:* 2 servings

Bancha Tea is good for the circulation; for relieving fatigue, weakness, heart conditions, gonorrhea, and syphilis; and for daily use. Also, it helps purify the blood by removing toxins, and helps to satisfy the craving for yin foods after a meal.

> ¼ cup bancha tea leaves
> 4 cups water

1. Bring tea and water to a boil in a porcelain or glass pot.
2. Simmer for 20 minutes.
3. Strain and serve hot.

Variations

With Gomashio

This variation is useful with menstrual problems or heartburn. Add 1 teaspoon Gomashio (see page 202) per cup of Bancha Tea.

With Grated Daikon

This variation is useful in cases of fainting. Add 1 tablespoon grated daikon mixed with 1 teaspoon soy sauce to ½ cup Bancha Tea. Use as directed in Part Two under the appropriate disorder.

With Salt

This variation is useful for mouth ulcers. It is also helpful in cases of epilepsy, gastritis, or stomach ulcers. Add ⅛ teaspoon sea salt to ⅔ cup Bancha Tea. Bancha Tea with Salt may be used to induce vomiting. In this case, add ½ teaspoon sea salt to ½ cup Bancha Tea.

BARLEY TEA

Preparation time: 2–3 minutes   *Yield:* 2 servings
Cooking time: 25–30 minutes

This tea is useful with lung problems, tetanus, tongue trouble, or blood poisoning. Purchase Barley Tea or mugicha already prepared or make it at home. Dry roast ⅓ cup unhulled barley in a skillet over medium heat until it is dark brown, almost black. Barley may also be spread on a cookie sheet and roasted slowly in a moderate oven.

> ⅓ cup roasted barley (mugicha)
> 6 cups cold water

1. Bring barley and water to a boil.
2. Simmer 20 minutes.
3. Strain and serve hot.

BLACK SOYBEAN TEA

Preparation time: 2–3 minutes   *Yield:* 1 serving
Cooking time: 1 hour

This tea is useful in cases of fish poisoning, whooping cough, or loss of voice. It is also helpful for professional singers.

> ⅓ cup black soybeans
> 6 cups water
> pinch sea salt

1. Clean and rinse soybeans.
2. Bring soybeans and water to a boil. Simmer about 1 hour until 2 cups of liquid remain.
3. Strain and add salt to the liquid. Reserve soybeans for another use.
4. Serve hot.

BROWN RICE BANCHA TEA

Cooking time: 5–10 minutes   *Yield:* 2–3 servings

This all-purpose tea is useful for weak people.

> 2 teaspoons brown rice
> 2 tablespoons bancha tea leaves
> 5 cups boiling water

1. Roast brown rice and mix with bancha tea leaves.
2. Put this mixture in boiling water in a porcelain pot. Let it steep for 3 to 5 minutes.
3. Strain and serve hot. The tea should be very fragrant.

BROWN RICE BROTH

Cooking time: 1 hour   *Yield:* 2–3 servings

Brown Rice Broth is useful to help induce urination in cases of kidney failure. It is also good in cases of leprosy, diphtheria, and diabetes.

> 1 cup brown rice
> 2 or 3 shiitake mushrooms
> 10 cups water

1. Cook ingredients together about 1 hour until volume is reduced to 7 cups.
2. Strain through a very fine colander.
3. Drink the liquid hot.

BROWN RICE CREAM TEA

Cooking time: 5–10 minutes   *Yield:* 1 serving

This tea is especially effective for people who have swollen legs (edema) caused by a weak heart.

> 1 tablespoon Brown Rice Cream with Oil (see page 199)
> 1/2 cup water

1. Add Brown Rice Cream with Oil to water.
2. Boil slightly.
3. Stir and drink hot.

BROWN RICE TEA

Cooking time: 50–60 minutes   *Yield:* 1 serving

Brown Rice Tea is an all-purpose beverage useful with all sicknesses, especially bladder infections, diarrhea, morning sickness, nervous system malfunction, and kidney failure.

> 1/3 cup brown rice
> 4 cups water
> 1 pinch sea salt

1. Roast rice about 10 minutes until it is well-browned.
2. Combine roasted rice with water in a porcelain or glass pot and bring to a rapid boil.
3. Add salt and simmer for 40 to 50 minutes or until volume is reduced to 2 cups.
4. Strain and serve hot.

Variations

With Dried Persimmon And Tangerine Skin

This tea is an anti-fever drink for those who cannot use Daikon Ginger Tea such as weak people, those with weak lungs, old people, and children. Add 1/2 of a tangerine skin and 1 dried persimmon when adding salt. Or, instead of the skins, you may use 3 dried plums or 3 to 4 dates. Bring to a boil and simmer, uncovered, for 20 minutes. Strain.

With Ginger

This variation is useful with a high fever, especially in cases of mumps or rheumatism. Add 1/4 teaspoon of ginger when adding salt. Strain.

With Kumquat Leaves

This variation is useful in cases of severe whooping cough. Add 5 to 6 kumquat leaves when adding salt. Simmer until only 3 cups of tea remain. Strain. This tea will taste bitter so, if desired, sweeten it with a little rice syrup or apple juice.

With Lotus Root and Shiitake Mushrooms

This variation is useful with high fever, especially in cases of bronchitis. Add 3 to 5 inches of fresh lotus root, finely chopped, and 2 or 3 shiitake mushrooms, soaked and sliced, when adding salt.

With Lotus Root and Shiso Leaves

This variation is useful in severe cases of whooping cough and in asthma attacks. Add 3 to 5 inches of fresh lotus root, chopped fine, and 2 or 3 dried beefsteak (shiso) leaves when adding salt. Strain.

With Lotus Root and Tangerine Skins

This variation is useful with coughs, especially in cases of measles. Add two 1/4-inch long, 2-inch-diameter pieces of lotus root and 1 teaspoon grated tangerine skin when adding salt. Strain.

With Shiitake Mushroom

This variation is useful in cases of high fever, thirst, or dry mouth. Add 2 to 3 shiitake mushrooms when adding salt. Strain.

With Soy Sauce

This variation is useful for those with a weak heart due to tuberculosis. Add ½ teaspoon soy sauce to ⅔ cup of tea.

With Umeboshi

This variation is useful for thirst or dry mouth. Add 1 umeboshi plum when adding salt.

BURDOCK BONITA TEA

Preparation time: 5–10 minutes   *Yield:* 1 serving

This tea is useful for promoting sweating, helping alkalize the body, and relieving fever from a cold.

> 1 tablespoon freshly grated burdock root
> 1 tablespoon bonita flakes
> ½–1 teaspoon barley miso
> ¾ cup boiling water

1. Combine ingredients.
2. Drink as directed in Part Two under the appropriate disorder.

Variation

With Baked Miso

A more fragrant and yangizing tea can be made by using baked miso. Roll approximately 1 tablespoon miso into a ball. Using a metal toaster, toast the ball over an open flame until the miso is slightly dried out, about 5 minutes. Mix ⅓ of the baked miso ball with ¾ cup boiling water and drink. Save excess baked miso for additional teas or eat it as a condiment.

BURDOCK CHICKWEED TEA

Preparation time: 3–5 minutes   *Yield:* 3 cups
Cooking time: 30–45 minutes

This tea is good in cases of appendix pain, especially when there is also constipation.

> ¾ cup finely chopped burdock root
> 1 handful chickweed
> 6 cups water

1. Combine ingredients in a porcelain or ceramic pot.
2. Bring to a boil and simmer 30 to 45 minutes, uncovered, until 3 cups of liquid remain.
3. Strain and drink as directed in Part Two under the appropriate disorder.

BURDOCK SEED TEA

Cooking time: 30–45 minutes   *Yield:* 1½ cups

Burdock Seed Tea can be helpful in reducing pain from skin infections such as boils.

> 1–2 teaspoons burdock seeds
> 3 cups water

1. Add burdock seeds to water.
2. Bring to a boil and simmer 30 to 45 minutes until 1½ cups of liquid remain.
3. Drink hot as directed in Part Two under the appropriate disorder.

CHERRY TREE BARK TEA

Cooking time: 25–30 minutes   *Yield:* 2½–3 cups

This tea is useful in cases of tuna poisoning.

> ½ cup chopped cherry tree bark or branches
> 3 cups water

1. Place chopped cherry tree bark or branches in water.
2. Bring to a boil and simmer 20 minutes.
3. Strain and serve hot as directed in Part Two under the appropriate disorder.

DAIKON GINGER TEA

Preparation time: 10 minutes   *Yield:* 1 serving

The main use of Daikon Ginger Tea is with fever and chills from any cause. If you have tuberculosis, lung problems, or are a weak person, use Brown Rice Tea with Dried Persimmon and Tangerine Skin (see page 233) instead of this tea to help reduce fever. Even if you are strong, use this tea only 3 times and no more unless otherwise directed in Part Two. This tea is also helpful for calming an excessive heartbeat; removing toxins; and relieving swelling, itchiness, or thirst.

> 3 heaping tablespoons grated daikon
> 1 teaspoon grated ginger
> 1½–2 tablespoons soy sauce
> 2–3 cups boiling Bancha Tea (see page 232)

1. Combine all ingredients.
2. In cases of fever, drink all at once.
3. Cover yourself completely with heavy blankets and quilts. If you don't begin to sweat after 10 minutes, try drinking another cup of this tea. After sweating 40 minutes, wipe off the perspiration with towels.

DAIKON MEASLES TEA

Preparation time: 5–10 minutes   *Yield:* 1 serving

This tea is used for one purpose only, to help induce a measles rash.

For children less than 1 year old:
    ¼ teaspoon daikon juice
    1 drop ginger juice
    1 drop soy sauce
    1 drop honey or rice syrup
    1 teaspoon warm water

For children 1 to 3 years old:
    1 teaspoon daikon juice
    3 drops ginger juice
    1 tablespoon warm Bancha Tea (see page 232)
    2–3 drops soy sauce
    1–2 drops honey or rice syrup

For children 3 to 5 years old:
    1 tablespoon daikon juice
    3–4 drops ginger juice
    ¼ cup warm Bancha Tea (see page 232)
    4–7 drops soy sauce
    ½ teaspoon honey or rice syrup

For children 5 years and older:
    2 tablespoons daikon juice
    6–7 drops ginger juice
    ½ cup warm Bancha Tea (see page 232)
    8–12 drops soy sauce
    1 teaspoon honey or rice syrup

1. Mix ingredients.
2. Give as directed in Part Two for measles.

DAIKON SEED COUGH DRINK

Preparation time: 10–15 minutes   *Yield:* 1 serving

This drink is good for people who have persistent coughs, including whooping cough.

    ¼ cup daikon seeds
    ½ cup cool water

1. Roast daikon seeds until fragrant and grind them to powder in a suribachi or blender.
2. Mix 1 tablespoon of powder with ½ cup cool water. (This powder can also be put in a capsule and swallowed.)
3. Drink as directed in Part Two under the appropriate disorder.

DAIKON SOY SAUCE TEA

Preparation time: 5–10 minutes   *Yield:* 1 serving

This tea is useful in cases of heartburn or tempura poisoning.

    1 heaping tablespoon grated daikon
    1 teaspoon soy sauce
    ½ cup boiling water

1. Combine ingredients.
2. Serve hot.

DAIKON TEA

Preparation time: 10–15 minutes   *Yield:* 3 cups

This tea is used to stimulate urination in cases of weak kidneys. Use only until urination occurs, then stop. It is also useful with edema, bladder infections, or peritonitis.

    1 cup daikon juice
    2 cups water
    pinch sea salt

1. Combine daikon juice, water, and salt. Boil slightly.
2. Drink hot, ¼ cup at a time. Drink approximately 1 to 1½ cups of tea per day, depending on your weight. Larger persons may drink up to 3 cups per day. If you are using Daikon Ginger Tea for fever, wait 30 minutes before drinking Daikon Tea.

Variation

With Soy Sauce

This variation is useful for abnormal urination such as in uremia. Add a very small amount of soy sauce when serving.

ENMEI TEA

Cooking time: 20 minutes   *Yield:* 3½ cups

Enmei Tea is good for people who have high blood pressure, high cholesterol, or yang cancer. It is also an enjoyable beverage. Children like it, too.

1 enmei tea bag
4 cups water

1. Put tea bag in water and boil for 20 minutes in a ceramic or glass pot.
2. Remove tea bag and drink tea hot.

GRAIN COFFEE

Preparation time: 5–10 minutes   *Yield:* 1 serving
Cooking time: 35–45 minutes

Grain Coffee is good with bladder infections, loss of appetite, anemia, weak digestion, nervous debility, or constipation. This ideal drink promotes clear thinking and a feeling of freshness.

> 1 cup whole grain (brown rice, rye, barley, wheat, oats, corn, buckwheat, millet, or any combination of grains)
> 1/3 cup azuki beans
> 1 tablespoon grain coffee powder or yannoh may be substituted for above
> 1 1/2 cups water

1. Roast grains and azuki beans separately until they are uniformly dark brown in color.
2. Mix together and grind as you would flour.
3. Add 1 tablespoon of powder to 1 1/2 cups water and bring to a boil. Retain extra powder for future use. (If using purchased grain coffee powder, add 1 tablespoon powder to 2/3 cup boiling water and drink.)
4. Simmer for 20 minutes.
5. Strain if desired or drink the whole mixture.

Variation

With Kuzu

This variation is good to drink when you need to concentrate well, such as before an exam or presentation, and when you have loss of appetite. After simmering Grain Coffee for 20 minutes, soften kuzu in cold water. Add kuzu to the Grain Coffee and bring to a boil, stirring constantly. Turn off heat and serve.

GRAIN MILK OR KOKKOH

Preparation time: 5–10 minutes   *Yield:* 1 serving
Cooking time: 30–45 minutes

This drink is good for babies when the mother's milk is insufficient. However, because some of the enzymes of the grains are lost in the roasting process, a better sub-

stitute is Rice Milk (see page 239). Grain Milk is also a delicious snack for adults or children and is good for digestion and a weak stomach.

> 3/4 cup sweet brown rice
> 3/4 cup brown rice
> 1 tablespoon sesame seeds
> pinch sea salt
> 1 cup water

1. Roast grains and seeds separately and grind finely.
2. Mix 1 teaspoon grain milk powder and a pinch of sea salt with 1 cup water. Retain extra powder for future use.
3. Simmer for 20 to 30 minutes.
4. Serve hot.

GREEN TEA

Preparation time: 5–10 minutes   *Yield:* 2–3 cups
Standing time: 10 minutes

Green Tea is useful in cases of stomachache, beriberi, or nocturnal emissions and is an excellent source of vitamin C. It should be avoided in cases of gallstones or kidney stones.

> 1 tablespoon green tea leaves
> 2–3 cups water

1. Boil water.
2. Remove from heat and let stand 5 minutes.
3. Place tea leaves in a ceramic tea pot and pour water over tea leaves. Allow tea to steep for 5 minutes.
4. Serve hot.

HABUCHA TEA

Cooking time: 20–30 minutes   *Yield:* 7 cups

Habucha Tea is useful for people who have acne, appendicitis, kidney failure, beriberi, mouth ulcers, syphilis, or blood poisoning.

> 1/4 cup habucha tea powder
> 8 cups cold water

1. Bring tea and water to a boil and cook 20 minutes.
2. Strain.

HATOMUGI TEA

Cooking time: 20–30 minutes *Yield:* 5½ cups

Hatomugi Tea is useful to help dissolve corns and remove warts. If Hatomugi Tea is unavailable, you may use Barley Tea (see page 232). However, Hatomugi Tea is quicker and may be used all year, whereas Barley Tea is recommended only in the summertime, unless you have a very yang condition.

⅓ cup hatomugi
6 cups cold water

1. Bring hatomugi and water to a boil in a ceramic pot.
2. Simmer, uncovered, for 20 minutes.
3. Strain and serve hot.

KOMBU TEA

Preparation time: 5 minutes *Yield:* 7½ cups
Cooking time: 20–30 minutes

This tea is good for the thyroid gland and the regulation of hormones. It helps improve blood circulation, lower high blood pressure, and renew blood vessels. A small amount of warm Kombu Tea can be taken every day in cases of loss of voice, high blood pressure, hemorrhoids, asthma, or sore throat.

1 piece kombu, 3 inches by 6 inches
8 cups water
¼ cup Bancha Tea (see page 232)

1. Cut kombu in 4 pieces.
2. Roast kombu in a dry pan until it is fragrant.
3. Combine roasted kombu, water, and bancha tea in a glass or porcelain pot.
4. Bring ingredients to a boil and allow to simmer for 20 minutes.
5. Strain and serve hot. (Use the cooked kombu in salad or nitsuke.)

KOREN TEA

Cooking time: 20 minutes *Yield:* 1 serving

This preparation may be used if you have no fresh or dried lotus root from which to make Lotus Root Tea. Koren Tea is also useful in cases of laryngitis.

2 tablespoons powdered lotus root (koren)
1 pinch sea salt
2 cups water

1. Mix tea ingredients.
2. Boil, uncovered, for about 20 minutes or until only 1 cup of liquid remains.
3. Serve hot.

KUZU BANCHA TEA

Yield: 1 serving

This tea is useful for the intestines, especially in cases of diarrhea. It is also useful in cases of appendicitis, laryngitis, or whooping cough. Buy good-quality kuzu; some brands are made from potatoes. Add more Bancha Tea or use less kuzu to make light Kuzu Bancha Tea.

1 teaspoon kuzu
1 tablespoon cold water
1 cup boiling Bancha Tea (see page 232)
1 pinch sea salt

1. Dissolve kuzu in a small amount of cold water.
2. Add boiling Bancha Tea and salt.
3. When kuzu turns from a milky color to clear, it is ready to drink.

Variation

With Ginger

This variation is useful if you have a cough from bronchitis or poor elimination from diarrhea. Substitute ½ teaspoon soy sauce for salt. After the kuzu turns clear, add ¼ teaspoon juice from freshly grated ginger.

LOTUS ROOT DAIKON TEA

Preparation time: 10–15 minutes *Yield:* 2 cups

This drink is beneficial for the lungs, especially in cases of pneumonia.

1 tablespoon lotus root juice
1 teaspoon ginger juice
1 tablespoon grated daikon
1½ tablespoons soy sauce
2 cups boiling water

1. Combine all ingredients.
2. Serve hot or warm.

LOTUS ROOT TEA

Preparation time: 5–10 minutes *Yield:* 1 serving

Lotus root is effective for all respiratory problems, especially for coughs, including whooping cough. It is also helpful in reducing a child's fever.

For children:

> 1 tablespoon lotus root juice*
> 2–3 drops ginger juice
> pinch sea salt
> 1/2 cup water

For adults:

> 3 tablespoons lotus root juice*
> 1 teaspoon ginger juice
> pinch sea salt
> 1 cup water

1. Combine ingredients and boil slightly.
2. Serve hot or warm.

MORNING TEA

Preparation time: 5–10 minutes   *Yield:* 1 serving

This tea is beneficial when drunk every morning. It is especially good when there is a lack of gastric juice. It also strengthens the digestive organs.

> 1 teaspoon kuzu
> 1 teaspoon water
> 1/2 teaspoon soy sauce
> 1/4–1/3 umeboshi plum
> 1/4 teaspoon ginger juice
> 2/3 cup boiling Bancha Tea (see page 232)

1. In a cup, dissolve kuzu in water.
2. Add soy sauce and umeboshi plum and mash together.
3. Add ginger juice.
4. Pour boiling tea over the ingredients in the cup and drink when it becomes clear.

MU TEA

Cooking time: 15–20 minutes   *Yield:* 1 serving

Mu tea is useful to improve your circulation, to help cleanse your body, to relieve numbness or pain from hysteria, and as a beverage for many other disorders.

> 1 mu tea bag
> 2 cups water

---

1. Place tea bag in 2 cups water and simmer for 15 minutes.
2. Remove the tea bag and retain it for later use. (To reuse the tea bag, place it in 2 cups water and boil until only 1 cup of liquid remains. Remove and discard the tea bag.)
3. Serve hot.

MU TEA WITH BLACK SOYBEANS

Preparation time: 2–3 minutes   *Yield:* 3 cups
Cooking time: 1 hour

This drink is good in cases of insomnia and helps cleanse the body by removing old medications. It also helps regenerate liver, skin, and kidneys that have been damaged by long-time drug use.

> 1/3 cup black soybeans
> 6 cups water
> 1 mu tea bag

1. Wash and drain soybeans.
2. Combine beans, water, and contents of tea bag.
3. Bring to a boil and simmer about 1 hour, uncovered, until 3 cups of liquid remain.
4. Strain and serve hot.

MUGWORT TEA

Cooking time: 20 minutes   *Yield:* 3 to 3 1/2 cups

This tea helps clean up parasites in the body and strengthens the heart, stomach, and liver.

> 5–7 fresh mugwort leaves or 1–2 small pinches
>   of dried mugwort per cup of water
> 4 cups water
> 1 pinch sea salt

1. Boil mugwort, water, and salt in a porcelain or glass pot for 20 minutes.
2. Strain and serve hot.

ORANGE PEEL TEA

Cooking time: 20–25 minutes   *Yield:* 1 serving

This tea is useful in cases of tempura poisoning.

> 1 orange peel (lemon or tangerine skins
>   are equally effective)
> 2 cups water

---

* Fresh lotus root is most effective for therapeutic use but dried lotus root can be used. Bring 2 dried lotus root slices to a boil in 1 cup water. Allow to cool slightly, and drink. If you have no fresh or dried lotus root, use Koren Tea (see page 237).

1. Peel an orange and bring the pieces to a boil in water.
2. Simmer for 20 minutes.
3. Strain and drink hot.

PERSIMMON CAP TEA

Cooking time: 20–30 minutes *Yield:* 2½ cups

This tea is useful for those who have swelling due to kidney failure.

> ¼–½ cup persimmon caps
> 3 cups water

1. Add persimmon caps to water.
2. Bring to a boil and simmer for 20 minutes.
3. Strain and drink hot.

POMEGRANATE BARK TEA

Cooking time: 20–30 minutes *Yield:* 3½ cups

This tea is good in cases of tapeworms. Do not drink this tea if you are pregnant.

> ¼–½ cup pomegranate bark
> 4 cups water

1. Dry pomegranate bark in a shady place.
2. Chop the bark.
3. Add ¼ cup chopped bark to water and simmer for 20 minutes.
4. Strain and serve hot.

RANSHO DRINK

Preparation time: 3–5 minutes *Yield:* 1 serving

Ransho Drink is good for people who have yin heart disease such as a weak pulse, palpitations, shortness of breath, dizziness, and for those who have poisonous snakebites since Ransho Drink helps makes the heart strong. However, in cases of yang heart diseases, drinking ransho may cause more pain, so use only with yin heart conditions.

> 1 organic fertile egg
> 1–1½ tablespoons natural soy sauce
>   (soy sauce may be measured
>   as ¼ of an eggshell)

1. Beat egg and mix well with soy sauce.
2. Except in an emergency, drink ransho just before going to bed.

RICE MILK

Preparation time: 5 minutes *Yield:* 8–10 cups
Cooking time: 2 hours

Rice Milk is often used as a substitute for mother's milk when breastfeeding is not possible. However, it is important to consult with your health-care advisor to make sure the baby is getting adequate nutrition. This drink is also useful in cases of thrush.

> 1 cup brown rice
> 1 cup sweet brown rice
> 20 cups water
> amasake or rice syrup to sweeten
>   Rice Milk, if desired

1. Add all rice to water.
2. Bring to a boil and simmer over medium heat for 2 hours.
3. Strain and reserve grain for use in bread or pancakes. The juice is Rice Milk.
4. Serve hot or warm.

ROASTED BROWN RICE TEA

Preparation time: 5 minutes *Yield:* 4 cups
Cooking time: 2–2½ hours

This tea is good for lowering a fever if you have already unsuccessfully tried Daikon Ginger Tea, apple juice, or Shiitake Tea. Roasted Brown Rice Tea is also good for cancer patients who have no appetite and for people with debilitating nervous conditions.

> 1 cup brown rice
> 8 cups water

1. Wash brown rice.
2. Roast rice over medium-high heat about 30 minutes until it becomes black.
3. When rice begins to smoke and stick to pan, remove it from heat and allow rice to continue roasting in hot pan.
4. Place water and roasted rice in a pot and bring to a boil.
5. Cook about 1½ hours, uncovered, over medium heat until 4 cups of liquid remain.
6. Strain and serve hot.

SALTWATER DRINK

Preparation time: 1–3 minutes *Yield:* 1 serving

This drink is useful for inducing vomiting, stopping nosebleeds or coughing up of blood, and relieving food poisoning. The proportion of salt to water varies with the usage.

- To help induce vomiting, mix 1 teaspoon of salt with ½ cup water. Drink.
- In cases of nosebleeds or coughing up of blood, strong salt water is drunk. Adults may use 1 teaspoon of salt with 1 cup water. Children may use ¼ teaspoon of salt with ½ cup of water. Drink as much of this as needed; it is okay not to finish it.
- In cases of food poisoning or stomach pain, mix ¼ teaspoon of salt with 1 cup of boiling water. Drink.

SCALLION BANCHA TEA

Preparation time: 5–10 minutes   *Yield:* 1 serving

This tea is useful with colds and fever because it promotes sweating and helps alkalize the body.

> 1 heaping tablespoon chopped scallions
>   (white part only)
> ¾ cup boiling Bancha Tea (see page 232)
> pinch of sea salt

1. Combine ingredients.
2. Serve hot or warm.

SCALLION MISO TEA

Preparation time: 5–10 minutes   *Yield:* 1–2 cups

This tea is useful for people who have colds or fevers.

> ½ cup chopped scallions
> 1 teaspoon miso
> 1–2 cups boiling water

1. Combine ingredients in a bowl.
2. Drink when tea is hot.

SHIITAKE DAIKON TEA

Preparation time: 2–3 minutes   *Yield:* 1 serving
Cooking time: 35 minutes

This tea is useful to help stop bleeding due to a stroke.

> 2 pieces daikon, 1-inch thick
> 5 or 6 dried shiitake mushrooms
> ⅛ teaspoon soy sauce
> 4 cups water

1. Bring ingredients to a boil and simmer for 35 minutes.
2. Drink all the tea at one time.

SHIITAKE DAIKON LOTUS ROOT TEA

Preparation time: 3–5 minutes   *Yield:* 1 serving
Cooking time: 1 hour

This tea is useful in cases of headaches, sore throats, weak stomachs, colds, or flu.

> 4 or 5 dried shiitake mushrooms
> 2 pieces lotus root, ½-inch thick
> 2 pieces daikon, ½-inch thick
> 2 cups water
> soy sauce

1. Combine mushrooms, lotus root, daikon, and water.
2. Bring to a boil and simmer for 1 hour.
3. Add a small amount of soy sauce to taste.
4. Drink hot.

SHIITAKE TEA

Cooking time: 30–40 minutes   *Yield:* 1 serving

Shiitake Tea is useful with fevers or headaches if Daikon Ginger Tea does not work. It is also used for itchy skin.

> 5 or 6 dried shiitake mushrooms
> 2 cups water
> ⅛ teaspoon soy sauce

1. Bring shiitake mushrooms and water to a boil and simmer for 30 minutes.
2. Remove mushrooms and add soy sauce.
3. Strain and drink hot.

SHO-BAN TEA

Preparation time: 5 minutess   *Yield:* 1 serving

This all-purpose beverage is useful for all yin disorders. It is a stimulating drink that is good for fatigue or anemia. It is good for a weak person to drink Sho-Ban Tea before or after a bath. Hard-working people can drink this once a day when tired. It is also useful for regaining strength after fainting, preventing epilepsy or dizziness, controlling heart palpitations or a rapid heartbeat, stopping nosebleeds and uterine bleeding, inducing vomiting, and relieving pain, thirst, or nausea.

2/3 cup boiling Bancha Tea (see page 232)
1 teaspoon soy sauce

1. Add boiling tea to soy sauce.
2. Adjust amounts to make tea stronger or weaker as desired. To induce vomiting, make salty Sho-Ban Tea with 2 teaspoons soy sauce and 1/2 cup Bancha Tea.
3. Drink hot.

Variation

With Grated Daikon

This variation is useful for heartburn. Add 1 tablespoon grated daikon to the tea.

SOYBEAN POWDER TEA

Preparation time: 10 minutes   *Yield:* 1 serving

This tea is useful in cases of tuna poisoning.

1 teaspoon roasted soybean powder
1 cup hot water

1. Combine ingredients.
2. Drink hot or warm.

UME EXTRACT TEA

Preparation time: 1–2 minutes   *Yield:* 1 serving

Ume Extract Tea is useful for people who have canker or cold sores, dysentery, acute intestinal or stomach pain, appendix or vaginal pain, typhoid or scarlet fever, erysipelas (St. Anthony's fire), or tuberculosis. Also, it helps stop the coughing of pleurisy.

For adults:
2–3 soybean-sized balls of ume extract
1/2 cup warm water

For children:
1–2 azuki-bean-sized balls of ume extract
1/2 cup warm water

1. Combine ingredients.
2. Drink 3 times per day after meals or at least 30 minutes before eating.

UMEBOSHI TEA

Preparation time: 5–10 minutes   *Yield:* 1 serving

Umeboshi Tea is useful in cases of cholera, dysentery,

enteritis, water poisoning, or motion sickness. Omit the ginger in cases of motion sickness.

1 umeboshi plum
3–4 drops ginger juice
1/2 cup hot water

1. Crush the umeboshi.
2. Combine ingredients.
3. Drink hot or warm.

UMESHO BANCHA TEA

Preparation time: 3–5 minutes   *Yield:* 1 serving
Cooking time: 7–10 minutes

This tea is useful with diseases of the digestive system, stomachaches, all cancers, and fatigue. It is good for improving blood circulation, strengthening weak pulse or slowing the heart beat, and is often given to a mother at the time her baby is delivered. Drink Umesho Bancha Tea if there is discomfort after fasting or long-time illness. Those with a thin lower body should use thin teas (a higher proportion of Bancha Tea). Those with a heavy upper body should use thicker teas (a lower proportion of Bancha Tea).

2/3 cup Bancha Tea (see page 232)
1/2 umeboshi plum
1/2 teaspoon soy sauce
1/4 teaspoon ginger juice

1. Place Bancha Tea and umeboshi in a porcelain or glass pot.
2. Bring to a boil and cook 5 minutes.
3. Remove from heat.
4. Add soy sauce and ginger juice.
5. Serve hot.

Variation

With Grated Daikon

This variation is useful for gallstones or kidney stones. Make thick Umesho Bancha Tea and mix 1 cup with 1 tablespoon grated daikon. For sharp pain, use 2 tablespoons grated daikon.

UMESHO KUZU TEA

Preparation time: 5 minutes   *Yield:* 1 serving
Cooking time: 10–12 minutes

This tea is useful for diarrhea.

241

1 umeboshi plum
1⅓ cups water
1 tablespoon kuzu
3 tablespoons cold water
1 teaspoon soy sauce*
7 drops ginger juice

1. Break umeboshi plum into several pieces.
2. Add to water in a porcelain or glass pot. Bring to a boil.
3. Dissolve kuzu in cold water and add to pot.
4. Cook, stirring until the liquid becomes clear.
5. Add soy sauce and bring to a boil.
6. Remove from heat and add ginger juice. Serve immediately.

VEGETABLE BROTH

Preparation time: 10 minutes   *Yield:* 3½ cups
Cooking time: 20–25 minutes

This broth is useful with many yang disorders, especially lung, skin, and kidney problems and colon, stomach, small intestine, and lung cancers.

1 large onion
¼ cabbage
½ carrot
4 cups Kombu Stock (see page 216) or water
1 teaspoon sea salt

1. Mince onion, cut cabbage in 1-inch squares, slice carrot in thin quarter moons.
2. Layer onions, cabbage, and carrot in a pot. Add stock or water and salt.
3. Cover and cook for 20 minutes.
4. Strain and serve broth hot. Vegetables may be used in another dish.

WATERMELON RIND TEA

Preparation time: 10 minutes   *Yield:* 3 cups
Cooking time: 30–40 minutes

This tea is useful for helping to induce urination when there are kidney problems. It is used in the summertime when watermelons are available. If the melons are unavailable, use Watermelon Syrup (see page xxx).

2 cups watermelon rind, white inner part only
5 cups water

1. Cut watermelon rind into 1-inch squares.
2. Add to water and bring to a boil.
3. Simmer about 30 minutes until only 3 cups liquid remain.
4. Strain and drink hot.

WINTER SQUASH AND WALNUT TEA

Preparation time: 2–3 minutes   *Yield:* 1 serving
Cooking time: 30–40 minutes

This tea is useful for mild cases of whooping cough.

⅓ cup winter squash seeds
⅓ cup walnuts
3 cups water

1. Dry-roast squash seeds.
2. Combine ingredients in a porcelain or glass pot.
3. Bring to a boil and simmer about 30 minutes until 1½ cups of liquid remain.
4. Strain and drink hot.

---

* Use less soy sauce and more kuzu for children.

Glossary

Acid-Forming Foods. Foods that when digested cause the bodily fluids to become more acidic. Examples include animal foods, grains, beans, nuts, sugar, alcohol, and most chemicals and drugs. See *Acid and Alkaline* by Herman Aihara (listed in Suggested Reading, pages 249–250) for more information.

Agé. Deep-fried tofu, often made in a bag-shaped pouch. Agé can be made at home (see page 215) or may be purchsed from some natural food stores. Use only agé made from nigari tofu.

Albi (also satoimo or taro). This Asian root vegetable or tuber is similar to a small potato and has a sticky interior. It is usually grated for topical applications and is most often used as an external plaster. Albi is available in Asian food stores and some natural food stores.

Alkaline-Forming Foods. Foods that when digested cause the bodily fluids to become more alkaline. Examples include salt and salt products, vegetables, fruits, seeds, nonchemicalized teas, and coffee. See *Acid and Alkaline* by Herman Aihara (listed in Suggested Reading, page 249) for more information.

Amasake. Liquid sweetener made by fermenting cooked sweet brown rice with koji enzyme; used to make desserts or as a beverage. Amasake is available in natural food stores or may be made at home (see Suggested Reading, page 249, for *The Do of Cooking*).

Arame. A sea vegetable similar in appearance to hijiki but more closely related to wakame and kombu. It is useful for treatment of the spleen, pancreas, female disorders, and high blood pressure, and is available in natural food stores or from mail-order suppliers (see pages 253–254).

Azuki Beans (also adzuki, adsuki, or aduki). An easily assimilated legume, the azuki bean is a good carbohydrate-source of phosphorus, potassium, iron, and calcium and an excellent protein complement to whole grains. In macrobiotic thinking, the azuki is considered to have excellent healing properties for the kidneys because of its diuretic quality. These beans are available in natural food stores or from mail-order suppliers (see pages 253–254).

Bancha Tea. Made from twigs and leaves from the tea plant that is at least three years old before harvesting. It has a low caffeine content, about one-fifth as much as green tea. The optimum proportion of twigs to leaves is considered to be six parts twigs to four parts leaves. Tea that is 100 percent twigs is called kukicha twig beverage. Bancha tea is available in natural food stores or from mail-order suppliers (see pages 253–254).

Beefsteak Leaves. The leaves of the beefsteak plant, a popular Japanese herb that is purple-red in color. The leaves are used in the making of umeboshi plums. *See also* Shiso.

Bonita Flakes. A dried fish product made by steaming, sun-drying, smoking, and then fermenting a fish of the mackerel family. The flakes are available from natural food stores, mail-order suppliers (see pages 253–254), and Japanese markets.

Brown Rice. Brown rice is a staple of the whole-grain macrobiotic approach. Although there are many varieties, short-grain, whole rice from which only the hull has been removed is rich in nutrients, easy to digest, and most beneficial for healing purposes. Pressure-cooked brown rice (see page 197) is used most often, especially for yin conditions. For more yang conditions, the rice is either boiled (see page 197) or prepared with more water to make a softer rice. As with all whole grains, the greatest benefit is achieved by thoroughly chewing each mouthful. Brown rice is available in natural food stores or from mail-order suppliers (see pages 253–254). The so-called brown rice found in most grocery stores is white rice colored brown and is not recommended.

Brown Rice Mochi. Mochi made with brown sweet rice; it is available in natural food stores.

Buckwheat Groats. The hulled and cracked seeds of the buckwheat plant, a relative of rhubarb. Botanically, buckwheat is a fruit, but it is often grouped with grains because of its looks and use in flour. Buckwheat groats are available in natural food stores in roasted and unroasted varieties.

Buckwheat Noodles. Noodles made from buckwheat and usually some percentage of wheat, also known as soba. Better quality buckwheat noodles are darker in color; lighter ones have more wheat flour added. The best quality buckwheat noodles are made from 100 percent buckwheat, but these are hard to find. These noodles are available in natural food stores and from mail-order suppliers (see pages 253–254).

Burdock. A long dark root vegetable. One of the most yang vegetables, it is especially good for the kidneys and sexual organs, and for purifying the blood. It is available in natural food stores and Japanese markets.

Burdock Seeds. Seeds from the burdock plant are useful for skin infections and are available from Japanese grocery, gift, or hardware stores, or through mail-order seed companies.

Chirimen Iriko. *See* Small Dried Fish.

Chuba Iriko. *See* Small Dried Fish.

Cotton Bandage. A strip of cloth made of 100 percent cotton used to bind or cover an injured part of the body. Any piece of cotton such as one from an old sheet or shirt may be used after cleaning it thoroughly, or purchase material from a fabric store.

Cotton-Flannel Cloth. A loosely woven, napped fabric made of 100 percent cotton. This cloth is available from fabric stores, or you may use an old shirt made of 100 percent cotton flannel. Clean the shirt thoroughly before using.

Daikon. A long white Japanese radish similar in shape to a carrot. Daikon is a member of the cabbage family and is used medicinally as a digestant. It is available in natural food stores, Japanese markets, and some grocery stores.

Dentie. Made from charcoaled eggplant and sea salt, dentie is used as a tooth powder and is very beneficial for pyorrhea and children's toothaches. It is available in natural food stores or Japanese markets, and from mail-order suppliers (see pages 253–254).

Dried Seitan (fu). Wheat gluten that has been cooked and then dried. Dried seitan is available in natural food stores or Japanese markets, and from some mail-order suppliers (see pages 253–254).

Eggplant Caps. The calyx or top gray or green fibrous stem of the eggplant.

Enema Syringe. A tube used to inject liquid into the rectum. An enema syringe is available from drug stores.

Enmei Tea. Tea popular in Japan made from five herbs: enmeiso, hatomugi, habuso, kuko, and kumasasa. Enmei means longevity. The tea is available from Asian markets or at many natural food stores.

Far-Infrared Sauna. A type of sauna that uses very long-wave far-infrared radiant heat to penetrate and dissolve fat deposits beneath the skin. The far-infrared sauna is assumed to be safer for the aged and for people with weak hearts because the user sweats at much lower temperatures than with water-type saunas. Far-infrared saunas are available by mail order (see pages 253–254).

Flame-Spreader. A flat metal disc with punched holes that is placed between a pan and the burner to diffuse the heat and to help keep the food from sticking to the bottom of the pan and burning. Flame-spreaders are available from grocery stores and natural food stores.

Food Mill. Specialized machine with a hand crank used to make purées and sauces. Food mills are available at some natural food stores and from some mail-order suppliers (see pages 253–254).

Gomashio. A condiment made from roasted and ground sesame seeds (goma) and sea salt (shio). Gomashio may be purchased in natural food stores or from mail-order suppliers (see pages 253–254) but is best when made fresh at home (see page 215).

Grain Mill. A machine for grinding grain. Grain mills are available in hand-operated and electric varieties. The best mills are made with natural stones and are available from natural food stores and mail-order suppliers (see pages 253–254).

Habucha. Herbal tea popular in Japan made from the seeds of the habuso plant. Habucha is available in natural food stores or Asian stores.

Hatomugi. A special type of barley that grows in China, hatomugi is available in Japanese and natural food stores and from some mail-order suppliers (see pages 253–254).

Hijiki. Dark stringy sea vegetable belonging to the brown algae family and very rich in minerals. Because of its high calcium and iron content, it is very useful during pregnancy. Hijiki grows deep under the sea in darkness and under the heavy pressure of the sea water. This is how it develops so strong a life power. Hijiki is available in natural food stores and from mail-order suppliers (see pages 253–254).

Hokkaido Squash. Type of winter squash that has the highest sugar content. Although the Japanese named this squash after Japan's most northern island, it originated in the United States. It is also known as Hokkaido pumpkin and kabucha and is available in natural food stores and at some farmers markets. Hokkaido squash grows well in backyard gardens.

Incense. A substance that is burned to produce a pleasant odor. A stick of incense burns slowly when lit and provides a source of heat that can be placed close to the skin. It is available from some natural food stores and gift shops.

Japanese Grater. A grater that shreds food so finely that juice can be extracted from the shreds. There are many varieties in different shapes and sizes. Porcelain and stainless steel graters are best. They can be purchased from Asian food stores, many natural food stores, and mail-order suppliers (see pages 253–254). A fine American grater may be used but it is more difficult to obtain juice than with the Japanese grater.

Kabocha. *See* Hokkaido Squash.

Kayu. Grain cooked for a long time in a lot of water until it is soft and creamy.

Koji. Enzyme used in fermentation of traditional Japanese foods. Packaging often includes directions for making homemade amasake and/or other fermented products. Koji is available in natural food stores and from some mail-order suppliers (see pages 253–254).

Kokkoh. Grain milk made from sweet brown rice, brown rice, sesame seeds, sea salt, and water. It is available in natural food stores or can be made at home (see page 236).

Kombu. Sea vegetable of the brown algae family grown in long streamers that lie along the sea bottom in deep intertidal waters. Kombu contains high amounts of potassium, iodine, and calcium and is often used in soups and bean dishes. It is available in natural food stores and from some mail-order suppliers (see pages 253–254).

Kukicha Twig Beverage. *See* Bancha Tea.

Kuzu (Japanese arrowroot). Starch extracted from the root of a Japanese wild plant. It is extremely good in cases of sharp intestinal pains, diarrhea, dysentery, cholera, and intestinal tuberculosis because of its strong contracting quality. It is also used as a thickener in cooking. Kuzu is available in natural food stores, from mail-order suppliers (see pages 253–254), and in Japanese grocery stores.

Lotus Root. The root of the lotus plant—a plant with edible blossoms, leaves, roots, and seeds that grows in tropical paddies. The roots grow under the pressure of muddy water and are a good-quality starch. They are available in some natural food stores and in Japanese markets, especially in fall or winter. Dried lotus root is available in most natural food stores and from mail-order suppliers (see pages 253–254).

Miso. Miso is made from fermented soybeans, salt, and barley (or other grain). Used as a flavoring agent, miso is useful for people who have heart conditions, diabetes, rheumatism, polio, asthma, tuberculosis, and skin problems. It is available in natural food stores or from mail-order suppliers (see pages 253–254).

Mochi. Steamed sweet (glutinous) rice that has been pounded and formed into balls or cakes.

Moxa. Short for "moxabustion," a process in which dried mugwort is placed on the skin and heated (burned) to stimulate energy. Dried mugwort is available in some natural food stores, Japanese hardware stores, or from acupuncturists.

Mu Tea. Created by George Ohsawa, Mu Tea is a full-bodied blend of from nine to sixteen herbs. It is useful for relieving menstrual cramps and fatigue, and is good for weak stomachs and mucus-thick coughs. Use the kind made from sixteen herbs, available at natural food stores and from some mail-order suppliers (see pages 253–254).

Mugicha. A tea made from roasted unhulled barley and water, mugicha is available from some natural food stores and from Japanese grocery stores.

Mugwort. A plant that grows in early spring. Mugwort is good in cases of anemia (since it is high in iron) and for ridding the body of parasites. It can be slightly bitter; gather only the young leaves as they are sweetest. Pick them in the spring and dry in a shady place. Mugwort will keep for the rest of the year in a glass jar. Soak the dried mugwort before using it.

Mugwort may be found in some natural food stores or in health food stores that carry herbs.

Mugwort Mochi. Brown rice mochi with mugwort added during processing. It is available in natural food stores.

Natto. Fermented soybean product that has an unusual taste, faintly resembling roquefort cheese, and is typically prepared with a special enzyme. An excellent source of protein, natto is available in Japanese markets and many natural food stores. It can also be made at home. (See Suggested Reading on page 249 for *The Do of Cooking* in which a recipe for natto appears.)

Natural Caviar. The salted roe of a sturgeon or other large fish, processed with only natural ingredients. Available in some natural food stores, natural caviar, when eaten in small amounts at a time, is useful for those with yin types of cancer, gallstones, and other disorders.

Nigari. Bitter liquid that drips from damp sea salt, traditionally used to solidify tofu. Nigari is available at some natural food stores.

Nishime. Style of cooking in which vegetables are cut in fairly large pieces and boiled slowly over low heat for a long time.

Nitsuke. Style of cooking in which vegetables are cut in fairly small pieces and boiled for a short time.

Nori. Sea vegetable of the red algae family that is delicate, leafy, and brownish in color. It is cultivated in Japan and is available in thin sheets after natural processing. It is useful in helping with the digestion of fats and is very high in vitamins (especially vitamin A) and minerals. Nori is available in natural food stores and from mail-order suppliers (see pages 253–254).

Okara. Soybean pulp that remains after the milk has been extracted to make tofu. Okara may be purchased in a Japanese market or from a maker of tofu.

Organic. Scientifically, any carbon-containing compound; in referring to food, organic means grown without the use of chemicalized fertilizers, pesticides, or additives. Organically-grown food is becoming more available and may be found in natural food stores, farmers markets, and some grocery stores.

Organic Fertile Eggs. Fertile eggs from chickens fed with organic food. These are available from many natural food stores.

Otoshibuta. Wooden lid that fits inside a pan and lies directly on top of vegetables. These lids are available from some natural food stores, Japanese markets, and some mail-order suppliers (see pages 253–254).

Peppermint Leaves. Lance-shaped leaves from a plant of the mint family. Seeds for growing your own may be found in seed stores. Dried ground peppermint is available from some natural and health food stores that carry herbs.

Persimmon Caps. Cap-like green part between stem and fruit. Persimmon trees grow in southern climates. If you have no persimmon trees where you live, try looking for dried persimmon caps in natural and health food stores that carry herbs.

Pickle Press. Special tool (usually plastic) used to make pickles by pressure. Also called a salad press when used to make salads. These presses are available from many natural food stores and mail-order suppliers (see pages 253–254).

Plantain. Plantain is a wild plant that is good for asthma, arthritis, stomach diseases, female sexual organ disorders, uterus pain after delivery, heart disease, weak nerves, headaches, brain diseases, sinusitis, and lower back pain. Plantain can be gathered during August in the early morning before the bright sunlight hits it. It is a weed with broad oval leaves and spikes of small greenish flowers. Pull out the whole plant, including the roots and flowers. Wash and dry in a shady place. Store in a paper bag in a cool place. Plantain may be found in some natural and health food stores that carry herbs.

Pyrethrum Flowers. The white, purplish, or red flowers from a variety of chrysanthemum with long stems. The flowers are available from nurseries or florists.

Rice Bran. The outer hull of brown rice, removed in the process of making white rice. It is used for making pickles and for baths and is available from some mail-order suppliers (see pages 253–254) or from rice farmers.

Rice Paddle. A flat, wooden tool used to serve rice. Rice paddles are available from natural food stores, Japanese gift and hardware stores, and many mail-order suppliers (see pages 253–254).

Rice Paper. A thin, delicate paper made of fiber from a particular tree bark. Rice paper is available from Japanese gift shops or bookstores and some natural food stores.

Rice Syrup. Natural sweetener made from milled, cooked sweet brown rice and dried sprouted barley. Also referred to as yinnie syrup or yinnie rice syrup. Rice syrup is available from natural food stores and mail-order suppliers (see pages 253–254).

Rice Vinegar. Seasoning made from whole-grain brown rice and water, aged for three years, and then filtered through cotton. Make certain the kind you buy contains only these ingredients. Rice vinegar is available from natural food stores or mail-order suppliers (see pages 253–254).

Rubbing Alcohol. Type of alcohol (usually isopropyl) used *exclusively* for external purposes. It is available from drug stores and many supermarkets.

Saké. Japanese rice wine. Saké is available from some Japanese food stores or from liquor stores.

Salad Press. Special tool (usually plastic) used to make pressed salads by the use of pressure. Also called a pickle press when used to make pickles. The presses are available from many natural food stores and mail-order suppliers (see pages 253–254).

Satoimo. *See* Albi.

Sea Vegetables. Sea vegetables are high in minerals, especially iodine and calcium. Examples include wakame, hijiki, kombu, nori, dulse, and arame. Sea vegetables are good for those with arteriosclerosis, asthma, hernia, and prolapsus. Make sure to buy sea vegetables that are of good quality and not dyed. They may be obtained from natural food stores and mail-order suppliers (see pages 253–254).

Seitan. Wheat gluten sautéed with soy sauce and ginger. Seitan is becoming increasingly available from natural food stores. It can also be made at home (see Suggested Reading, pages 249–250, for macrobiotic cookbooks).

Sesame Oil. Oil extracted from sesame seeds. Sesame oil contains 87 percent unsaturated fats and is considered the most healthful oil by macrobiotic practitioners. Dark sesame oil is made by roasting the seeds before extracting the oil. Light and dark sesame oils are available from natural food stores and mail-order suppliers (see pages 253–254).

Shio Kombu. Condiment made from kombu (see also) cut into small pieces and cooked with soy sauce for a long time.

Shiso. An iron-rich herb *(Iresine herbistii)*. Shiso is known as the beefsteak plant in the United States. Its seeds and leaves are used for their tangy flavor. The leaves are often pickled during the umeboshi-making process. It is available from natural food stores or mail-order suppliers (see pages 253–254) as a powdered condiment, which is good in cases of anemia.

Shiso Leaves. *See* Beefsteak Leaves.

Shiitake. Type of large Japanese mushroom usually available in dried form. These mushrooms are helpful in reducing blood serum cholesterol but are usually expensive. They are available at Japanese and natural food stores or from some mail-order suppliers (see pages 253–254).

Sho-ban. Tea made from Bancha Tea and soy sauce. A recipe appears on page 240.

Small Dried Fish. These can be found in Asian and macrobiotic markets under the names chuba iriko and chirimen iriko and are similar to small, dried sardines. They can be roasted in a skillet with a little oil to prevent sticking and are eaten whole. If you have difficulty eating them whole, grind them and use them in soup or in gomashio as a condiment. They are very high in calcium and are a good source of vitamin B12.

Soba. *See* Buckwheat Noodles.

Sour Apple. Any variety of edible apple that is sour or tart to the taste, such as Granny Smith, Cortland, Newton, Pippen, and Jonathan. Available in grocery stores, sour apples are useful for diarrhea and for helping reduce children's fevers.

Soy Sauce. A soybean product fermented with salt, water, and wheat koji, containing about one-seventh as much sodium as sea salt. (Also mistakenly known by the names shoyu and tamari.) For healing purposes, the best quality natural product without chemicals or preservatives is the most desirable. Natural soy sauce is available from natural food stores and mail-order suppliers (see pages 253–254).

Sulfur. A pale-yellow, nonmetallic chemical element used in making products such as paper, gun powder, and insecticides. It is available by special order at most pharmacies. Sulfur is for external use only.

Suribachi. Bowl with ridged inner surface, it is used with a suricogi (wooden pestle) for grinding seeds and other foods. Suribachis are available from natural food stores and mail-order suppliers (see pages 253–254), or from Japanese food, gift, or hardware stores.

Sushi. Rice rolled into rounds with vegetables, fish, or pickles, then wrapped with nori, and sliced into rounds. It is available at some restaurants although the quality varies. The best quality sushi is made at home using brown rice and fresh vegetables, fish, or homemade pickles.

Sweet Brown Rice. A variety of rice that is slightly sweeter in taste, stickier in consistency when cooked, and higher in protein than other varieties of rice. It is used to make brown rice mochi and amasake and is available in natural food stores or from mail-order suppliers (see pages 253–254).

Takuan Pickles. Dried daikon pickles made in rice bran in the winter. Takuan pickles can be purchased in natural food stores and are useful for all yin types of diseases. Recipes for making your own takuan pickles can be found in *Macrobiotic Kitchen* and other macrobiotic cookbooks (see Suggested Reading, pages 249–250).

Taro. See Albi.

Tekka Miso. A condiment made by cooking minced burdock, carrot, and lotus root with miso until the mixture is crumbly and dry. Tekka miso is available from natural food stores and mail-order suppliers (see pages 253–254) and a recipe appears on page 226.

Tempura. Style of cooking in which vegetables or fish are dipped in batter and deep-fried.

Tofu. A soybean product that is becoming increasingly popular and is available in most supermarkets. For eating, a natural tofu made with nigari is preferred, but any tofu will do for topical applications. Nigari tofu is available at natural food stores.

Tororo Kombu. Fine shreds of the sea vegetable kombu (see also), seasoned with rice vinegar and used in soups or as a condiment. Tororo kombu is available in natural food stores.

Udon. Large, flat white or whole-wheat noodles, often served in soup. It is available in natural food stores and from mail-order suppliers (see pages 253–254).

Ume. Japanese plum. A sour green fruit that looks like an unripened apricot.

Ume Extract. Strong concentrate made from Japanese plums (ume) without adding salt. It is very alkalizing when eaten, usually in very small amounts. Ume extract is available in natural food stores and from mail-order suppliers (see pages 253–254); a recipe appears on page 227.

Ume Zu (umeboshi vinegar). Pink liquid that results from fermenting Japanese plums (ume). Available from some natural food stores and mail-order suppliers (see pages 253–254), ume zu has a sour taste and can be substituted for vinegar and/or salt in any recipe.

Umeboshi. Japanese plums pickled with salt and beefsteak leaves. Used for seasoning and for therapeutic reasons, it is very salty. It can be purchased as the whole plum, plum paste, or plum extract from natural food stores or mail-order suppliers (see page 253).

Wakame. Kelp-type sea vegetable of the brown algae family, native of Japan and very tender. Often used in soup or ground as a condiment. It is high in iron and calcium and, just like hijiki (see also), is valuable during pregnancy. Wakame is available in natural food stores and from mail-order suppliers (see pages 253–254).

Wood Ashes. The residue from burning wood. Wood ashes may be obtained by burning any nonchemically-treated wood such as oak, pine, or cedar in a fireplace.

Yang Foods. Yang foods are those foods that make the body more yang (contractive) and, in general, if consumed in excess, cause yang types of diseases. Examples of yang foods listed generally from most yang to least yang are: salt, salted products (umeboshi, miso, and soy sauce), eggs, red meat, poultry, salted cheeses, fish, shellfish, natural grain beverages, whole grains, and certain root vegetables.

Yannah. Grain coffee made from roasted whole grains and roasted azuki beans. It is available in natural food stores or may be made at home (see recipe on page 236).

Yin Foods. Yin foods are those foods that make the body more yin (expansive) and, in general, if consumed in excess, cause yin type diseases. Examples of yin foods listed generally from most yin to least yin are: chemicalized foods and drugs, refined sugar, candy, soft drinks, alcoholic drinks, honey, coffee, herb teas, dairy foods, Bancha Tea, fruits, beans, nuts, seeds, and vegetables.

Yinnie Rice Syrup. *See* Rice Syrup.

SUGGESTED READING

INTRODUCTORY MACROBIOTIC THEORY

Aihara, Herman. *Basic Macrobiotics*. New York: Japan Publications, 1985.

Heidenry, Carolyn. *Making the Transition to a Macrobiotic Diet*. Garden City Park, NY: Avery Publishing Group, 1984.

Ohsawa, George and Herman Aihara. *Macrobiotics: An Invitation to Health and Happiness*. Oroville, CA: George Ohsawa Macrobiotic Foundation, 1971.

Ohsawa, George. *Zen Macrobiotics*. Oroville, CA: George Ohsawa Macrobiotic Foundation, 1965.

MACROBIOTIC PHILOSOPHY/THEORY

Aihara, Herman. *Acid and Alkaline*. 5th ed. Oroville, CA: George Ohsawa Macrobiotic Foundation, 1986.

Aihara, Herman. *Kaleidoscope*. Oroville, CA: George Ohsawa Macrobiotic Foundation, 1986.

Aihara, Herman. *Learning from Salmon*. Oroville, CA: George Ohsawa Macrobiotic Foundation, 1980.

Gagne, Steve. *The Energetics of Food*. Santa Fe: Spiral Sciences, 1990.

Kotzsch, Ronald E. *Macrobiotics Beyond Food*. New York: Japan Publications, 1988.

Kushi, Michio and Aveline. *Macrobiotic Diet*. New York: Japan Publications, 1985.

Kushi, Michio. *Macrobiotic Way*. Garden City Park, NY: Avery Publishing Group, 1985.

Ohsawa, George. *The Art of Peace*. Oroville, CA: George Ohsawa Macrobiotic Foundation, 1990.

Ohsawa, George. *Macrobiotics: The Way of Healing*. Oroville, CA: George Ohsawa Macrobiotic Foundation, 1981.

Ohsawa, George. *The Order of the Universe*. Oroville, CA: George Ohsawa Macrobiotic Foundation, 1986.

Ohsawa, George. *Philosophy of Oriental Medicine*. Oroville, CA: George Ohsawa Macrobiotic Foundation, 1991.

BEGINNING MACROBIOTIC COOKING

Aihara, Cornellia. *How to Prepare a Macrobiotic Meal*. Produced and directed by Vega Study Center, 75 minutes. Oroville, CA: George Ohsawa Macrobiotic Foundation, 1990.

Esko, Wendy. *Introducing Macrobiotic Cooking*. New York: Japan Publications, 1988.

Ferré, Julia. *Basic Macrobiotic Cooking*. Oroville, CA: George Ohsawa Macrobiotic Foundation, 1987.

Turner, Kristina. *Self-Healing Cookbook*. Grass Valley, CA: Earthtones Press, 1987.

MACROBIOTIC COOKBOOKS

Aihara, Cornellia. *The Calendar Cookbook*. Oroville, CA: George Ohsawa Macrobiotic Foundation, 1979.

Aihara, Cornellia. *The Do of Cooking*. Oroville, CA: George Ohsawa Macrobiotic Foundation, 1982.

Aihara, Cornellia, ed. *The First Macrobiotic Cookbook*, Revised ed. Oroville, CA: George Ohsawa Macrobiotic Foundation, 1985.

Aihara, Cornellia. *Macrobiotic Kitchen*. New York: Japan Publications, 1982.

Albert, Rachel. *Cooking with Rachel*. Oroville, CA: George Ohsawa Macrobiotic Foundation, 1989.

Colbin, Annemarie. *The Book of Whole Meals*. New York: Ballantine Books, 1979.

Colbin, Annemarie. *The Natural Gourmet*. New York: Ballantine Books, 1989.

Henkel, Pamela and Lee Koch. *As Easy As 1, 2, 3*. Oroville, CA: George Ohsawa Macrobiotic Foundation, 1990.

Jacobs, Barbara and Leonard. *Cooking with Seitan*. New York: Japan Publications, 1986.

Kushi, Aveline. *Complete Guide to Macrobiotic Cooking*. New York: Warner Books, 1985.

Kushi, Aveline and Wendy Esko. *The Changing Seasons Macrobiotic Cookbook*. Garden City Park, NY: Avery Publishing Group, 1985.

Kushi, Aveline and Wendy Esko. *The Good Morning Macrobiotic Breakfast Book*. Garden City Park, NY: Avery Publishing Group, 1991.

Kushi, Aveline and Wendy Esko. *The Macrobiotic Cancer Prevention Cookbook*. Garden City Park, NY: Avery Publishing Group, 1988.

Kushi, Aveline and Wendy Esko. *The Quick and Natural Macrobiotic Cookbook*. Chicago: Contemporary Books, 1989.

Lerman, Andrea Bliss. *The Macrobiotic Community Cookbook*. Garden City Park, NY: Avery Publishing Group, 1989.

Levin, Cecile Tovah. *Cooking for Regeneration*. New York: Japan Publications, 1988.

McCarty, Meredith. *American Macrobiotic Cuisine*. Eureka, CA: Turning Point Publications, 1986.

McCarty, Meredith. *Fresh from a Vegetarian Kitchen*. Eureka, CA: Turning Point Publications, 1989.

Ohsawa, Lima. *Macrobiotic Cuisine*. New York: Japan Publications, 1984.

Saltzman, Joanne. *Amazing Grains*. Tiburon, CA: H. J. Kramer, 1990.

Wood, Rebecca. *Quinoa—the Super Grain*. New York: Japan Publications, 1989.

WELL-BEING

Aihara, Cornellia. *Macrobiotic Child Care*. Oroville, CA: George Ohsawa Macrobiotic Foundation, 1979.

Briscoe, David and Charlotte Mahoney-Briscoe. *A Personal Peace: Macrobiotic Reflections on Mental and Emotional Recovery*. New York: Japan Publications, 1989.

Colbin, Annemarie. *Food and Healing*. New York: Ballantine Books, 1986.

Esko, Edward, ed. *Doctors Look at Macrobiotics*. New York: Japan Publications, 1988.

Hashimoto, Keizo. *Sotai Natural Exercise*. Oroville, CA: George Ohsawa Macrobiotic Foundation, 1981.

Kushi, Michio. *The Cancer Prevention Diet*. New York: St. Martin's Press, 1983.

Kushi, Michio with Alex Jack. *Diet for a Strong Heart*. New York: St. Martin's Press, 1985.

Kushi, Michio. *How to See Your Health*. New York: Japan Publications, 1980.

Kushi, Michio. *The Macrobiotic Approach to Cancer*. Garden City Park, NY: Avery Publishing Group, 1991.

Kushi, Michio and Aveline Kushi. *Macrobiotic Child Care and Family Health*. New York: Japan Publications, 1986.

Kushi, Michio and Marc van Cauwenberghe, M.D. *Macrobiotic Home Remedies*. New York: Japan Publications, 1985.

Kushi, Michio and Martha C. Cottrell, M.D., with Mark Mead. *AIDS, Macrobiotics, and Natural Immunity*. New York: Japan Publications, 1990.

Monte, Tom. *The Way of Hope*. New York: Warner Books, 1989.

Muramoto, Noboru. *Healing Ourselves*. New York: Avon Books, 1973.

Muramoto, Noboru. *Natural Immunity: Insights on Diet and AIDS*. Oroville, CA: George Ohsawa Macrobiotic Foundation, 1988.

Nussbaum, Elaine. *Recovery from Cancer to Health*. New York: Japan Publications, 1986.

Ohsawa, George. *Macrobiotic Guidebook for Living*. Oroville, CA: George Ohsawa Macrobiotic Foundation, 1985.

Sattilaro, Anthony with Tom Monte. *Recalled by Life*. New York: Avon Books, 1982.

EDUCATIONAL RESOURCES

MACROBIOTIC RESIDENTIAL PROGRAMS

Herman and Cornellia Aihara direct the Vega Study Center in Northern California. Ongoing live-in programs feature hands-on macrobiotic cooking classes, lectures, home remedies, and more. Programs are designed to meet the needs of all, from those new to macrobiotics to those seeking professional development, and to address all areas of concern, from healing to informal weekends of relaxation and rejuvenation. The center also maintains a current list of other macrobiotic educational centers around the world.

Here is a list of some major macrobiotic educational centers. There are numerous other educational centers and counsellors who can provide macrobiotic information. Contact the Vega Study Center or any of these centers for further information regarding your area.

Australian School of Macrobiotics
P.O. Box 705
Glebe 2037
Australia
02-660-1199; fax 02-692-0908

Community Health Foundation
188 Old Street
GB-19 London
Great Britain
071-251 40 76

Toronto East West Center
90 Barton Ave..
Toronto, Ontario
Canada M6G 1P6
(416) 530-1571

International Macrobiotic Institute
Kientalerhof
CH-3723 Kiental
Switzerland
033-76 26 76; fax 033-76 12 41

Kushi Institute of the Berkshires
Box 7, Leland Road
Becket, MA 01223
United States
(413) 623-5742; fax (413) 827-8827

Macrobiotic Foundation of Florida
2977 McFarlane Road, No. 305
Coconut Grove, FL 33133
United States
(305) 448-6625

Nippon C. I.
11-5 Ohyama-machi-cho
Shibuya-ku
Tokyo, Japan 151
03-469 7631

Vega Study Center
1511 Robinson Street
Oroville, CA 95965
United States
(916) 533-7702; fax (916) 533-7908

PUBLICATIONS

The Aiharas also founded the George Ohsawa Macrobiotic Foundation, now in its fourth decade of providing complete macrobiotic educational services in conjunction with the Vega Study Center. The publication department publishes many books of George Ohsawa, Herman and Cornellia Aihara, and others and publishes *Macrobiotics Today*, a popular bimonthly magazine providing timely articles and news of macrobiotic interest and activities. *Macrobiotics Today* contains the Natural Living Directory, a listing of macrobiotic persons and businesses.

Here is a list of some of the English-language macrobiotic periodicals. For a curent complete list, including periodicals in foreign languages, contact *Macrobiotics Today* or the Vega Study Center.

Macro News
243 Dickinson Street
Philadelphia, PA 19147
(215) 551-1430

Macrobiotics Today
P.O. Box 426
Oroville, CA 95965
(916) 533-7702; fax (916) 533-7908

One Peaceful World Newsletter
P.O. Box 10
Becket, MA 01223
(413) 623-2322; fax (413) 623-8827

Spectrum Wholistic News Magazine
61 Dutile Road
Belmont, NH 03220
(603) 528-4710

CAMPS AND CONFERENCES

Herman and Cornellia Aihara host the annual French Meadows Summer Camp near Lake Tahoe in the Sierra Nevada each July. This outdoor camping experience is an excellent way to learn from macrobiotic teachers from around the world. Health Classics are held at hotels in Florida in February, southern California in October, and elsewhere. The Kushi Summer Conference is held at a New England college campus in August each year. There are many camps and conferences held throughout the world. The summer camp department of the Vega Study Center maintains a list of phone numbers of current camps and conferences in the United States.

French Meadows Summer Camp
1511 Robinson Street
Oroville, CA 95965
(916) 533-7702; fax (916) 533-7908

Health Classics
1223 Wilshire Blvd, #H
Santa Monica, CA 90403
(800) 275-3722

Kushi Foundation Summer Conference
P.O. Box 390
Becket, MA 01223
(413) 623-2103

Further information may be obtained with one phone call or letter; call or write:

Vega Study Center
1511 Robinson Street
Oroville, California 95965
(916) 533-7702; fax (916) 533-7908

If writing, be sure to specify the information you want to receive.

☐ Vega Study Center brochure
☐ List of macrobiotic educational centers in your area
☐ *Macrobiotics Today* subscription
☐ Complete macrobiotic book catalog
☐ French Meadows Summer Camp flyer
☐ List of current camps and conferences in the United States

SOURCES OF SUPPLIES

LOCAL SOURCES

Most macrobiotic foods are available from natural food stores. Health food stores usually sell mostly vitamin supplements but do have some natural foods. Many supermarkets now have health food sections that contain some useful products. Most natural food stores and some health food stores will order food items and begin to stock items for which they see a demand, so don't hesitate to tell them of your needs.

Japanese and Asian food stores or markets are a source for some of the harder-to-find foods. However, unless you live on the West Coast or in New York City, Japanese or Asian stores may be hard to find or nonexistent. If you do shop in Japanese or Asian food stores, you must be careful because most processed food contains chemical additives and preservatives and labels can be hard to read.

Many natural food stores also carry the kitchenware and utensils necessary for a macrobiotic approach to life and health as do all of the mail-order suppliers listed below. Japanese and Asian hardware, gift, and grocery stores are a good source, especially for the more specialized Japanese items.

Consult your local phone book and/or library for the location of natural food stores, health food stores, herb shops, nurseries, florists, seed companies, and liquor stores. If you are unable to find what you need, you can approach the lack of local sources in several ways. One way is to order via the mail. Another is to ask existing stores to begin carrying macrobiotic foods and supplies. A third option is to put up a sign on public notice boards or an ad in the newspaper stating that you are interested in joining or starting a macrobiotic support group. Or simply announce a macrobiotic or vegetarian potluck and then discuss the need for better sources of supply with those who attend or contact you.

MAIL-ORDER SUPPLIERS

There are several excellent macrobiotic mail-order suppliers and these offer not only a convenient way to shop from home but are also vital for those living in rural areas or areas with no other source of supply. Here is a list of the major ones to get you started. Write or call them for information or for a catalog.

Gold Mine
Natural Food Company
1947 30th Street
San Diego, CA 92102
(800) 475-3663

Mountain Ark
Trading Company
P.O. Box 3170
Fayetteville, AR 72702
(800) 643-8909

Granum, Inc.
2901 NE Blakeley
Seattle, WA 98105
(800) 882-8943

Natural Lifestyle Supplies
16 Lookout Drive
Asheville, NC 28804
(800) 752-2775

Since mail-order companies change and new ones are established all the time, contact the George Ohsawa Macrobiotic Foundation for a current list of suppliers or for the name of someone close to you who might be able to help with local sources of supply. The foundation mail-orders some hard-to-find items, the far-infrared sauna, and a product price list.

George Ohsawa Macrobiotic Foundation
Sales Department
1511 Robinson Street
Oroville, California 95965
(916) 533-7702; fax 533-7908

If writing, be sure to specify the information you want to receive.

☐ Product price list and complete macrobiotic book catalog
☐ Far-infrared sauna information
☐ Name and number of the macrobiotic contact person nearest to you
☐ List of current mail-order suppliers

If writing, be sure to specify the information you want to receive.

☐ Product price list and complete macrobiotic book catalog

☐ Far-infrared sauna information
☐ Name and number of the macrobiotic contact person nearest to you
☐ List of current mail-order suppliers

BIBLIOGRAPHY

Balch, James F., M.D., and Phyllis A. Balch, C.N.C. *Prescription for Nutritional Healing*. Garden City Park, NY: Avery Publishing Group, 1990.

Dorland's Illustrated Medical Dictionary, 25th ed. Philadelphia: W. B. Saunders, 1974.

Griffith, H. Winter, M.D. *Complete Guide to Symptoms, Illness, and Surgery*. Tucson: The Body Press, 1985.

Guyton, Arthur C., M.D. *Textbook of Medical Physiology*, 4th ed. Philadelphia: W. B. Saunders Company, 1971.

Kiester, Edwin, Jr., ed. *New Family Medical Guide*. Des Moines, IA: Better Homes and Gardens Books, 1982.

Miller, Benjamin F., M.D. and Lawrence Galton. *The Family Book of Preventive Medicine*. New York: Simon and Schuster, 1971.

Miller, Sigmund Stephen, ed. *Symptoms: The Complete Home Medical Encyclopedia*. New York: Thomas Y. Crowell Company, 1976.

Shadman, Alonzo J., M.D. *Who Is Your Doctor and Why*. City not given: Lanesville Publishing Company, 1971.

Van Amerongen, C. *The Way Things Work—Book of the Body*. New York: Simon and Schuster, 1973.

West, Edward Staunton, Ph.D. *Textbook of Biochemistry*, 4th ed. New York: The Macmillan Company, 1967.

Wood, Rebecca. *The Whole Foods Encyclopedia*. New York: Prentice Hall Press, 1988.

Wright, John W., ed. *The Universal Almanac*. New York: Andrews and McMeel, 1989.

Index